Psychiatry for the Neurologist

Guest Editor

SILVANA RIGGIO, MD

NEUROLOGIC CLINICS

www.neurologic.theclinics.com

Consulting Editor
RANDOLPH W. EVANS, MD

February 2011 • Volume 29 • Number 1

SAUNDERS an imprint of ELSEVIER, Inc.

W.B. SAUNDERS COMPANY
A Division of Elsevier Inc.

1600 John F. Kennedy Boulevard ● Suite 1800 ● Philadelphia, Pennsylvania 19103-2899

http://www.theclinics.com

NEUROLOGIC CLINICS Volume 29, Number 1
February 2011 ISSN 0733-8619, ISBN-13: 978-1-4557-0470-5

Editor: Donald Mumford

Neurologic Clinics (ISSN 0733-8619) is published quarterly by Elsevier Inc., 360 Park Avenue South, New York, NY 10010–1710. Months of issue are February, May, August, and November. Periodicals postage paid at New York, NY, and additional mailing offices. Subscription prices are $264.00 per year for US individuals, $441.00 per year for US institutions, $130.00 per year for US students, $332.00 per year for Canadian individuals, $530.00 per year for Canadian institutions, $368.00 per year for international individuals, $530.00 per year for international institutions, and $184.00 for Canadian and foreign students/residents. To receive student/resident rate, orders must be accompanied by name of affiliated institution, date of term, and the *signature* of program/residency coordinator on institution letterhead. Orders will be billed at individual rate until proof of status is received. Foreign air speed delivery is included in all *Clinics* subscription prices. All prices are subject to change without notice. **POSTMASTER:** Send address changes to *Neurologic Clinics*, Elsevier Health Sciences Division, Subscription Customer Service, 3251 Riverport Lane, Maryland Heights, MO 63043. **Customer Service: Telephone: 1-800-654-2452 (U.S. and Canada); 314-447-8871 (outside U.S. and Canada). Fax: 314-447-8029. E-mail: journalscustomerservice-usa@elsevier.com (for print support); journalsonlinesupport-usa@elsevier.com (for online support).**

Reprints. For copies of 100 or more of articles in this publication, please contact the Commercial Reprints Department, Elsevier Inc., 360 Park Avenue South, New York, New York, 10010-1710; Tel.: (+1) 212-633-3812; Fax: (+1) 212-462-1935, and E-mail: reprints@elsevier.com.

Neurologic Clinics is also published in Spanish by Nueva Editorial Interamericana S.A., Mexico City, Mexico.

Neurologic Clinics is covered in *Current Contents/Clinical Medicine, MEDLINE/PubMed (Index Medicus), EMBASE/Excerpta Medica, and PsycINFO, and ISI/BIOMED.*

Printed and bound in the United Kingdom

Transferred to Digital Print 2011

Contributors

CONSULTING EDITOR

RANDOLPH W. EVANS, MD
Clinical Professor, Department of Neurology, Baylor College of Medicine, Houston, Texas

GUEST EDITOR

SILVANA RIGGIO, MD
Professor, Departments of Psychiatry and Neurology, Mount Sinai School of Medicine, New York; Director of Consultation Liaison Service, James J. Peters Veterans Affairs Medical Center, Bronx, New York

AUTHORS

SELIM R. BENBADIS, MD
Director of Epilepsy, Tampa General Hospital; University of South Florida, Tampa, Florida

E. CABRINA CAMPBELL, MD
Associate Professor, Department of Psychiatry, The Veterans Affairs Medical Center; University of Pennsylvania School of Medicine, Philadelphia, Pennsylvania

STANLEY N. CAROFF, MD
Professor, Department of Psychiatry, The Veterans Affairs Medical Center; University of Pennsylvania School of Medicine, Philadelphia, Pennsylvania

ALAN CARSON, MB,ChB, MPhil, MD, FRCP
Consultant Neuropsychiatrist and Part Time Senior Lecturer, Department of Clinical Neurosciences, University of Edinburgh, Western General Hospital; Department of Rehabilitation Medicine, Astley Ainslie Hospital; Department of Psychiatry, University of Edinburgh, Royal Edinburgh Hospital, Edinburgh, United Kingdom

CHRISTOPHER M. FILLEY, MD
Director, Behavioral Neurology Section; Professor of Neurology and Psychiatry, University of Colorado School of Medicine, Aurora; Neurology Service Chief, Denver Veterans Affairs Medical Center, Denver, Colorado

MARK W. GREEN, MD
Professor of Neurology and Anesthesiology, Director of Headache and Pain Medicine, Mount Sinai School of Medicine, New York, New York

BRIAN HAINLINE, MD
Clinical Associate Professor of Neurology, New York University School of Medicine; Chief, Neurology and Integrative Pain Medicine, ProHEALTH Care Associates, Lake Success, New York

IRENE HURFORD, MD
Assistant Professor, Department of Psychiatry, The Veterans Affairs Medical Center; University of Pennsylvania School of Medicine, Philadelphia, Pennsylvania

DAN V. IOSIFESCU, MD, MSc
Director, Mood and Anxiety Disorders Program, Associate Professor of Psychiatry and Neuroscience, Mount Sinai School of Medicine, New York, New York; Consultant in Psychiatry, Massachusetts General Hospital; Lecturer in Psychiatry, Harvard Medical School, Boston, Massachusetts

ANDRES M. KANNER, MD
Professor, Departments of Neurological Sciences and Psychiatry, Rush University Medical Center, Rush Medical College at Rush University; Director, Laboratory of EEG and Video-EEG-Telemetry; Associate Director, Section of Epilepsy and Rush Epilepsy Center, Rush University Medical Center, Chicago, Illinois

KIMBERLY L. KJOME, MD
Assistant Professor, Department of Psychiatry and Behavioral Sciences, University of Texas Health Science Center at Houston, Houston, Texas

W. CURT LAFRANCE Jr, MD, MPH
Director of Neuropsychiatry and Behavioral Neurology, Rhode Island Hospital; Assistant Professor of Psychiatry and Neurology (Research), Brown Medical School, Providence, Rhode Island

SCOTT D. LANE, PhD
Professor, Department of Psychiatry and Behavioral Sciences, University of Texas Health Science Center at Houston, Houston, Texas

KYLE A.B. LAPIDUS, MD, PhD
Department of Psychiatry, Mount Sinai School of Medicine, New York, New York

TERESA LIM, MD, MSc
Resident, Department of Psychiatry, Mount Sinai School of Medicine, New York, New York

JANICE LYBRAND, MD
Staff Psychiatrist, Department of Psychiatry, The Veterans Affairs Medical Center, Philadelphia, Pennsylvania

DEBORAH B. MARIN, MD
Associate Professor of Psychiatry, Department of Psychiatry, Mount Sinai School of Medicine; Associate Professor of Geriatrics and Palliative Medicine, Department of Geriatrics and Palliative Medicine, Mount Sinai School of Medicine, New York, New York

F. GERARD MOELLER, MD
Professor, Department of Psychiatry and Behavioral Sciences, University of Texas Health Science Center at Houston, Houston, Texas

KENNETH PODELL, PhD
Division of Neuropsychology, Henry Ford Health System; Clinical Associate Professor, Department of Psychiatry and Behavioral Neurosciences, Wayne State University, Detroit, Missouri

SILVANA RIGGIO, MD
Professor, Departments of Psychiatry and Neurology, Mount Sinai School of Medicine, New York; Director of Consultation Liaison Service, James J. Peters Veterans Affairs Medical Center, Bronx, New York

LAILI SOLEIMANI, MD, MSc
Department of Psychiatry, Mount Sinai School of Medicine, New York, New York

JON STONE, MB,ChB, PhD, FRCP
Consultant Neurologist and Honorary Senior Lecturer, Department of Clinical Neurosciences, University of Edinburgh, Western General Hospital, Edinburgh, United Kingdom

KAREN TORRES, PsyD
Neuropsychology Fellow, Department of Psychiatry, Cambridge Health Alliance/Harvard Medical School, Cambridge, Massachusetts

Contents

The complex phenomenology of white matter dementia and many neuro-psychiatric disorders implies that they originate from involvement of distributed neural networks, and white matter neuropathology is increasingly implicated in the pathogenesis of these network disconnection syndromes. White matter disorders produce functional asynchrony of interdependent cerebral regions subserving normal cognitive and emotional functions. Accumulating evidence suggests that white matter dementia primarily reflects disturbed frontal systems connectivity, whereas disruption of frontal and temporal lobe systems is implicated in the pathogenesis of neuropsychiatric disorders. Continued study of normal and abnormal white matter promises to help resolve challenging problems in behavioral neurology and neuropsychiatry.

The phenotypic expression of neuropsychological deficits can have very different genotypic etiologies. Understanding the causes of various neuropsychological deficits is tantamount in developing the appropriate treatments. The literature on mood disorders as a risk factor for dementia is reviewed as well as common neuropsychological patterns in dementia and mood disorders. A brief discussion on chronic traumatic encephalopathy is provided.

The physician must explain the treatment or procedure in detail including risks, benefits, and alternative options; the patient's choice must be voluntary; the patient must demonstrate his or her ability to understand the risks and benefits of their choice; and the patient must be able to manipulate information in a logical way. These criteria must be met in order for the process of informed consent to be valid.

Drug-induced movement disorders have dramatically declined with the widespread use of second-generation antipsychotics, but remain important in clinical practice and for understanding antipsychotic pharmacology. The diagnosis and management of dystonia, parkinsonism, akathisia, catatonia, neuroleptic malignant syndrome, and tardive dyskinesia are reviewed in relation to the decreased liability of the second-generation antipsychotics contrasted with evidence from the Clinical Antipsychotic Trials of Intervention Effectiveness (CATIE) Schizophrenia Trial. Data from the CATIE trial imply that advantages of second-generation antipsychotics in significantly reducing extrapyramidal side effects compared with haloperidol may be diminished when compared with modest doses of lower-potency first-generation drugs.

FORTHCOMING ISSUES

RECENT ISSUES

THE CLINICS ARE NOW AVAILABLE ONLINE!

Access your subscription at:
www.theclinics.com

Preface

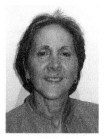

Silvana Riggio, MD
Guest Editor

It is with great pleasure that I accepted the role of editor for this issue of *Neurologic Clinics* on "Psychiatry for the Neurologist." As a psychiatrist and a neurologist, with a strong interest in the neurobehavioral sequelae of neurological disease, in particular as it pertains to seizures and traumatic brain injury, I found this project exciting and challenging. I am firmly convinced that the fields of psychiatry and neurology cannot exist as two separate disciplines, but rather are intimately intertwined. Indeed, in my opinion, a comprehensive approach to the neurologic and psychiatric assessment, to diagnostic testing, and to behavioral and pharmacologics interventions is needed to maximize patient outcomes.

Neurology and psychiatry, once a unified specialty, have drifted apart over the years. The separation has resulted in the loss of a vital connection between treating the body and the mind, a connection which is critical to caring for patients with neuro-psychiatric disease. Without this understanding, a comprehensive treatment plan cannot be reached.

Contributors to this issue include experts in neurology, psychiatry, and neuropsy-chology. Articles focus on areas of common interest and controversy. Topics were chosen to accentuate the importance of the multidisciplinary collaboration. This collaboration is essential to understanding the complex relationship between brain and behavior and the challenges that both fields present to one another.

One of the goals of this issue of *Neurologic Clinics* is to promote a clearer under-standing of the neurology/psychiatry interface. Topics include neurobehavioral mani-festations as they relate to pain, pain, aggression, movement disorders, depression, seizures, panic attacks, traumatic brain injury, and dementia. The reader is presented with a wide variety of challenges that the psychiatrist and neurologist are confronted with every day.

It is commonly thought that the psychiatrist is best equipped to address the behav-ioral sequelae of neurological diseases and the neurologist is best equipped to corre-late anatomic lesion with neurological signs and symptoms. The neuropsychologist, on the other hand, can integrate both information, help quantify the impairment, and provide both the neurologist and the psychiatrist with a better understanding of the

Neurol Clin 29 (2011) xi–xii
doi:10.1016/j.ncl.2010.11.003
0733-8619/11/$ – see front matter © 2011 Elsevier Inc. All rights reserved.

neurologic.theclinics.com

extent of the deficit and its impact on functionality. Ultimately the success of each in caring for the patient is dependent on the other.

My hope is to provoke the reader to reflect on the interface between neurologic and psychiatric illness. Topics were chosen to increase awareness of the complex processes that go beyond the anatomic lesion itself; to provide a deeper understanding of brain and behavior and their interrelationship. To reach an insightful perspective on the controversies and challenges we are confronted with daily, an understanding of the pathophysiology is required; unfortunately, science has yet to fully elucidate many of the mechanisms involved and the multifactorial components of illness expression challenges the skill of the best clinician. However, without engaging the challenge and addressing all facets of the clinical presentation, outcomes can be compromised. In doing so, it is of fundamental importance that we understand the "whole person," ie, the patient's response to their illness as it relates to the underlying personality structure, individual defense and coping mechanisms, social setting, including support or lack of, as well as physical or emotional impact of their illness. Ultimately, good outcome depends on a coordinated approach to the patient that ensures comprehensive management from the onset of the disease in question through recovery.

Silvana Riggio, MD
Departments of Psychiatry and Neurology
Mount Sinai School of Medicine
One Gustave L. Place, Box 1230
New York, NY 10029, USA

James J. Peters VA Medical Center
Bronx, NY, USA

E-mail address:
silvana.riggio@mssm.edu

Functional Neurologic Symptoms: Assessment and Management

Jon Stone, MB,ChB, PhD, FRCP[a,*],
Alan Carson, MB,ChB, MPhil, MD, FRCP[a,b,c]

KEYWORDS

- Psychogenic • Conversion disorder
- Dissociative motor disorder • Nonorganic • Hysteria
- Pseudoneurological • Functional weakness

INTRODUCTION AND TERMINOLOGY

This article provides a review of the symptoms and signs that may be useful in the diagnosis of functional neurologic symptoms. Management of the patients with functional symptoms often requires close collaboration between neurology and psychiatry, but there is much that a neurologist can usefully do before onward referral.

Terminology in this area is problematic and reflects many different ways of conceptualizing and approaching the problem of patients with symptoms that are unexplained by the disease. There is no perfect solution. The term used depends not only on how neurologists perceive the cause of these symptoms but also on how they wish to communicate the diagnosis to the patient (discussed later).

Conversion Disorder (DSM [Fourth Edition] 300.11)

Conversion disorder is based on the Freudian idea that intolerable psychological conflict leads to the conversion of distress into physical symptoms. The definition in DSM-IV requires that the patient is not feigning and psychological factors precede the initiation or exacerbation of the symptom or deficit. In the forthcoming revision of DSM (DSM-5), the need for these psychological factors to be present and the term conversion may be eliminated.[1]

Funding support: none.

Financial disclosures and conflicts of interest: none.

This article has been adapted from another article by the same authors in: Daroff, Fenichel, Jankovic, et al, editors. Neurology in clinical practice. 6th edition.

[a] Department of Clinical Neurosciences, University of Edinburgh, Western General Hospital, Crewe Road, Edinburgh EH4 2XU, UK

[b] Department of Rehabilitation Medicine, Astley Ainslie Hospital, Edinburgh EH9 2HB, UK

[c] Department of Psychiatry, University of Edinburgh, Royal Edinburgh Hospital, Edinburgh EH10 5HF, UK

* Corresponding author.

E-mail address: Jon.Stone@ed.ac.uk

Dissociative Seizure/Motor Disorder (Conversion Disorder) (International Classification of Diseases, Tenth Revision F44.4-9)

This term suggests dissociation as an important mechanism in symptom production.[2] Dissociation encompasses a variety of symptoms in which there is a lack of integration or connection of normal conscious functions. The difficulty with this term is that not all patients with functional symptoms describe dissociative symptoms (see section on history taking later in the article).

Somatization Disorder (DSM-IV 300.81)

Somatization disorder refers to a history of multiple symptoms unexplained by disease starting before the age of 30 years. The current definition requires the presence of at least 1 conversion symptom, 4 pain symptoms, 2 gastrointestinal symptoms (usually irritable bowel syndrome), and 1 sexual symptom (dyspareunia, dysmenorrhea, or hyper emesis gravidarum).

Hypochondriasis

The diagnosis of hypochondriasis is used in patients who demonstrate excessive and intrusive health anxiety about the possibility of serious disease that the patient has trouble controlling. Typically, the patient seeks repeated medical reassurance, which only has a short-lived effect. Health anxiety is often present to varying degrees in patients with psychogenic/functional symptoms but may be absent.

Factitious Disorder (DSM-IV 300.19)

This term describes symptoms that are consciously fabricated for the purpose of medical care or other nonfinancial gain.

Munchausen Syndrome

This syndrome describes someone with factitious disorder who wanders between hospitals, typically changing their name and story. There is a strong association with severe personality disorder.

Malingering

Malingering is not a psychiatric diagnosis but describes the deliberate fabrication of symptoms for material gain.

Terminology Used by Neurologists

Many neurologists, even when faced with clear evidence of a functional or psychogenic neurologic problem, usually make no diagnosis at all and simply conclude that there is no evidence of neurologic disease.[2] The term functional describes in the broadest possible sense a problem caused by a change in function (of the nervous system) rather than structure. Use of this term has the advantage of sidestepping the problems of determining the cause, but can be criticized for being too broad. Hysteria is an ancient term originating from the idea of the "wandering womb" causing physical symptoms and is generally viewed as pejorative. The terms psychogenic, psychosomatic, and somatization describe an exclusively psychological cause. The term medically unexplained superficially seems to be a neutral term but is often interpreted by patients and doctors as not knowing what the diagnosis is (rather than not knowing why they have the problem). Furthermore, many neurologic diseases have uncertain causes.

The authors' preferred terms for motor and sensory symptoms and blackouts unexplained by disease are "functional" and "dissociative" because they describe a mechanism and not a cause, they sidestep an illogical debate about whether symptoms are in the mind or the brain, and they can be used easily with patients. For simplicity, the term functional is used in this article, although it is recognized that the term psychogenic remains popular.[3]

EPIDEMIOLOGY OF FUNCTIONAL SYMPTOMS

Studies estimate that one-third of patients seen in outpatient neurology settings present with symptoms that are not caused by neurologic disease.[4–6] These figures mirror those in other medical specialties; **Table 1** lists functional symptoms and syndromes according to specialty.[4] Approximately half of these one-third of patients or 15% of patients seen in a neurology practice are ultimately diagnosed as having a functional disorder, and the other half are determined to have symptoms that are out of proportion to their disease.[5] Studies of patients with functional neurologic symptoms have shown that these patients report just as much physical disability and are more distressed than patients with neurologic disease. Patients with these symptoms are more likely to be out of work because of ill health than the general population.[6]

ETIOLOGY AND MECHANISM

The causes of functional symptoms are multifactorial and vary hugely between patients (**Box 1**). For example, in a systematic review, the frequency of childhood abuse in patients with nonepileptic attacks was 36% compared with 16% in epilepsy, which still leaves most patients studied without this risk factor.[7] Similarly, although in some studies life events are more common before symptom onset,[8] in others, they are no more common.[9]

The neural mechanisms of functional neurologic symptoms are not yet well understood, but functional imaging studies of functional motor symptoms combined with other neurophysiologic techniques are starting to help understand them.[10–12] These studies promise an understanding of these symptoms in parallel neurologic and psychiatric ways.

Table 1 Functional symptoms and syndromes in medical specialties	
Gastroenterology	Irritable bowel syndrome
Respiratory	Chronic cough, brittle asthma (some)
Rheumatology	Fibromyalgia, chronic back pain (some)
Gynecology	Chronic pelvic pain, dysmenorrhea (some)
Allergy	Multiple chemical sensitivity syndrome
Cardiology	Atypical/noncardiac chest pain, palpitations (some)
Infectious diseases	(Postviral) chronic fatigue syndrome, chronic Lyme disease (where the physician disagrees that there is ongoing infection)
ENT	Globus, functional dysphonia
Neurology	Dissociative (nonepileptic) attacks, functional weakness, and sensory symptoms
Psychiatry	Depression, anxiety

Box 1
A range of potential etiologic factors in patients with functional symptoms

Factors	Biologic	Psychological	Social
Factors acting at all stages	Organic Disease	Emotional disorder Personality disorder	Socioeconomic/ deprivation Life events and difficulties
	History of previous functional symptoms		
Predisposing	Genetic factors affecting personality Biologic vulnerabilities in nervous system?	Perception of childhood experience as adverse Personality traits Poor attachment/ coping style	Childhood neglect/ abuse Poor family functioning Symptom modeling (via media or personal contact)
Precipitating	Abnormal physiologic event or state (eg, hyperventilation, sleep deprivation, sleep paralysis) Physical injury/pain	Perception of life event as negative, unexpected Acute dissociative episode/panic attack	
Perpetuating	Plasticity in CNS motor and sensory (including pain) pathways Deconditioning Neuroendocrine and immunologic abnormalities similar to those seen in depression and anxiety	Illness beliefs (patient and family) Perception of symptoms as being caused by disease/ damage/without the scope of self-help Not feeling believed Avoidance of symptom provocation	The presence of a welfare system Social benefits of being ill Availability of legal compensation Stigma of mental illness in society and from medical profession Ongoing medical investigations and uncertainty

CLINICAL ASSESSMENT

A useful way to begin the assessment of the patient with suspected functional neurologic symptoms is to quickly create a list of their physical symptoms, which helps build a rapport early in the interview. Patients should be questioned about fatigue, pain, sleep disturbance, dizziness, and memory and concentration symptoms. The patient's complaints of dizziness may in fact be of dissociative symptoms such as being spaced out or unreal. The onset is sudden in about half the patients with weakness and movement disorders. Physical injury, pain, or an attack with acute symptoms of dissociation or panic is common in this situation. More gradual-onset symptoms are often associated with fatigue.

It is essential at some point to find out the patients own understanding of what they think is wrong and what should be done and if they have any fears about any specific neurologic disease. Beliefs about irreversibility or damage seem to be important prognostic factors[13] and important targets for treatment.

The initial assessment need not be overburdened with attempts at a full psychiatric evaluation. Patients with functional symptoms do have high rates of depression and anxiety but are often wary of questions about their emotions, which, if handled carelessly, risk alienating the patient. It is often wise to leave questions about emotions until later in the consultation or a follow-up visit. **Box 2** lists interviewing strategies for detecting emotional disorder in this patient group.

Psychiatric findings and stressful life events are common, but many patients with functional symptoms do not have either. Avoiding a diagnosis of functional symptoms in someone just because they seem "normal" is as much an error as making the diagnosis simply because the patient has obvious psychological comorbidity. "La belle indifference" (smiling indifference to disability) was once thought to be a useful sign in functional symptoms but occurs in disease at a similar frequency and is not of discriminating value.[9]

The diagnosis of functional neurologic symptoms should be made from physical symptoms demonstrating internal inconsistency or incongruity with neurologic disease. In addition, the clinician must be careful to consider the possibility of comorbid neurologic disease and be aware of the unusual nature of some neurologic disorders, for example, frontal lobe seizures.

Pain or fatigue is often present with functional symptoms disorder, and fatigue may be ultimately the most limiting symptom. Chronic persistent fatigue in the absence of a defined disease process has been labeled in many ways including chronic fatigue syndrome (CFS), neurasthenia, and myalgic encephalomyelitis.

Weakness

Weakness as a functional symptom is more common in women and typically presents in the mid-30s. Estimates of incidence are 5 of 100,000, comparable with that of multiple sclerosis.[8,14] Comorbidity with other functional symptoms, especially fatigue and pain, is common. The most common presentation is unilateral weakness, followed by monoparesis and paraparesis. Complete paralysis is usually temporary and less common.[14] The onset of functional weakness is sudden in around 50% of patients.

Box 2
Interviewing strategies for exploring emotional health in patients with suspected functional disorder

For depression: Ascertain if there are activities that give the patient pleasure; if there are no such activities, the patient may have anhedonia. Inquire if there are friends and family the patient looks forward to seeing. Assess the patient's overall appearance, facial expression, and presence of eye contact. Ask if their physical symptoms make them feel depressed rather than if they themselves are depressed. Depression is likely when there is persistent anhedonia or low mood most of the time, with 4 or more of the following: fatigue, sleep disturbance, suicidal ideation, poor memory or concentration, psychomotor retardation/agitation, and feelings of worthlessness/guilt and/or suicidal ideation.

For anxiety: Ask whether their physical symptoms make them worried rather than if they feel anxious. Look for 3 of the following 6 symptoms: restlessness/nervousness, insomnia, fatigue, irritability, poor concentration, and tense muscles combined with a history of worry that is persistent and hard to control. Worry is often primarily focused on health.

For panic attacks: Ask the patients if they ever have "attacks of symptoms occurring all at once" rather than asking about "panic attacks." Look for 4 of the following: palpitations, sweating, trembling/shaking, shortness of breath, choking sensation, chest pain/pressure, nausea/feeling of imminent diarrhea, dizziness, derealization/depersonalization, fear of going crazy/losing control, fear of dying, tingling, flushes/chills. Panic is a common problem in patients with functional symptoms, especially nonepileptic attacks.

Subjectively, patients with functional weakness often report that the affected limb "doesn't feel as if it belongs" to them or, in extreme situations, as if it "is not there" or "is someone else's" limb. They commonly report that the leg "gives way" or that they drop things unexpectedly.

Box 3 lists signs and maneuvers that may be helpful in identifying functional weakness, none of which are foolproof but can be used together to build clinical confidence. The examiner must be especially careful to consider the possibility of comorbid organic weakness and take in to account the effect of pain or anxiety in the examination.

Movement Disorders

Functional movement disorders account for up to 10% of new referrals to movement disorder specialty clinics.[15] The onset of functional movement disorders, like that of weakness, is often sudden or may be accompanied by pain. The course may be unusual, with sudden remissions or relapses in different limbs. General clues to

---

Box 3
Physical signs that may be helpful in identifying functional weakness

- Global pattern of weakness: the limb is usually globally weak or may demonstrate the inverse of pyramidal weakness, with the flexors weaker in the arms and the extensors weaker in the legs.

- Inconsistency during the examination: for example, a patient who walks to the examination couch but cannot raise their leg against gravity on examination, a weakness of ankle movements when the patient can stand on tip toes or on their heels, or arm weakness in a patient who can remove their shoes or carry a bag.

- Hoover sign: this test is positive when weakness of hip extension returns to normal during contralateral hip flexion against resistance. The test is most easily done with the patient in a sitting position (**Fig. 1**), although it can also be done with the patient lying down and contralateral extension appreciated by holding the patient's heel. The results of this test may be false positive when there is cortical neglect.

- Hip abductor sign: a test similar to Hoover sign involves demonstrating weakness of hip abduction, which returns to normal with contralateral hip abduction against resistance.

- Dragging gait: if there is a moderate or severe unilateral leg weakness, the patient may walk with a dragging gait, in which the foot does not leave the ground. Often the hip is externally or internally rotated (**Fig. 2**).

- Give way weakness: this is a pattern of weakness in which the patient transiently has normal power, but then the limb gives way, sometimes just before it is touched. If the arm is weak, it may hover for a second before collapsing down. The difference between mild give way weakness and normal power can be shown by saying to the patient, "At the count of 3, push—1, 2, 3, push." This is a less-reliable sign and occurs more commonly in painful limbs or occasionally in myasthenia gravis.

- Facial weakness: pseudoptosis is recognized, in which the forehead appears weak with a depressed eyebrow. The problem is overactivity of the orbicularis oculi. A similar appearance of lower facial weakness can occur because of overactivity of the platysma. These features can be enhanced on examination by sustained voluntary contraction of facial or periocular muscles.

Occasionally, patients with functional weakness may have what appears to be an ankle clonus, which on closer inspection has features of a functional tremor. There may also appear to be reflex asymmetry if the patient is co-contracting agonist and antagonist muscles on one side of their body. The plantar response may be relatively mute on the affected side if there is marked sensory disturbance.

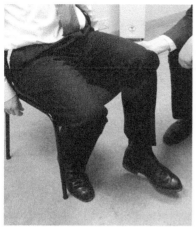 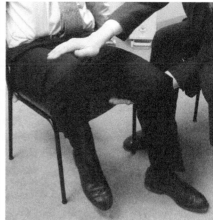

Test hip extension – it's weak | Test contralateral hip flexion against resistance – hip extension has become strong

Fig. 1. Hoover sign is most easily demonstrated in the sitting position. (*Reproduced from* Stone J. The bare essentials: functional symptoms in neurology. Pract Neurol 2009;9:179–89; with permission of BMJ publications.)

a functional movement disorder include improvement with distraction (many neurologic movement disorders get worse during distraction) and worsening with attention. Many organic movement disorders, especially gait disorders, can look bizarre. A careful and structured approach is essential to reach a clear diagnosis. Resolution of symptoms with placebo may be helpful but is not always diagnostic in that some neurologic movement disorders may temporarily improve with placebo.

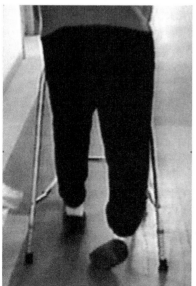 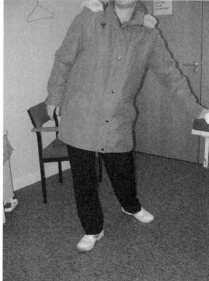

Fig. 2. A dragging gait with external or internal hip rotation is characteristic of functional weakness.

Tremor

Tremor is the most commonly encountered functional/psychogenic movement disorder. There are several positive clinical features, none of which are 100% reliable (**Box 4**). Slowness and postural instability in a patient with functional tremor can give the appearance of Parkinson disease, especially if the patient is also depressed, with diminished facial expression. The slowness is distractible and without the normal decrement seen in parkinsonism. There may be stiffness but with a quality of active resistance to it. Fluorodopa positron emission tomographic scanning or dopamine transporter *single photon emission computed tomographic* scanning should be normal in patients with functional movement disorder.

Myoclonus

Brief jerky movements may seem like myoclonus. More commonly, patients have complex hyperkinetic movements that are hard to accurately classify. Functional myoclonus may be stimulus sensitive, especially during deep tendon reflex testing, when myoclonus may occur even before the reflex hammer has made contact.[12] Functional myoclonus is often associated with a Bereitschaftpotential (BP) before the movement, which requires recording multiple events using an electroencephalogram and back averaging according to an electromyogram. The presence of a BP

Box 4
Findings and tests useful in making the diagnosis of a functional tremor

- Variable frequency: this test may include starting and stopping of the tremor and is more useful than variable amplitude, which can be found in organic tremor.

- Entrainment test: This test is performed by asking the patient to make a rhythmic tapping movement with their unaffected limb, preferably at around 3 Hz. The test can be improved if the patient is externally cued by having to copy a similar movement in the examiner. If the tremor is functional, then one of several things may happen: (1) the patient is unable to copy the simple tapping movement and cannot explain why, (2) the tremor in the affected limb stops, or (3) the tremor in the affected hand entrains to the same rhythm as the examiner's. False positive results in this test seem to be rare. False negative results, however, are more common, particularly if the tremor is longstanding (and hence more automatic) or if the tremor relies on mechanics (eg, a heel-tapping leg tremor in someone sitting with their foot plantarflexed on the ground is characteristic of a functional tremor).[16] Accelerometry, if available, can be helpful in recording the response to this test.

- Distractibility using mental tasks: other forms of distraction, such as being asked to calculate serial 7s, can temporarily abolish tremor.

- Ballistic movements: ask the patient to make sudden ballistic movements with their unaffected hand by touching the rapidly moving finger of the examiner. Functional tremor often stops briefly during the movement.

- Attempted immobilization: attempting to immobilize the affected limb often makes a functional tremor worse. Likewise, loading the limb with weights tends to make the tremor worse, whereas organic tremor tends to improve with this maneuver.

- Coactivation sign: most functional tremor is similar to voluntary tremor. Sometimes the mechanism of the tremor is different and relates to coactivation of agonist and antagonist muscles (like shivering).

- Coherence analysis: if functional tremor is present in more than one limb, it usually has the same frequency. In contrast, organic tremor usually has slightly different frequencies in different body parts. Therefore, demonstrating coherence of the tremor between different body parts can provide supportive evidence of a functional tremor.

does not provide evidence of a conscious intention to move but does indicate that the voluntary motor system is being used for the movement.

Dystonia

In the heyday of psychoanalysis, cervical dystonia was interpreted as a "turning away of responsibility" and writers cramp as evidence of sexual conflict. Nonetheless, there is now a consensus that dystonic movements, especially in fixed dystonia, in which the posture does not fluctuate, do occur as a functional/psychogenic phenomenon. The most common presentation is a clenched fist, sometimes with wrist-elbow flexion or an inverted and plantarflexed foot (**Fig. 3**).[17] Fixed dystonia is most frequently seen in association with limb pain; however, it can occur without pain, commonly in a limb with functional weakness. Neurophysiologic studies have found it impossible to distinguish functional dystonia and organic dystonia by neurophysiologic measures such as short and long intracortical inhibition, cortical silent period, and reciprocal inhibition in the forearm, although measures of cortical plasticity may be different.[16] It is perhaps with dystonia that traditional boundaries between functional and structural disorders are at their most blurred.

Gait disorders

In studies of misdiagnosis, gait disorders figure disproportionately in cases in which the initial diagnosis of a functional problem turned out to be wrong. Nonetheless, there are certain characteristic types of functional gait disorders[18,19]: (1) dragging gait (as described in functional weakness); (2) tightrope walker's gait, where the arms are outstretched like a tightrope walker, often with lurches to one side and the other but good recovery of balance; (3) astasia-abasia, where there is normal limb power and sensation on the bed but inability to stand and walk (this can occur in organic truncal ataxia and sensory ataxia); and (4) crouching gait, which requires better strength and balance than a normal gait. Patients with this gait can be frightened of falling, and this gait allows them to be closer to the ground; knee buckling gait is usually seen when the patient has unilateral functional weakness.

Sensory Symptoms

Functional sensory symptoms are common in patients with functional weakness and in patients with chronic unexplained limb pain. These symptoms occur on their own, although patients often have some signs of functional weakness on examination even in the absence of symptoms of weakness. Examination findings in functional sensory

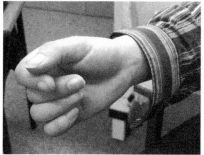 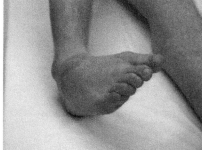

Fig. 3. Functional/psychogenic dystonia typically presents with a clenched fist or an inverted plantarflexed ankle. (*Reproduced from* Stone J. The bare essentials: functional symptoms in neurology. Pract Neurol 2009;9:179–89; with permission of BMJ publications.)

disturbance are much less reliable than motor signs, and it is best to rely on evidence of mild functional weakness if present. The following signs are sensitive but not specific:

- Alteration of vibration sense across the forehead or sternum
- Tests for complete sensory loss: complete sensory loss is rare so that tests such as "say yes when you feel it and no when you don't" and "close your eyes and touch your nose when I touch your hand" are rarely useful (and involve some physician deception anyway); the Bowlus maneuver requires patients to interlock their fingers behind their back and state whether the right or left finger is being touched
- Other sensory tests such as finding exact splitting of sensation at the midline and nondermatomal sensory loss are common but even less specific for functional sensory symptoms.

Visual Symptoms

There are several patterns of functional visual complaints. Intermittent blurred vision is often ipsilateral to functional weakness and hemisensory disturbance. Functional binocular diplopia is usually caused by convergence spasm, an asymmetrical overactivity of the normal convergence response. This condition can be demonstrated by testing convergence movements but holding the finger at a close distance for longer than usual. When convergence spasm is persistent, it can resemble a sixth nerve palsy. Monocular diplopia is usually functional but can be caused by ocular abnormality. Triplopia is usually related to an organic eye-movement abnormality but can be functional.[20]

Complete functional visual loss

When this is suspected, patients can be asked to put their fingers together or sign their name (not a problem if neurologically blind). Physicians can put out their hand as if they are expecting a handshake or watch the patients navigate around the room. Normal findings include pupillary response, menace reflex (sudden movements of the hand toward the eye), and optokinetic nystagmus with a rotating striped drum. There may be a convergence response to a mirror placed close in front of the face. The possibility of organic cortical blindness should always be considered.

Monocular/partial visual loss

At the bedside, many patients with functional monocular symptoms have a tubular field defect, such that the visual field at 2 m is the same width as that at 1 m. Normally, the visual field is conical, such that the visual field at 2 m is twice as large as that at 1 m. Another common finding is spiral, star-shaped or pinpoint visual fields on Goldmann perimetry. As the test proceeds, the patient tires and reports progressively constricted fields. A large variety of other tests exist to give an objective measure of acuity.[21] For example, in monocular visual problems, the fogging test involves gradually worsening acuity in the normal eye until the point when any acuity better than 6/60 must be from the affected eye. The stereoscopic test gives an estimate of the acuity based on the perception of varying stereoscopic images.

Speech and Swallowing Symptoms

Articulation

Functional dysarthria usually takes the form of intermittent slurred speech or stuttering speech, with difficulty starting words. Speech may be slow and with hesitations noticeably occurring in the middle of sentences when it is harder to interrupt. In this context, speech may become telegrammatic, missing the prepositions and conjunctions of normal speech. Just as functional weakness is at its worst when directly tested, functional speech problems are worst when having to repeat words or phrases to command and, like developmental stuttering, may resolve when the patient is singing or speaking about something that makes them feel emotional or angry. Complete mutism still occurs; the authors have seen a man who used a computer to speak for 4 years before making a good recovery.

Dysphonia

Functional dysphonia is a common presenting symptom to otolaryngologists but may be seen by neurologists in combination with other functional symptoms. Speech is usually a whisper and may follow on from a genuine or perceived episode of laryngitis. At least 6 randomized controlled trials (RCTs) in this field have suggested benefit of voice therapy.[22]

Globus

Globus describes the symptom of something being stuck in the throat, even when the patient is not swallowing anything. There is controversy regarding how often this symptom can be explained by gastroesophageal reflux disease.

Memory and Cognitive Symptoms

Cognitive symptoms are common among patients with functional neurologic symptoms. These symptoms may be attributable (by doctor or patient) to associated fatigue, anxiety, or low mood or become presenting symptoms in their own right. Anxiety about the cause can amplify the problem and lead to neurologic referral. A subgroup of patients in any memory clinic present without obvious anxiety, depression, or stress (apart from anxiety about their memory symptoms).[23]

Functional memory symptoms are typically those that many people might regard as normal, such as forgetting why they went upstairs, losing their keys, or losing track of conversation. A common feature is the report of variability in memory for familiar facts such as their own address, which they forget but recall in a short while. Difficulty in finding words may be present in patients with functional neurologic symptoms, although true dysphasia is rare.

In pure retrograde amnesia, patients present with an inability to recall extensive parts of their past life. In dissociative fugue, the disturbance is sudden and characterized by unexpected travel away from home or customary place of work.

Cognitive effort tests are simple tests that even patients with severe dementia or head injury should be able to perform well. For example, the "coin in the hand" test involves 10 trials of showing a patient which hand a coin is held in and asking them to close their eyes for 10 seconds and then choose the hand with the coin.[24] A score at chance indicates poor effort. A score below chance is sometimes used as evidence of factitious disorder/malingering, although in reality, these tests cannot distinguish between conscious or unconscious exaggeration.

INVESTIGATIONS

The presence of positive signs of a functional symptom does not exclude a comorbid underlying neurologic disease. Laboratory and/or radiologic tests are therefore often required. Wherever possible, the diagnosis of functional weakness/movement disorder should be indicated to the patient at the first visit, explaining that the physician expects the tests to be normal. Ideally tests should be performed quickly and in parallel rather than in series to avoid the agony of "diagnostic limbo."

MALINGERING

Malingering has always been closely associated with "hysteria" because the symptoms relate to the voluntary nervous system.[25] Distinguishing symptoms that are under conscious intentional voluntary control from those that are not is difficult because (1) the positive signs used to make a diagnosis of functional symptoms would be the same if someone was malingering, (2) doctors are not trained to detect deception, and (3) some patients may be in a state of self-deception. Clues to malingering include a documented history of lying in the past or using different names, major inconsistencies in the history given to different clinicians, and avoidance of investigations. The only definitive ways to be confident that malingering is an explanation for functional neurologic symptoms are (1) if patients are covertly observed doing something that is highly discrepant with what they have claimed to be able to do (eg, playing squash when they claim to be in a wheelchair) or (2) if they confess to malingering.[26]

MISDIAGNOSIS

Although neurologists tend to worry about malingering, doctors other than neurologists, especially psychiatrists, tend to be preoccupied by the opposite concern of misdiagnosis. Studies in the 1950s and 1960s suggested high rates of misdiagnosis of hysteria in up to 60% of patients.[27,28] The authors' systematic review of 27 studies including 1466 patients with a mean follow-up of 5 years found a frequency of misdiagnosis of about 4% since 1970, before the advent of computed tomographic scans and videotelemetry.[28] A recent study of 1144 patients in Scotland found an even lower misdiagnosis rate at 18 months of only 4 patients.[5]

PROGNOSIS

Long-term follow-up studies have suggested that functional neurologic symptoms persist in most patients and improve in roughly a third.[4,29–31] Sensory symptoms have a better prognosis than weakness, which in turn has a better outcome than fixed dystonia.[30] Good prognostic factors for functional neurologic symptoms from research studies include a willingness to accept the potential reversibility of the symptoms,[13] an acceptance that psychological factors may play a part in symptom formation, a good interaction with the doctor, a short duration of symptoms, a lack of other physical symptoms, the presence of concurrent anxiety and depression, and removal of stress or change in marital status (either divorce or marriage).[4]

    Poor prognostic factors include strong beliefs in lack of reversibility of symptoms/damage, anger at the diagnosis of a nonorganic disorder, delayed diagnosis, multiple other physical symptoms/somatization disorder, concurrent organic disease, personality disorder, older age, sexual abuse, receipt of financial benefits, and litigation. However, in most studies, these prognostic factors only explained a limited amount of the variance. In practice, some patients with poor prognostic factors respond well to treatment and some patients with good prognostic features do badly.

TREATMENT: EXPLANATION

The literature supports the premise that a good explanation of the symptoms to a patient with a functional disorder is a prerequisite to successful further treatment.[32] **Box 5** lists the components that may play a role in the explanation and provide a constructive basis for further treatment. The issue of whether patients are told that they have psychogenic symptoms, conversion disorder, functional symptoms, or dissociative symptoms is only one of these components, depends on how the

---

Box 5
Components of a successful explanation for patients with functional symptoms

Ingredient	Example
Explain what they do have	"You have 'functional weakness'" "You have dissociative (nonepileptic) attacks"
Emphasize the mechanism of the symptoms rather than the cause	Weakness: "your nervous system is not damaged, but it is not functioning properly" Attacks: "you are going into a trancelike state, a bit like someone being hypnotised"
Explain how you made the diagnosis	Show patients their Hoover sign, tremor entrainment, or dissociative attack video, explaining why it is typical of the diagnosis you are making
Explain what they do not have	"You do not have multiple sclerosis, epilepsy, and so on"
Indicate that you believe them	"I do not think you are imagining/making up your symptoms/mad"
Emphasize that it is common	"I see lots of patients with similar symptoms"
Emphasize reversibility	"Because there is no damage, you have the potential to get better"
Emphasize that self-help is a key part of getting better	"This is not your fault, but there are things you can do to help it get better"
Metaphors may be useful	"The hardware is alright, but there is a software problem," "it is like a car/piano that is out of tune"
Introducing the role of depression/anxiety	"If you have been feeling low/worried, that will tend to make the symptoms even worse" (often easier to achieve on a second visit)
Use written information	Send the patient their clinic letter. Give them a Web site address (eg, www.neurosymptoms.org)
Suggesting antidepressants when appropriate	"So-called antidepressants often help these symptoms even in patients who are not feeling depressed. They are not addictive."
Making the psychiatric referral when appropriate	"I do not think you are mad, but Dr X has a lot of experience and interest in helping people like you to manage and overcome their symptoms. Are you willing to overcome any misgivings about their specialty to try to get better?"
Involve the family/friends	Explain it all to them as well

physician conceives of the problem, and is not as important as the totality of the explanation. It is key that whatever terminology is used does not alienate the patient. Terms such as psychogenic are commonly interpreted by patients as meaning crazy or making symptoms up, so even if this term is preferred for theoretical reasons, it should be considered whether patients are translating the term into meanings that were never intended. The authors find that "functional" is a useful acceptable term,[32] which, along with dissociative, describes a mechanism and leaves the cause more open. These two terms have the advantage of allowing a more integrated description involving biologic, psychological, and social factors as stressors on neural function and allow treatment aimed at restoring nervous system function. A common criticism is that these terms are too broad and open to confusion. One option is to use a functional explanation by default and introduce discussion of psychological factors later if relevant or necessary. Ultimately the sincerity with which the diagnosis is delivered may be more important than the precise words used.

There are other barriers to successful explanation. Even when patients are comfortable with the diagnosis of functional symptoms, it is hard to explain the diagnosis to friends, family, and employers. Neurologists, for their part, are often not sure what to think about this whole area of their practice and may prefer to dodge the whole issue by simply explaining that there is no neurologic disease, which, however, avoids the key (and reasonable) need of the patient to know what they *do* have wrong with them.

Explanation may be usefully supplemented by online material. There is further free self-help information at www.neurosymptoms.org, written by the authors.

FURTHER TREATMENT

Traditionally, many neurologists terminate their involvement with a patient once a functional disorder is suspected, handing care back to the family doctor or referring on to a psychiatrist. However, neurologists can play an important role with further visits to reinforce the explanation and rationale for the diagnosis. If the patient gains trust in the treating physician, it becomes relatively easy to discuss any associated psychological factors and, if appropriate, a referral to a psychiatrist /psychologist with experience in this area. Because up to one-third of all neurology outpatients have functional symptoms to some degree, it is unlikely they could all access specialist psychological treatment; nor do of them need it. Patients with mild symptoms may just need to be steered in the right direction and given sensible information, and they will do the rest themselves.

Patients who struggle with disabling symptoms are likely to benefit from further treatment. A recent RCT in patients with psychogenic nonepileptic seizures showed benefit from cognitive behavioral treatment (CBT) compared with standard therapy over a 6-month period.[33] An RCT in somatization disorder showed similarly positive results.[34] Other uncontrolled studies have shown similar treatment effects for CBT in dissociative (nonepileptic) seizures[33] and for more broad-based psychotherapy in a range of functional neurologic symptoms.[35]

Psychiatrists and psychologists need to be familiar with the issues involved in the diagnosis of patients with functional symptoms to reinforce the rationale for diagnosis (ie, they are not just there because the test results are negative, there was positive evidence of the diagnosis on examination). It is important that the patient receives an explanation for their symptoms that is consistent with the one they received from the neurologist. A psychiatrist can also assess for comorbidities, such as depression, anxiety, or personality disorder. Once the diagnosis is reached, different treatment options are available.

Cognitive behavioral treatment involves developing the patient's diagnosis to change what they think about their symptoms and how they behave as a consequence of them (**Table 2**). It is an approach based in learning theory and aims to provide a detailed examination of the interactions between physical symptoms, thoughts, behavior, and mood. For example, a patient with back pain may rest at the first signs of exacerbation, removing the pain in the short term but leading to long-term poorer function. Illness and other beliefs also feature; patients may believe that an acute exacerbation of their back pain is a sign of damage and thus strive to avoid this and become fearful of it, which in

Table 2 Examples of changes in thoughts and behavior that can help in patients with functional symptoms			
	Dissociative Attacks	**Functional Weakness**	**Chronic Back Pain**
Old thought	"Oh no, what's happening to me. Am I going to die during one of these attacks?"	"I've got multiple sclerosis, I'm going to end up in a wheelchair. No one believes me"	"My spine is damaged, I must avoid moving too much in case it makes it worse"
New thought	"I'm going into a trancelike state a bit like a panic attack"	"Mmm… this is odd, but it looks as if I can get better. That doctor is right that when I'm not thinking about the leg it does seem to move better"	"My bones are fine, its my muscles that are stiff and out of condition"
Old behavior	Avoid going out. Worry constantly about attacks	Seeing lots of specialists. Not doing very much in case it makes it worse	Avoiding exercise/back movement
New behavior	Try out distraction techniques during warning symptoms	Gradually exercise trying not to focus on limb weakness, learn to expect relapses	Gradually exercise expecting exacerbations of pain

turn can result in increased muscle tension and poor posture, making the actual occurrence more likely. Such vicious circles are postulated as contributing to the genesis of many functional symptoms, and the therapy aims to unpick them.

Psychodynamic psychotherapies have been historically popular in the treatment of functional neurologic symptoms, but empirical support is lacking. There is, however, evidence of benefit of short psychodynamic psychotherapy in other somatic symptoms such as irritable bowel syndrome and chronic pain.[36] Such therapy is based on the premise that symptom development occurs as a means of escape from an interpersonal conflict. These conflicts are seen in the context of abnormally learned patterns of interpersonal relationships during childhood, which then go on to distort social interactions in adulthood. For example, a patient who has suffered an abusive upbringing may perceive the neutral comments of their physician as being attacking or aggressive because they identify the paternal role of the physician with their actual experience of an abusive father. The patient's behavior of either anger or extreme passivity can engender feelings of irritation in the physician bringing the fantasy view into reality. Therapy based on these principles includes learning to recognize these subconscious maladaptive patterns, allowing for a more mature and social-skilled approach to interpersonal conflict resolution and discarding the presumed psychic need to develop physical symptoms.

In addition to the aforementioned approach, some additional helpful measures include the following:

Physiotherapy is important for someone with a physical disability. For weakness, rather than paying a lot of attention to the weak limb, as one might do after a stroke, it may be helpful to use distraction techniques during movement to allow better movement. Principles of graded exercise as used in CFS are likely to be helpful. As with back pain, patients should be told to expect relapses as they increase activity. Mental imagery techniques and mirror therapy as used in complex regional pain syndrome may be useful.

Physical aids and appliances/sickness benefits: Patients with disability from functional symptoms may ask if they should have a wheelchair or receive health-related financial benefits. The advice here is not really different from that to any other patient with a disability that may improve. Wheelchairs and sickness benefits definitely improve independence and morale in some patients; they also create a further obstacle to rehabilitation by discouraging day-to-day movement and an early return to work.

Hypnosis is a treatment with a long association with functional neurologic symptoms especially suited to functional motor symptoms. Two RCTs found it to be of benefit in patients with motor symptoms.[37] Patients may be able to learn self-hypnosis and other relaxation techniques.

Sedation: Patients with prolonged paralysis or fixed dystonia may benefit from examination under sedation. Rather than interview the patient under sedation, the authors use it to demonstrate better function under sedation than during wakefulness and to kick start some improvement. An anesthetist administers an intravenous propofol infusion titrated to the point at which the patient is almost unconscious. The session is filmed to be later shown to the patient. A secondary function of the procedure is to look for evidence of contractures in patients with fixed dystonia. It is important for the patient to be given vigorous physiotherapy immediately afterward if they have made some improvement during the procedure.

Pharmacotherapy

There is little evidence to guide the use of antidepressant drugs for patients with functional neurologic symptoms, except for one recent trial of a selective serotonin reuptake inhibitor in 33 patients with nonepileptic attacks.[38] A systematic review found that antidepressants were effective for a range of functional symptoms in other specialities and that outcomes do not seem to be affected by the presence or absence of depressed mood.[39] If comorbid anxiety, depression, or panic is present, drug treatment can be discussed on its own merits. Similarly, there is evidence for the use of tricyclic antidepressants in pain or insomnia. Pharmacotherapy, when indicated, should be started at a low dose, and the dose is increased slowly. It is always good care to advise the patient of possible side effects and monitor them accordingly.

The Patient Who Does Not Improve

All patients with functional symptoms do not automatically get better. Neurologists should bear in mind that only 1 in 3 patients (or much < that for symptoms like fixed dystonia) improve spontaneously. It is important to maintain reasonable expectations of one's own therapeutic abilities in a situation in which only 1 of multiple powerful perpetuating factors is uncertainty about the diagnosis. If, despite best efforts, the patient does not really believe or cannot understand the diagnosis, then the physician has probably done what he or she can. Alternatively, the patient may be fully accepting of the diagnosis, but it may be too difficult for anyone to help. Patients can be told that they have done their best for the time being and their symptoms may improve in the future, but for now the management is to learn to work around the symptoms. In this situation, the patient's primary physician has an important role in recognizing vulnerability to symptoms, treating intercurrent mood and anxiety problems, and protecting them from unnecessary investigations and treatments in secondary care where possible.

SUMMARY

Functional and dissociative symptoms in neurology are common, disabling, and distressing. The diagnosis should be made from positive physical signs of inconsistency or incongruity combined with a sound knowledge of neurologic disease, not on psychological grounds. Neurologists are in a good position to alter the illness trajectories of many patients, with a careful and rational explanation of the diagnosis and onward appropriate referral.

Sources of self-help for patients: www.neurosymptoms.org, free self-help material designed specifically for the symptoms described in this article.

REFERENCES

1. Stone J, LaFrance WC, Levenson JL, et al. Issues for DSM-5: conversion disorder. Am J Psychiatry 2010;167:626–7.
2. Friedman JH, LaFrance WC Jr. Psychogenic disorders: the need to speak plainly. Arch Neurol 2010;67:753–5.
3. Espay AJ, Goldenhar LM, Voon V, et al. Opinions and clinical practices related to diagnosing and managing patients with psychogenic movement disorders: an international survey of Movement Disorder Society members. Mov Disord 2009;24:1366–74.
4. Crimlisk HL, Bhatia K, Cope H, et al. Slater revisited: 6 year follow up study of patients with medically unexplained motor symptoms. BMJ 1998;316:582–6.
5. Stone J, Carson A, Duncan R, et al. Symptoms 'unexplained by organic disease' in 1144 new neurology out-patients: how often does the diagnosis change at follow-up? Brain 2009;132:2878–88.
6. Carson A, Stone J, Hibberd C. et al. Disability, distress and unemployment in neurology outpatients with symptoms 'unexplained by disease'. J Neurol Neurosurg Psychiatry, in press.
7. Sharpe D, Faye C. Non-epileptic seizures and child sexual abuse: a critical review of the literature. Clin Psychol Rev 2006;26:1020–40.
8. Binzer M, Andersen PM, Kullgren G. Clinical characteristics of patients with motor disability due to conversion disorder: a prospective control group study. J Neurol Neurosurg Psychiatry 1997;63:83–8.
9. Roelofs K, Spinhoven P, Sandijck P, et al. The impact of early trauma and recent life-events on symptom severity in patients with conversion disorder. J Nerv Ment Dis 2005;193:508–14.
10. Cojan Y, Waber L, Carruzzo A, et al. Motor inhibition in hysterical conversion paralysis. Neuroimage 2009;47:1026–37.
11. Vuilleumier P, Chicherio C, Assal F, et al. Functional neuroanatomical correlates of hysterical sensorimotor loss. Brain 2001;124:1077–90.
12. Espay AJ, Morgante F, Purzner J, et al. Cortical and spinal abnormalities in psychogenic dystonia. Ann Neurol 2006;59:825–34.
13. Sharpe M, Stone J, Hibberd C, et al. Neurology out-patients with symptoms unexplained by disease: illness beliefs and financial benefits predict 1-year outcome. Psychol Med 2010;40:689–98.
14. Stone J, Warlow C, Sharpe M. The symptom of functional weakness: a controlled study of 107 patients. Brain 2010;133:1537–51.
15. Hallett M, Fahn S, Jankovic J, et al. Psychogenic movement disorders. Philadelphia: Lippincott Williams & Wilkins; 2006.
16. Hallett M. Physiology of psychogenic movement disorders. J Clin Neurosci 2010; 17:959–65.
17. Schrag A, Trimble M, Quinn N, et al. The syndrome of fixed dystonia: an evaluation of 103 patients. Brain 2004;127:2360–72.
18. Lempert T, Brandt T, Dieterich M, et al. How to identify psychogenic disorders of stance and gait. A video study in 37 patients. J Neurol 1991;238:140–6.

19. Baik JS, Lang AE. Gait abnormalities in psychogenic movement disorders. Mov Disord 2007;22:395–9.
20. Keane JR. Triplopia: thirteen patients from a neurology inpatient service. Arch Neurol 2006;63:388–9.
21. Chen CS, Lee AW, Karagiannis A, et al. Practical clinical approaches to functional visual loss. J Clin Neurosci 2007;14:1–7.
22. Ruotsalainen JH, Sellman J, Lehto L, et al. Interventions for treating functional dysphonia in adults. Cochrane Database Syst Rev 2007;3:CD006373.
23. Schmidtke K, Pohlmann S, Metternich B. The syndrome of functional memory disorder: definition, etiology, and natural course. Am J Geriatr Psychiatry 2008; 16:981–8.
24. Kapur N. The coin-in-the-hand test: a new "bed-side" test for the detection of malingering in patients with suspected memory disorder. J Neurol Neurosurg Psychiatry 1994;57:385–6.
25. Kanaan R, Armstrong D, Barnes P, et al. In the psychiatrist's chair: how neurologists understand conversion disorder. Brain 2009;132:2889–96.
26. Sharpe M. Distinguishing malingering from psychiatric disorders. In: Halligan PW, Bass C, Oakley DA, editors. Malingering and illness deception. Oxford: OUP; 2003.
27. Stone J, Hewett R, Carson A, et al. The 'disappearance' of hysteria: historical mystery or illusion? J R Soc Med 2008;101:12–8.
28. Stone J, Smyth R, Carson A, et al. Systematic review of misdiagnosis of conversion symptoms and "hysteria". BMJ 2005;331:989.
29. McKenzie P, Oto M, Russell A, et al. Early outcomes and predictors in 260 patients with psychogenic nonepileptic attacks. Neurology 2010;74:64–9.
30. Stone J, Sharpe M, Rothwell PM, et al. The 12 year prognosis of unilateral functional weakness and sensory disturbance. J Neurol Neurosurg Psychiatry 2003;74:591–6.
31. Jankovic J, Vuong KD, Thomas M. Psychogenic tremor: long-term outcome. CNS Spectr 2006;11:501–8.
32. Carton S, Thompson PJ, Duncan JS. Non-epileptic seizures: patients' understanding and reaction to the diagnosis and impact on outcome. Seizure 2003; 12:287–94.
33. Goldstein LH, Chalder T, Chigwedere C, et al. Cognitive-behavioral therapy for psychogenic nonepileptic seizures: a pilot RCT. Neurology 2010;74(24):1986–94.
34. Allen LA, Woolfolk RL, Escobar JI, et al. Cognitive-behavioral therapy for somatization disorder: a randomized controlled trial. Arch Intern Med 2006;166(14): 1512–8.
35. Reuber M, Burness C, Howlett S, et al. Tailored psychotherapy for patients with functional neurological symptoms: a pilot study. J Psychosom Res 2007;63:625–32.
36. Abbass A, Kisely S, Kroenke K. Short-term psychodynamic psychotherapy for somatic disorders. Systematic review and meta-analysis of clinical trials. Psychother Psychosom 2009;78:265–74.
37. Moene FC, Spinhoven P, Hoogduin KA, et al. A randomised controlled clinical trial on the additional effect of hypnosis in a comprehensive treatment programme for in-patients with conversion disorder of the motor type. Psychother Psychosom 2002;71:66–76.
38. LaFrance WC Jr, Keitner GI, Papandonatos GD, et al. Pilot pharmacologic randomized controlled trial for psychogenic nonepileptic seizures. Neurology 2010;75:1166–73.
39. O'Malley PG, Jackson JL, Santoro J, et al. Antidepressant therapy for unexplained symptoms and symptom syndromes. J Fam Pract 1999;48:980–90.

Neuropathic Pain: Mind-body Considerations

Brian Hainline, MD[a,b]

KEYWORDS

• Neuropathic • Nociceptive • Mind-body • Limbic

MIND-BODY MEDICINE OVERVIEW

Traditional neurology focuses on obtaining a history of the present illness, and separately obtaining a past medical history, family history, and social history. Although the past medical history, family history, and social history may be relevant to the history of the present illness, they are generally not incorporated into the proposed pathophysiology of the patient's condition. The history of the present illness, coupled with the physical examination and pertinent imaging studies, form the basis of first localizing a lesion or lesions in the nervous system, and then deriving a differential diagnosis of medical processes that may cause such lesion or lesions. Ultimately, traditional neurology focuses on reductionist thinking in which the disease state is associated with a lesion or lesions of the nervous system.[1] The patient's perceptions, family and social situation, and environmental factors are usually not at the forefront of localizing the lesion and forming a differential diagnosis.

Psychiatry and neurology were previously unified fields of study. Several social and medical forces led to a separation of these 2 fields, and a particularly strong force was the emergence of psychoanalytical theory.[2] For example, at the turn of the twentieth century, schizophrenia was described neuroanatomically, genetically, and behaviorally,[3] but the emergence of psychoanalytical theory led to schizophrenia being considered a mind or psychiatric condition.[4] Because emerging neuroscience clearly points to abnormalities in brain function in schizophrenia, this condition is now more properly considered a neuropsychiatric condition. Using schizophrenia as a model, some have argued that the current boundary between psychiatry and neurology is, in essence, a baseless cleavage of brain-based disorders into 2 separate medical specialties with 2 separate conceptual frameworks for understanding pathophysiology and management.[5–8]

Psychiatry and neurology are not the only example of how the mind and body have been cleaved in the practice of medicine. In the middle of the twentieth century,

[a] Department of Neurology, New York University School of Medicine, NY, USA
[b] ProHEALTH Care Associates, Neurology and Integrative Pain Medicine, 3 Delaware Drive, Lake Success, NY 11042, USA
E-mail address: bhainline@prohealthcare.com

Neurol Clin 29 (2011) 19–33
doi:10.1016/j.ncl.2010.10.007
0733-8619/11/$ – see front matter © 2011 Elsevier Inc. All rights reserved.

psychosomatic medicine was becoming a respectable field, both in Europe and in America.[2] Psychosomatic medicine was a challenge to more mechanistic and reductionistic thinking in medical practice. In essence, the practice of psychosomatic medicine places the patient at the center of the medical encounter, rather than focusing on pathogens that could cause a disease state in the patient. Psychosomatic medicine incorporated the effects of chronic repressed emotions and stress in the underlying manifestation of disease, with an understanding that chronic, repressed emotions could target vegetative organs such as the cardiovascular system, pulmonary system, and gastrointestinal system.[9] However, by the 1980s, psychosomatic medicine was considered alternative and no longer within the mainstream of modern medicine. In this setting, the mind-body dialog no longer assumed primary importance.

Even as mind-body medicine lost its importance relative to mainstream medicine, the importance of trauma in producing disease took a significant leap forward when the American Psychiatric Association recognized posttraumatic stress disorder as a valid clinical entity.[2] This diagnosis paved the way for the acceptance in traditional medicine that war, rape, and other types of physical and emotional abuse could lead to the development of physical and mental symptomatology that could be recognizable and managed in a clinical setting. The emergence of posttraumatic stress disorder as a recognizable clinical entity is especially pertinent to neuropathic pain because clinical manifestations and functional brain imaging studies of patients who suffer with chronic posttraumatic stress disorder and chronic neuropathic pain are similar.[10,11]

DEFINITIONS

The International Association for the Study of Pain defines pain as an unpleasant sensory and emotional experience associated with actual or potential tissue damage, or described in terms of such damage.[12] It is clear from this definition that pain is both a physical and an emotional experience. Using this definition as a springboard, it is useful to differentiate pain into either nociceptive pain or neuropathic pain.[13]

Nociceptive pain is pain that is appropriate to an inciting event, and is generated by activation of peripheral nerves called nociceptors. Neuropathic pain is defined as pain initiated or caused by a primary lesion or dysfunction in the nervous system.[12] Neuropathic pain is defined as a nervous system lesion or dysfunction that is no longer dependent on activation of primary afferent nociceptors. Thus, neuropathic pain takes on a life of its own, independent of an ongoing inciting event. As an example, if someone places a hand in a fire, the appropriate nociceptive response is immediate hand withdrawal coupled with the perception of pain. If tissue damage occurs as a result of the fire, the patient will experience ongoing nociceptive pain that is appropriate to ongoing tissue damage. However, if the patient continues to manifest with pain months after the tissue has healed appropriately, then there no longer exists an inciting event to account for the pain response. This condition enters the domain of neuropathic pain, because the pain is caused either by a lesion or dysfunction of the nervous system.

The controversy about the definition of neuropathic pain has to do with dysfunction.[1] Neurologic diseases are commonly defined in terms of lesion localization. Thus, if nerve damage can be identified as a result of placing a hand in a flame, then the nerve damage becomes a lesion that can account for an ongoing clinical manifestation. If no such lesion is identified and the patient has neuropathic pain, then such pain is a manifestation of nervous system dysfunction. However, if we insist on identifying a lesion and cannot accept nervous system dysfunction as a cause of pain, then we assume the pain has no basis in organicity and is simply from the mind; such thinking creates a mind-body split. In this article, neuropathic pain is defined as pain initiated or caused by a primary lesion or dysfunction in the nervous system. Patients who suffer with neuropathic pain complain of physical, emotional, cognitive, and social suffering. Neuropathic pain is therefore an example of a transformation from an inciting event with an appropriate response to a more complex behavioral manifestation. Given this framework, it is appropriate to consider neuropathic pain as a neuropsychiatric condition. Failure to appreciate the multidimensional nature of neuropathic pain will lead to failure in managing this condition appropriately.

PATHOPHYSIOLOGY
Pain Pathways

Nociceptive pain processing begins in the peripheral nervous system in primary afferent neurons called nociceptors, which may be mechanical, thermal, or chemical. Nociceptors distinguish noxious from innocuous events. Once threshold activation is achieved in these afferent neurons, pain-appropriate afferent transmission occurs through lightly myelinated or unmyelinated nerves, primarily through the dorsal root of the spinal cord, although there is also a ventral root pathway.[14]

In the simplistic view of pain processing, nociceptive-specific pathways ascend the spinal cord by the neocortical spinothalamic tract to the contralateral thalamus, and then end in the primary and secondary somatosensory cortices. Such pathway activation is critical for the protective response to a potential physical threat. However, at the level of the spinal cord, nociceptive input can be modified. Spinal cord wide dynamic range cells can amplify nociceptive afferent input,[14] which can lead to more widespread ascending pathways from the spinal cord to the brain.

In addition, 3 critical descending pathways influence nociceptive afferent input at the level of the spinal cord: the endogenous opioid system, the serotonergic system, and the adrenergic system. The endogenous opioid system originates in the midbrain periaquaductal gray matter. Endogenous opioids are endorphins and enkephalins that not only regulate the pain response but also homeostasis, immune function, and the stress response. If the periaquaductal gray matter is activated, the dorsal horn neurons become inhibited, leading to relative analgesia. The endogenous opioid system interacts with the dorsal raphe nucleus, which is the origin of the serotonergic pain system. Activation of the dorsal raphe nucleus similarly leads to inhibition at the spinal cord level. The locus ceruleus is the origin of the descending noradrenergic pathway, which also inhibits pain perception at the spinal cord level. These brain stem centers are modified by cortical, subcortical, and limbic pathways. Thus, even acute nociceptive pain can be modified based on prior experiences of pain coupled with emotional and cognitive interpretation of pain.[15,16]

In addition to these 3 primary descending brain pathways, there are numerous other endogenous neurotransmitter systems that can modulate nociceptive pain, including acetylcholine, γ-aminobutyric acid (GABA), vasoactive intestinal polypeptide, oxytocin, somatostatin, cholecystokinin, vasopressin, histamine, prolactin, and cannabinoids.[17–19] Thus, even nociceptive pain is not a simple reflex arc in which a given unit of pain perception develops as a result of a given unit or threshold activation of nociceptive afferent neurons. Nociceptive pain is not simply sensory-discriminative perception. Because of the involvement of multiple brainstem and subcortical regions, limbic pathways, and both ipsilateral and contralateral cortical brain regions, nociceptive pain perception also involves affective-motivational perception and cognitive perception.[20,21]

Even though nociceptive pain is influenced by multiple brain regions that subserve cognition and emotions, it is still possible on clinical grounds to establish a link between an inciting event and the response to pain that is consistent with such an inciting event. For example, placing a hand in a fire will lead to an immediate withdrawal response and perception of pain. The degree of pain and the emotions associated with that pain may vary, but, in essence, the nociceptive pain response can be linked in a reasonable manner to an inciting event.

Take again the example of an individual who places a hand in a flame. A prior traumatic experience with fire may lead to a markedly exaggerated pain response, with associated cognitive and emotional overlay. Take as another example the familiar wartime story of an individual who is considerably injured, but perceives no pain until he or she is taken safely out of danger. In this case, the imminent threat to the person's life overrides the normal protective response to pain. Even the experience of acute, nociceptive pain can vary considerably, based not only on activation of the ascending pathways, thalamus, and primary and secondary somatosensory cortex but also based on the patient's prior experience and perception of that experience.

The primary and secondary somatosensory cortex is but 1 aspect of the conscious experience of pain. Through functional brain imaging studies (primarily positron emission tomography and functional magnetic resonance imaging) the pain neuromatrix has been mapped out.[21–24] This includes the primary and secondary somatosensory cortices, which mediate sensory-discriminative features of pain; the anterior cingulate cortex and insular cortex, which mediate affective-motivational components of pain; and the prefrontal cortex, which mediates cognitive aspects of pain. The thalamus serves as the gateway between the cortical pain neuromatrix and the brainstem and spinal cord pathways.

Functional Brain Imaging

Functional brain imaging studies have revealed that patients who suffer with neuropathic pain have an increase in regional blood flow in the primary and secondary somatosensory cortices, and this response is often bilateral.[23,25] Brain metabolism is diminished in the orbitofrontal and insular cortices.[21] Functional brain imaging studies further reveal that pain perception in patients with neuropathic pain is mediated primarily by the anterior cingulate gyrus.[21,23] Such brain metabolism is distinct from that of acute nociceptive pain, in which alterations are not noted in orbitofrontal, insular, and anterior cingulate gyrus. In addition, bilateral activation of the somatosensory cortex is not the rule in processing of acute nociceptive pain. The essential question is what takes place in transforming nociceptive pain to neuropathic pain. To date, there has not been a single study that can predict the transformation from nociceptive to neuropathic pain based on a lesion or disease affecting the somatosensory system.

In patients who develop neuropathic pain, cortical reorganization develops in addition to changes in brain metabolism.[21,24] Such reorganization is an example of brain plasticity, which is the ability of the central nervous system to adapt or to reorganize in response to new internal or external environmental requirements.[26] This reorganization is the hallmark of neuropathic pain. It is not clear whether this reorganization is causative or adaptive.[27–29] For example, patients who suffer with complex regional pain syndrome show considerable reorganization of the somatotopic map within the primary somatosensory cortex. In this reorganization, the contralateral hand representation shrinks, and the head position shifts toward the mouth. The somatotopic reorganization correlates with the clinical experience of the patient, in which pain is perceived along a broad region of the body. Such changes have also been noted in patients with neuropathic pain who have such pain in conjunction with carpal tunnel syndrome and herpes simplex virus infections.[21,24] When patients improve, whether by therapeutic injections, pharmacologic strategies, or behavioral strategies, or some combination of all 3, the somatotopic reorganization reverses.[30,31]

Functional brain imaging studies have shown that neuropathic pain is not mediated by a simplistic and prolonged sensory-discriminative activation. Neuropathic pain is mediated and maintained by dysfunction in pathways that mediate affect, motivation, and cognition. Again, there is no cause-and-effect explanation for how neuropathic pain becomes transformed, or how neuropathic pain is maintained. However, functional brain imaging studies do show that neuropathic pain develops as a manifestation of brain plasticity.

Reversal of somatotopic reorganization as a result of any number of interventions tells us that the brain and environment communicate interactively and bidirectionally.[7,27-29] Functional brain imaging studies show that changes in the brain can be affected by any combination of interventions, including psychological or pharmacologic interventions, or by way of direct therapeutic injections. Such studies show that pain must not be considered simplistically, and dysfunction must be understood within the mind-body continuum.

Genetics

Similar to functional brain imaging studies, genetic data indicate that neuropathic pain may commingle with pathways that were formerly believed to mediate emotions. Genetic data must be interpreted with caution. For example, genetic factors may increase the risk of psychiatric morbidity, but do not necessarily code for a psychiatric disorder. These genetic factors are referred to as endophenotypic traits, which affect circuitry for affective function, cognition, and the stress response.[32]

Some genes modulate human nociception, and alterations in these genes may be a risk factor for impaired pain processing and neuropathic pain.[33,34] Genes identified to date include those that code for opioid receptors, transient receptor potential cation channels, fatty acid, amino hydrolase, guanosine triphosphate cyclohydrolase, and spinal cord N-methyl-D-aspartic acid receptors.[35-37] Alterations in genes that code for the D4 dopamine receptor predispose patients to the development of fibromyalgia, which is a neuropathic pain condition.[32] Alternations in the gene that encodes the sodium channel Nav1.7 can affect pain perception: mutations can lead to either the inability to perceive pain, or to enhanced pain perception and the development of erythromelalgia, which is also a neuropathic pain condition.[38] The s allele of the 5-HTTLPR gene alters the perception of pain. Individuals who carry the s allele of the 5-HTTLPR gene and the met-BDNF allele may have a protective effect against depression in the context of environmental adversity earlier in life, and the protective effect also extends to the gray matter volume in the anterior cingulate cortex, the area of the brain that mediates both neuropathic pain and depression.[33,34]

Clinical Pathophysiology

Clinical data bring us closer to understanding the implications of functional brain imaging studies and genetic data. For example, depression and anxiety are almost universal features in patients with neuropathic pain, and this makes sense because functional brain imaging studies and genetic data show that emotional pathways and neuropathic pain commingle.[10,11,39-44] It would be wrong to conclude from these data that there is a cause-and-effect relationship in either direction. For now, it is simply understood that there is a commingling of emotional and pain pathways in patients with neuropathic pain.

Depression is virtually universal in patients who suffer with neuropathic pain, with some studies suggesting a rate approaching 100%.[39] Depression is not an independent risk factor for the development of neuropathic pain, but patients suffering with depression report higher levels of pain than patients without depression.[40,41] Depression amplifies the pain response in patients who suffer with neuropathic pain.[39] Studies have shown that it is extremely difficult to successfully treat neuropathic pain if depression is not treated successfully itself.[39] In essence, is difficult to treat pain when patients are depressed, and it is difficult to treat depression when patients continue to suffer with pain.

Anxiety also commingles with neuropathic pain. It is difficult, if not impossible, to differentiate functional brain imaging studies of patients with chronic posttraumatic stress disorder and chronic neuropathic pain.[10,42–44] Chronic anxiety, especially chronic posttraumatic stress disorder, may provide an important window to understanding the transformation into neuropathic pain. Patients who have suffered with prior traumatic experiences and who have developed chronic maladaptive behavioral strategies may be at risk of developing neuropathic pain years later in response to an adverse inciting event. The speculation is that the inciting event is linked emotionally and cognitively to the prior traumatic experience, and this emotional and cognitive link intermingles with the recurrent pain experience. This linkage may lead to an augmentation of a pain experience even if the inciting event seems to be innocuous. Such clinical data, coupled with other scientific evidence, helps us to understand why the pain experience of some patients may be profound.[45]

If the entire experience of the patient is not taken into consideration, and if the patient's experience is not accepted as being real, the patient will simply be treated as an object and his or her life experience invalidated, which may be particularly relevant in the clinical expression of neuropathic pain. For example, in 100 patients having spinal surgery, 95% had successful outcomes if they had no prior history of physical, sexual, or emotional trauma. Only 15% of patients who had 3 or more prior traumatic events had successful surgical outcomes.[46] It is postulated that such patients have already developed transformed pain, which should properly be considered neuropathic pain. In such cases, further surgery may augment the pain response, because the patient may perceive the surgery as another traumatic event.[45] In the simplistic and reductionistic view of treating the patient as an object, the prolonged postoperative pain would be viewed as either a mechanical failure of surgery, or as a psychological weakness in the patient. However, if a mind-body perspective is retained and the patient's entire life experience considered, it is understood that the patient's expression of chronic pain should not have been addressed surgically.

Other studies have shown that prior trauma may predispose to neuropathic pain. Patients who have been victims of childhood abuse have an increased risk of developing neuropathic pain relative to controls.[47–50] These studies do not implicate a causal relationship between childhood abuse and neuropathic pain, but suggest that prolonged posttraumatic stress shares important neural pathways that are also critical in the development of neuropathic pain.[51]

MANAGEMENT

It is important to distinguish nociceptive pain from neuropathic pain on clinical and pathophysiologic grounds. It is a mistaken notion by too many neurologists and other clinicians to view all pain in nociceptive terms; that is, to view pain as an appropriate response of the body to an ongoing mechanical, thermal, or chemical stimulus. If this were the case, then pain medicine could more simplistically be viewed as the use of therapeutic injections and medications to alleviate ongoing nociceptive pain. It is also important that the patient understands that his or her chronic pain is not simply the result of a simplistic nociceptive pain pathway that can be managed with a therapeutic injection or medication. A misperception by both the treating clinician and patient can only compound a therapeutic failure.[52]

The hallmark of effective management for patients with neuropathic pain is a recognition that neuropathic pain is a transformed pain syndrome in which patients suffer in a multidimensional manner: physically, emotionally, cognitively, and socially. The clinical pathophysiologic data make it clear that neuropathic pain is not simple nociceptive pain, and it is not described or experienced in a simplistic sensory-discriminative manner. Patients who suffer with neuropathic pain have developed a pain syndrome in which neural dysfunction is more widespread, involving limbic and prefrontal pathways. A singular focus on trying to manage the pain as nociceptive pain will not be successful. Successful management depends on a mind-body approach in which the multiple dimensions of pain and sufferings are addressed by the treating physician.

The foundation for appropriate management lies in securing a diagnosis. It is important to determine whether the patient is presenting with nociceptive pain, neuropathic pain, or both. Nociceptive pain should have a clear-cut, active irritation or entrapment along a defined dermatome or within the musculoskeletal system.[13] For example, a patient with nociceptive pain from a lumbar disc herniation that is compressing the L5 nerve root will complain of pain along the posterolateral leg of the affected nerve. Generally, there will be positional components in which the pain is better, and other positional components in which the pain is worse. It is possible for lumbar radicular pain to become transformed and, in this scenario, the pain becomes more constant, without precipitating or palliative features. In addition, the patient's leg pain becomes more disruptive to the patient's well-being, with associated psychological comorbidities such as depression or anxiety.[13]

In some cases, transformed neuropathic pain can be associated with nociceptive components. For example, a patient with neuropathic pain in the leg from a prior lumbar disc herniation may have active mechanical components of facet pain, with low back pain associated with standing that is relieved with sitting. Once the physician identifies the underlying pathophysiology of pain, treatment is directed accordingly. Treatment of facet-generated pain can be directed appropriately at the level of the facet, whereas treatment of prolonged neuropathic leg pain must consider that such pain is now generated from the central nervous system pathways, and the focus on the leg or nerve root itself will not lead to pain alleviation. Thus, a careful history and physical examination are the first steps in appropriate management.[53]

Psychological Therapies

Patients who suffer with neuropathic pain have a high prevalence of depression and anxiety, and the limbic neural circuitry is a major component of maintaining pain. This neuropathic origin does not make the pain any less real or physical; it means that addressing the patient's underlying emotionality will lead to addressing a major component of the pain.[54,55] It is important to stress to patients that psychological therapies are important because they help to manage depression, anxiety, and coping skills, and may uncover a previously underdiagnosed traumatic life event.[45]

The hallmark of psychological intervention for patients with neuropathic pain is cognitive-behavioral therapy, which helps patients to understand the interplay of pain perception, emotions, and daily thought patterns.[45] This type of therapy focuses on the development of positive thoughts, and uses techniques such as relaxation training and biofeedback. Group therapy benefits patients who have had prolonged suffering, because it enables the patients to develop skills as a group, and helps patients understand that they are not alone in their pain experience. Family therapy is useful in helping other family members understand that neuropathic pain is a real medical condition. Psychiatric intervention may become necessary, both from the point of view of psychopharmacologic strategies in managing depression and anxiety, and in the acute management of patients who develop sudden flashbacks from previously unrecognized trauma.[13]

Pharmacologic Therapy

Pharmacologic therapy relies primarily on the use of anticonvulsants, antidepressants, and opioid medicine.[56] Anticonvulsants are first-line medications in treating patients with neuropathic pain.[57–61] They reduce neuronal hyperexcitability, reduce neuronal influx of sodium and calcium, and can have direct effects on GABA and glutamate. The choice of drugs should be based on physician familiarity and relative indications and contraindications. Anticonvulsants can be used in conjunction with other medications. Only gabapentin and pregabalin are approved by the US Food and Drug Administration for treating neuropathic pain, specifically postherpetic neuralgia and the pain of diabetic peripheral neuropathy.

Antidepressants are also a first-line pharmacologic treatment of neuropathic pain.[53] Tricyclic antidepressants have been the mainstay of treatment for many years, although new antidepressants have been developed that have fewer side effects.[57,60,62–64] Antidepressants should be prescribed based on physician familiarity and relative indications and contraindications. Antidepressants are extremely useful in patients who additionally suffer with depression and anxiety.[65–67]

Opioid medicines are the most important prescription analgesics. There remains a fear amongst physicians of prescribing opioid medicines,[13] especially with recent data indicating that prescription medicines have become widely abused drugs by students at high school and college.[68,69] It is common practice for pain medicine physicians to ask patients to sign a controlled substance agreement if they are to begin opioid medicine. These agreements help provide clarity regarding the intent of opioid usage for the manner in which medications will be prescribed and used.[70] It is appropriate to begin with short-acting opioid medicines and, once the medication need is discerned, to switch to a long-acting medication. Short-acting medicines are used only intermittently for breakthrough pain.[13]

Other pharmacologic strategies include topical analgesics,[71–73] antispasticity agents, and muscle relaxers. These drugs are adjunct medicines that are used according to the patients' symptoms.[57]

Interventional Strategies

Pain interventionalists include anesthesiologists, neurologists, physiatrists, and others who have obtained fellowship training in interventional pain medicine. Interventional strategies should not be used as the sole treatment strategies for patients with neuropathic pain. Although this approach may be successful for nociceptive pain, a singular focus is unsuccessful in treating multidimensional suffering in patients with neuropathic pain.[74] Sympathetic blocks can help break the cycle of pain in the early manifestations of complex regional pain syndrome.[75–77] Epidural, transforaminal, and facet corticosteroid injections may benefit patients who have an ongoing mechanical or nociceptive component to conditions such as lumbar disc herniation, lumbar stenosis, or lumbar degenerative disc disease with facet dysfunction.[76,78,79]

Spinal cord stimulation is akin to pacemaker placement in the dorsal spinal cord. It is believed that stimulation to the posterior spinal cord blocks central pain processing from a peripheral pain generator.[80] Spinal cord stimulators work best in patients who have well-localized extremity or axial pain. They should always be considered as part of a multidisciplinary strategy.[13]

Intrathecal administration of opioid analgesics take advantage of spinal cord opioid centers receptors having a higher affinity for intrathecal opioid medicine. In essence,

1/100 of the normal oral dosage is used, thus minimizing systemic side effects. Intrathecal opioid medicine is particularly useful in patients who have shown a positive effect to oral opioid medicine, but who have reached a limit in this medicine because of systemic side effects.[81] These medicines can be combined with baclofen and clonidine.

Physical Therapy

Physical therapy is extremely important in patients with neuropathic pain. Most of these patients have developed maladaptive physical manifestations, which leads to worsening pain. It is particularly common for patients with postlaminectomy syndrome and associated chronic neuropathic back pain to manifest concomitantly with multifidus atrophy and dysfunction.[13,82–84] These patients are unable to properly activate their multifidus muscles, which worsens any type of prolonged axial loading. Other intuitive physical therapy strategies, such as myofascial release and craniosacral technique, help some patients to develop a better awareness of the link between their pain presentation and their underlying physiology.[13]

Complementary Strategies

Complementary strategies include acupuncture, massage therapy, and nutritional counseling.[85,86] Some patients with neuropathic pain cannot tolerate acupuncture because they are hypersensitive to the insertion of small needles. However, there are several studies showing the efficacy of acupuncture in treating different types of nerve pain.[85] Nutritional counseling should focus on developing good eating habits. Many patients with chronic pain, depression, and anxiety develop poor eating habits by choosing foods that have immediate gratifying effects, which becomes a form of self-treating of underlying anxiety and depression. Massage therapy can help to desensitize areas of hyperalgesia, and also can help to alleviate muscular and emotional stress.[87]

Some studies have shown the effectiveness of mirror therapy for treating patients with neuropathic pain, especially phantom limb pain and complex regional pain syndrome.[88,89] The patients are positioned so that they are in a rectangular box with a mirror placed vertically and sagittally. The limb with neuropathic pain is on the nonreflecting side of the mirror, and the normal limb is placed on the reflecting side. When the patient is told to move the normal limb, there is the visual impression that the painful limb is being moved, and this leads to the perception that the neuropathic limb has been restored. It is possible that visual stimuli can override tactile and proprioceptive stimuli, which may lead to the efficacy of mirror therapy.

CASE REPORT

A 35-year-old man presented with low back and left leg pain. He first developed back and leg pain after he fell as one of the first responders for 9/11. He completed his work that day, but the next day developed increasingly severe pain in the left lower back radiating into the left posterolateral leg. Bed rest and over-the-counter nonsteroidal antiinflammatory drugs were unhelpful. He was treated by an orthopedic surgeon who recommended physical therapy and continued use of nonsteroidal antiinflammatory drugs, but pain persisted. He underwent magnetic resonance imaging of the lumbar spine, which showed an acute-appearing disc herniation at L4-L5, central lateral to the left, with compression of the left L5 nerve root. He then underwent a lumbar epidural corticosteroid injection and, although he obtained some relief, pain recurred 1 month later. Subsequent lumbar epidural and transforaminal corticosteroid injections were unhelpful. Ongoing physical therapy led to no relief. He then underwent lumbar laminectomy, L4-L5, with removal of the extruded disc fragment, without spine fusion. There were no operative complications, but the patient did not develop meaningful pain relief. Subsequent studies revealed some degenerative disc changes at L4-L5, with no recurring disc herniation, and with no L5 nerve root entrapment. Continued physical therapy and repeat epidural injections were unhelpful.

The patient developed increasing pain, and the quality of the pain changed. Although he initially described leg pain as sharp and stabbing, and it clearly worsened with standing and walking, and was better lying supine, he later described burning leg pain that was essentially constant. This condition was associated with almost constant burning pain across the lower back. He stated that the burning was intense, and that he sometimes felt as if gasoline was being poured onto a flame in his leg. He was begun on opioid medicine, and although this initially provided partial relief, escalating doses of opioid medicine provided limited therapeutic effect. The patient was referred to a pain anesthesiologist, who performed transforaminal lumbar nerve root injections and lumbar facet injections to no avail. He then underwent placement of a spinal cord stimulator, but could not tolerate its effects. The patient perceived that the spinal cord stimulator only worsened the burning leg pain.

The patient was next evaluated by another spine surgeon, who recommended lumbar spine fusion. This recommendation was despite the patient exhibiting no symptoms of spinal instability (considerable back pain on first standing in the morning or with positional changes, relative relief of back pain with steady walking), and also despite the patient having no ongoing signs of nerve root entrapment. Instead, his leg pain was constant and worsening with time, with a burning and hypersensitivity quality. The patient's pain worsened following posterior spine fusion with placement of pedicle screws and rods. Back pain spread over a larger region, and he now had a sense of more global leg pain, no longer in a radicular pattern. He had no change in skin color or temperature. He was diagnosed with complex regional pain syndrome despite never having had signs of autonomic instability in the affected limb. Lumbar sympathetic blockade was unsuccessful. He was then referred to a multidisciplinary pain center.

The patient was initially resistant to any type of psychological therapy. He was treated with escalating doses of gabapentin, and this provided partial relief. He was converted to a long-acting opioid medicine, and was told that the dose would not be changed. Once he agreed to psychological therapy, it became clear that the patient suffered with considerable anxiety. He had witnessed the deaths of 2 colleagues during the 9/11 rescue efforts, and he feared for his own life at the time that he injured himself. Treatment became directed at posttraumatic stress disorder and, in this setting, the patient developed better coping skills and had a better sense of control of his pain. He then had a retrial of physical therapy, and ultrasound of his multifidus muscles showed considerable atrophy, with inability to activate these muscles on command. Once he developed insight into multifidus function and activation, the patient's back pain began to improve. He then became engaged in group therapy and cognitive-behavioral therapy, and, in this setting, the patient obtained improvement in leg pain. For the first time he was able to actively express his fears as well as his considerable loss from 9/11. He came to understand that the inciting event led to the disc herniation and was also filled with profound psychic trauma that had never been addressed. Long-term, the patient was weaned from opioid medicine, and had considerably improved quality of life on moderate-dose gabapentin, ongoing psychological therapy, and a regular exercise program.

This case report shows a common failure in managing patients with neuropathic pain. The patient initially presented with seemingly straightforward nociceptive pain.

Once treatment of nociceptive pain became ineffective, and the pain developed a transforming character, the treatment should have changed. Rather than escalating treatment of an apparent nociceptive cause, it would have been more fruitful for the patient to be engaged in multidisciplinary treatment. The transformation to neuropathic pain became clear clinically when the pain seemingly developed a life of its own. There was no longer a positional component to pain, and the expressions of pain became more complex. Ultimately, multidisciplinary treatment uncovered that the inciting event was not a simple physical trauma; treating the patient as if he had a simple physical trauma represented a mind-body split and a failure in appropriate medical management.

SUMMARY

Neuropathic pain is a neuropsychiatric condition that represents dysfunction of the central nervous system. This dysfunction may or may not be traced to an identifiable lesion, but can be understood as a complex commingling of perception and pain. Neuropathic pain is best managed in a multidisciplinary setting in which the mind and body are treated as a whole.

REFERENCES

1. Treede R-D, Jensen TS, Campbell JN, et al. Neuropathic pain: redefinition and a grading system for clinical and research purposes. Neurology 2008;70:1630–5.
2. Harrington A. The body that speaks . The cure within: a history of mind-body medicine. New York: WW Norton; 2008. p. 67–101.
3. Engstrom EJ, Weber MM. Making Kraepelin history: a great instauration? Hist Psychiatry 2007;18:267–73.
4. Falzeder E. The story of an ambivalent relationship: Sigmund Freud and Eugen Bleuler. J Anal Psychol 2007;52:343–68.
5. Yudofsky SC, Hales RE. The reemergence of neuropsychiatry: definition and direction. J Neuropsychiatry Clin Neurosci 1989;1:1–6.
6. Yudofsky SC, Hales RE. Neuropsychiatry and the future of psychiatry and neurology. Am J Psychiatry 2002;159:1261–4.
7. Geschwind N. The borderland of neurology and psychiatry: some common misconceptions. In: Benson DF, Blumer D, editors. Psychiatric aspects of neurologic diseases. New York: Grune & Stratton; 1975. p. 1–9.
8. Price BH, Adams RD, Coyle JT. Neurology and psychiatry: closing the great divide. Neurology 2000;54:8–14.
9. Dunbar HF. Emotions and bodily change: a survey of literature on psychosomatic interrelationships. New York: Columbia University Press; 1935.
10. Otis JD, Keane TM, Kerns RD. An examination of the relationship between chronic pain and posttraumatic stress disorder. J Rehabil Res Dev 2003;40: 397–405.
11. Liberizon I, Phan KL. Brain-imaging studies in posttraumatic stress disorder. CNS Spectr 2003;8:641–50.
12. Merskey H, Bogduk N, editors. Classification of chronic pain: descriptions of chronic pain syndromes and definitions of pain terms. 2nd edition. Seattle (WA): IASP Press; 1994. p. 209–14.
13. Hainline B. Back pain understood. Leonia (NJ): Medicus Press; 2007.
14. Woolf CJ, Fitzgerald M. The properties of neurons recorded in the superficial dorsal horn of the rat spinal cord. J Comp Neurol 1983;221:313–28.

15. Basbaum AI, Jessell TM. The perception of pain. In: Kandel ER, Schwartz JH, Jessell TM, editors. Principles of neural science. New York: McGraw-Hill; 2000. p. 472–91.
16. Basbaum AI, Fields HL. Endogenous pain control systems: brainstem spinal pathways and endorphin circuitry. Annu Rev Neurosci 1984;7:309–38.
17. Duggan AW, Weihe E. Central transmission of impulses in nociceptors: events in the superficial dorsal horn. In: Basbaum AI, Besson JM, editors. Toward a new pharmacotherapy of pain. Chichester (UK): John Wiley; 1991. p. 35–67.
18. Hokfelt T, Johansson O, Ljungdahl A. Peptidergic neurons. Nature 1980;284:515–21.
19. Meng ID, Manning BH. An analgesia circuit activated by cannabinoids. Nature 1998;394:381–3.
20. Dubois MY, Gallagher RM, Lippe PM. Pain medicine position paper. Pain Medicine 2009;10:972–1000.
21. Seifert F, Maihofner C. Central mechanisms of experimental and chronic neuropathic pain: findings from functional imaging studies. Cell Mol Life Sci 2009;66: 375–90.
22. Chen FY, Tao W, Li YJ. Advances in brain imaging of neuropathic pain. Chin Med J (Engl) 2008;121:653–7.
23. Stephenson DT, Arneric SP. Neuroimaging of pain: advances and future prospects. J Pain 2008;9:567–79.
24. Vartiainen N, Kirveskari E, Kallio-Laine K, et al. Cortical reorganization in primary somatosensory cortex in patients with unilateral chronic pain. J Pain 2009;10: 854–9.
25. Witting N, Kupers RC, Svennson P, et al. A PET activation study of brush-evoked allodynia in patients with nerve injury pain. Pain 2006;120:145–54.
26. Shih JJ, Cohen LG. Cortical reorganization in the human. Neurology 2004;63: 1772–3.
27. Mayberg HS. Limbic-cortical dysregulation: a proposed model of depression. J Neuropsychiatry Clin Neurosci 1997;9:471–81.
28. Hubel DH, Weisel TN. Binocular interaction in striate cortex of kittens reared with artificial squint. J Neurophysiol 1965;28:1041–59.
29. Leshner AI. Addiction is a brain disease and it matters. Science 1997;278:45–7.
30. Maihofner C, Handwerker HO, Neundorfer B, et al. Cortical reorganization during recovery from complex regional pain syndrome. Neurology 2004;63:693–701.
31. Pleger B, Tegenthoff M, Ragert P, et al. Sensorimotor retuning in complex regional pain syndrome parallels pain reduction. Ann Neurol 2005;57:425–9.
32. Maletic V, Raison CL. Neurobiology of depression, fibromyalgia and neuropathic pain. Front Biosci 2009;14:5291–338.
33. Apkarian AV, Bushnell MC, Treede RD, et al. Human brain mechanisms of pain perception and regulation in health and disease. Eur J Pain 2005;9:463–84.
34. Baliki MN, Geha PY, Apkarian AV. Spontaneous pain and brain activity in neuropathic pain: functional MRI and pharmacologic functional MRI studies. Curr Pain Headache Rep 2007;11:171–7.
35. Sery O, Hrazdilova O, Matalova E, et al. Pain research update from a genetic point of view. Pain Pract 2005;5:341–8.
36. Buskila D. Genetics of chronic pain states. Best Pract Res Clin Rheumatol 2007; 21:535–47.
37. Lotsch J, Geisslinger G. Current evidence for a modulation of nociception by human genetic polymorphisms. Pain 2007;132:18–22.
38. Cox JJ, Reimann F, Nicholas AK, et al. An SCN9A channelopathy causes congenital inability to experience pain. Nature 2006;444:894–8.

39. Romano JM, Turner JA. Chronic pain and depression: does the evidence support a relationship? Psychol Bull 1985;97:18–34.
40. Keefe FJ, Wilkins RH, Cook WA, et al. Depression, pain, and pain behavior. J Consult Clin Psychol 1986;54:665–9.
41. Krause SJ, Wiener RL, Tait RC. Depression and pain behavior in patients with chronic pain. Clin J Pain 1994;10:122–7.
42. Grande LA, Loeser JD, Ashleigh OJ, et al. Complex regional pain syndrome as a stress response. Pain 2004;110:295–498.
43. Frayne SM, Seaver MR, Loveland S, et al. Burden of medical illness in women with depression and posttraumatic stress disorder. Arch Intern Med 2004;164:1306–12.
44. Asmundson GJ, Wright KD, Stein MB. Pain and PTSD symptoms in female veterans. Eur J Pain 2004;8:345–50.
45. Lebovits AH. Trauma and the treatment of pain. In: Carll EK, editor, Trauma psychology: issues in violence, disaster, health, and illness, vol. 2. Westport (CT): Praeger Publishers; 2007. p. 47–62.
46. Schofferman J, Anderson D, Hines R, et al. Childhood psychological trauma correlates with unsuccessful lumbar spine surgery. Spine 1992;17:S138–44.
47. Katan W, Egan K, Miller D. Chronic pain: lifetime psychiatric diagnoses and family history. Am J Psychiatry 1984;142:1156–60.
48. Dickinson LM, de Gruy FV, Dickinson WP, et al. Health-related quality of life and symptom profiles of female survivors of sexual abuse. Arch Fam Med 1999;8:35–43.
49. Fillingim RB, Wilkinson CS, Powell T. Self-reported abuse history and pain complaints among young adults. Clin J Pain 1999;15:85–91.
50. Goldberg RT, Goldstein R. A comparison of chronic pain patients and controls on traumatic events in childhood. Disabil Rehabil 2000;22:756–63.
51. Nicholson B, Verma S. Co-morbidities in chronic neuropathic pain. Pain Med 2004;5:S9–27.
52. Meldrum ML. Brief history of multidisciplinary management of chronic pain, 1900–2000. In: Schatman ME, Campbell A, editors. Chronic pain management: guidelines for multidisciplinary program development. New York: Informa Healthcare; 2007. p. 1–14.
53. Irving GA. Contemporary assessment and management of neuropathic pain. Neurology 2005;64:S21–7.
54. Palermo TM, Eccleston C, Lewandowski AS, et al. Randomized controlled trials of psychological therapies for management of chronic pain in children and adolescents: an updated meta-analytic review. Pain 2010;148(3):387–97.
55. Eccleston C, Williams AC, Morley S. Psychological therapies for the management of chronic pain (excluding headache) in adults. Cochrane Database Syst Rev 2009;2:CD007407.
56. Dworkin RH, O'Connor AB, Backonja M, et al. Pharmacologic management of neuropathic pain: evidence-based recommendations. Pain 2007;132:237–51.
57. Namaka M, Gramlich CR, Ruhlen D, et al. A treatment algorithm for neuropathic pain. Clin Ther 2004;26:951–79.
58. Wiffen P, Collins S, McQuay H, et al. Anticonvulsant drugs for acute and chronic pain. Cochrane Database Syst Rev 2000;3:CD001133.
59. Tremont-Lukats IW, Megeff C, Backonja MM. Anticonvulsants for neuropathic pain syndromes: mechanisms of action and place in therapy. Drugs 2000;60:1029–52.
60. O'Connor AB, Dworkin RH. Treatment of neuropathic pain: an overview of recent guidelines. Am J Med 2009;122:S22–32.

61. Jensen TS, Madsen CS, Finnerup NB. Pharmacology and treatment of neuro-pathic pains. Curr Opin Neurol 2009;22:467–74.
62. Max MB, Lynch SA, Muir J, et al. Effects of desipramine, amitriptyline and fluox-etine on pain in diabetic neuropathy. N Engl J Med 1992;326:1250–6.
63. Max MB, Culnane M, Schafer SC, et al. Amitriptyline relieves diabetic neuropathy pain in patients with normal or depressed mood. Neurology 1987;37:589–96.
64. Wong M, Chung JW, Wong TK. Effects of treatments for symptoms of painful dia-betic neuropathy: systematic review. BMJ 2007;335:87–90.
65. Ansari A. The efficacy of newer antidepressants in the treatment of chronic pain: a review of current literature. Harv Rev Psychiatry 2000;7:257–77.
66. Goldstein D, Iyengar S, Mallinckrodt C, et al. A potential new treatment for depressed patients with co-morbid pain. Pain Med 2002;3:177–81.
67. Delgado PL. Common pathways of depression and pain. J Clin Psychiatry 2004; 65:S16–9.
68. Monitoring the future: national survey results on drug use, 1975–2008, volume I: secondary school students. Bethesda: National Institute on Drug Abuse/National Institutes of Health/US Department of Health & Human Services; 2008.
69. Monitoring the future: national survey results on drug use, 1975–2008, volume II: college students & adult ages 19–50. Bethesda: National Institute on Drug Abuse/ National Institutes of Health/US Department of Health & Human Services; 2008.
70. Staats PS, Argoff CE, Brewer R, et al. Neuropathic pain: incorporating new consensus guidelines into the reality of clinical practice. Adv Stud Med 2004;4: S550–66.
71. Wilhelm IR, Tzabazis A, Likar R, et al. Long-term treatment of neuropathic pain with a 5% lidocaine medicated plaster. Eur J Anaesthesiol 2010;27:169–73.
72. Backonja M, Wallace MS, Blonsky ER, et al. NGX-4010, a high-concentration capsaicin patch, for the treatment of postherpetic neuralgia: a randomized, double-blind study. Lancet Neurol 2008;7:1106–12.
73. Simpson DM, Brown S, Tobias J. Controlled trial of high-concentration capsaicin patch for treatment of painful HIV neuropathy. Neurology 2008;70:2305–13.
74. Scadding JW. Treatment of neuropathic pain: historical aspects. Pain Med 2004; 5:S3–8.
75. Boas RA. Sympathetic nerve blocks: in search of a role. Reg Anesth Pain Med 1998;23:292–306.
76. Varrassi G, Paladini A, Mariinangeli F, et al. Neural modulation by blocks and infu-sions. Pain Pract 2006;6:34–8.
77. Hartrick CT, Kovan JP, Naismith P. Outcome prediction following sympathetic block for complex regional pain syndrome. Pain Pract 2004;4:222–8.
78. Eckel TS, Bartynski WS. Epidural steroid injections and selective nerve root blocks. Tech Vasc Interv Radiol 2009;12:11–21.
79. Stone JA, Bartynski WS. Treatment of facet and sacroiliac joint arthropathy: steroid injections and radiofrequency ablation. Tech Vasc Interv Radiol 2009;12:22–32.
80. Hassenbusch SJ, Stanton-Hicks M, Covington EC. Spinal cord stimulation versus spinal infusion for low back and leg pain. Acta Neurochir Suppl 1995;64:109–15.
81. Smith HS, Deer TR, Staats PS, et al. Intrathecal drug delivery. Pain Physician 2008;11:S89–104.
82. Hides J, Stokes M, Saide M, et al. Evidence of lumbar multifidus muscle wasting ipsilateral to symptoms in patients with acute/subacute low back pain. Spine 1994;19:165–72.
83. Rantanen J, Hurme M, Falck B, et al. The lumbar multifidus muscle five years after surgery for a lumbar intervertebral disc herniation. Spine 1993;18:568–74.

84. Jemmet RS. Rehabilitation of lumbar multifidus dysfunction in low back pain: strengthening versus a motor re-education model. Br J Sports Med 2003;37:91.

85. Rosman SM, Hainline B. Complementary and alternative medicine. In: Hainline B, Devinsky O, editors. Neurological complications of pregnancy. 2nd edition. Philadelphia: Lippincott Williams & Wilkins; 2002. p. 307–16.

86. Dallman MF, Pecoraro N. Chronic stress and obesity: a new view of "comfort food". Proc Natl Acad Sci U S A 2003;100:11696–701.

87. Hasson D, Arnetz B. A randomized clinical trial of the treatment effects of massage compared to relaxation tape recordings on diffuse long-term pain. Psychother Psychosom 2004;73:17–24.

88. Cacchio A, De Blasis E. Mirror therapy for chronic complex regional pain syndrome type 1 and stroke. N Eng J Med 2009;361:634–6.

89. Ramachandran VS, Altschuler EL. The use of visual feedback, in particular mirror visual feedback, in restoring brain function. Brain 2009;132:1693–710.

Traumatic Brain Injury and Its Neurobehavioral Sequelae

Silvana Riggio, MD[a,b,*]

KEYWORDS

- Traumatic brain injury • Postconcussive syndrome
- Neuropsychiatric disorders • Frontal lobe seizures

The development of neurobehavioral sequelae (NBS) associated with traumatic brain injury (TBI) is a multifactorial process. NBS is characterized by somatic and/or neuropsychiatric symptoms (**Box 1**). These clusters of symptoms have also been referred to in the literature as postconcussive symptoms, syndrome, or disorder, but because these symptoms are not restricted to patients with concussion but instead to TBI of all severities, the term, *NBS of TBI*, is more appropriate.

Evaluating TBI patients who present with neurobehavioral complaints requires a systematic history and physical that carefully defines the complaints and places them in the context of the injury, premorbid health, and postinjury circumstances. Somatic symptoms associated with NBS consist mostly of fatigue, lack of energy, sleep disturbances, dizziness, nausea, and headaches. Neuropsychiatric symptoms include cognitive and behavioral changes (ie, impairment of attention and/or memory, executive dysfunction, aggression, poor impulse control, irritability, anhedonia, and apathy). The complex of symptoms seen in TBI patients overlaps with several psychiatric disorders and/or neurologic disorders or medical disorders. Complicating the presentation and diagnosis of TBI patients with suspected NBS are seizures. In particular, seizures of frontal lobe origin can be associated with bizarre behavioral manifestations and repetitive motor activity (RMA), which at times can be mistaken for a psychiatric manifestation.[1]

Evaluation of patients for NBS of TBI requires a structured history, including onset, duration, and severity of symptoms, environmental and social stressors, medical

[a] Departments of Psychiatry and Neurology, Mount Sinai School of Medicine, One Gustave L. Levy Place, Box 1230, New York, NY 10029, USA
[b] James J. Peters VA Medical Center, Bronx, NY, USA
* Corresponding author. Department of Psychiatry, Mount Sinai School of Medicine, One Gustave L. Levy Place, Box 1230, New York, NY 10029.
E-mail address: silvana.riggio@mssm.edu

Neurol Clin 29 (2011) 35–47
doi:10.1016/j.ncl.2010.10.008
0733-8619/11/$ – see front matter © 2011 Published by Elsevier Inc.

neurologic.theclinics.com

> **Box 1**
> **Neurobehavioral sequelae of traumatic brain injury**
>
> Neuropsychiatric
>
> - Cognitive (eg, deficits in attention, memory, and executive function)
> - Behavioral[a]: aggression, irritability, poor impulse control, anhedonia, apathy, depressed mood, and affective disorders
> - Exacerbation of a primary psychiatric disorder (eg, affective disorders)
> - Other
>
> Somatic (eg, sleep disturbance, fatigue, dizziness, vertigo, headaches, visual disturbances, nausea, sensitivity to light and sound, hearing loss, and seizures)
>
> [a] Behavioral changes can be secondary to a primary psychiatric disorder versus possible underlying personality disorders and/or frontal/temporal lobe dysfunction or any central nervous system dysfunction secondary to the TBI.

comorbidities, medications, and recreational drug use. It is key to delineate physiologic dysfunction and place deficits in the context of a patient's pre- and postinjury psychiatric status. A careful physical examination is needed to establish the neurologic baseline and identify deficits that may be contributing to the presenting complaint. For example, a subtle fourth or sixth cranial nerve injury (the most common neurologic injuries in TBI patients) may contribute to headaches, difficulty concentrating, or sustaining attention. The physical examination must also include a comprehensive neurologic and psychiatric mental status evaluation. It is only after a complete history and physical examination is performed that a clinician decides which additional diagnostic studies are indicated (eg, neuroimaging, neurophysiologic, and/or neuropsychological testing).

The evolution or resolution of the symptoms over time is dependent on several variables, thus predicting prognosis can be difficult.[2] Symptoms can vary, depending on the localization and lateralization of the injury, extent of the injury, medical and psychiatric comorbidities, and pre- and postpsychosocial factors. In addition, individual coping mechanisms play a significant role in recovery.

This article explores the NBS that may occur after TBI. A focus in this article is on demonstrating the overlap of NBS with other conditions and providing a framework for developing a diagnostic and management strategy. The strategy must keep in mind acute and long-term goals. Although pharmacotherapy is important in select cases, it can also be associated with side effects that may interfere with a patient's function. Early rehabilitation, psychotherapy (eg, supportive, family, group, and behavioral), and cognitive rehabilitation are some of the measures that must be tailored to individuals.

CLINICAL OVERVIEW

Almost all TBI patients report some NBS in the acute phase after injury.[3] It is estimated that 30% to 80% of patients with mild to moderate TBI experience some NBS, which can persist for up to 3 months.[2] In adults, cognitive deficits are common in the acute stage, and the majority of studies indicate that in mild TBI complete recovery occurs within 3 to 12 months.[2] In up to 15% of patients with mild TBI, NBS persist beyond 3 months and may contribute to long-term social and occupational difficulties; however, when this occurs, the clinician should aggressively look for contributing factors.[3–5] Cognitive dysfunction (eg, impaired attention, memory, and executive function) may play a predominant role in patients who experience persistent symptoms.[6] Identifying these deficits and developing an effective intervention plan may be critical to the successful recovery of patients. Risk factors for persisting symptoms, in addition to structural injury, include female gender, advanced age, pain, and prior affective or anxiety diagnoses.[7]

According to the World Health Organization Collaborating Centre Task Force on Traumatic Brain Injury, a diagnosis of TBI-related NBS requires the presence of 3 or more of the following 8 symptoms[2]:

- Headache
- Dizziness
- Fatigue
- Irritability
- Insomnia
- Concentration
- Memory difficulties
- Intolerance to stress, emotion, or alcohol.

The overlap of NBS symptoms with primary affective disorders or cognitive disorders as well as other medical and neurologic disorders makes differentiating the entities difficult. It takes a carefully designed evaluation to sort out these conditions. Factors that help distinguish one diagnosis from another include time of onset, duration of symptoms, and characteristic of the symptoms.

NEUROBEHAVIORAL SEQUELAE

Neurobehavioral consists of a spectrum of neuropsychiatric and somatic symptoms which can be present after a traumatic brain injury. The neuropsychiatric symptoms include cognitive and behavioral/psychiatric disorders.

NEUROPSYCHIATRIC SYMPTOMS
Cognitive Disorders

Cognitive complaints after TBI include impairment of attention/concentration, memory, and/or executive function.[8] There may be difficulties performing preinjury tasks and jobs or following instructions that would ordinarily be routine. Patients often report difficulty sustaining attention, planning, switching parameters, organizing, or sequencing, especially in the setting of a frontal lobe injury. These deficits may result in frustration and be expressed in the form of increased irritability, anxiety, apathy, or depression. The clinician must determine if these symptoms are the result of the injury per se or a manifestation of the frustration with not performing at premorbid baseline.

The post-TBI evaluation of cognitive function must determine if performance problems are due to deficits in attention versus memory. If attention is impaired, there is difficulty retaining information with obvious impact on memory and thus performance. If a patient has an underlying affective disorder, attention can also be impaired due to lack of interest and/or distractibility. Therefore, the assessment of memory must be placed in context of attention and other disorders that may interfere with performance.

Persistence of cognitive deficits is related to some degree to severity of injury. In a systematic review of the literature, Dikmen and colleagues[8] reported that penetrating, moderate, and severe TBIs were associated persisting cognitive deficits. Patients with mild TBI are a more difficult population to understand, but the authors concluded that there is insufficient evidence to associate mild TBI with cognitive deficits persisting beyond 6 months after the TBI. Studies in the sports medicine literature demonstrate that cognitive deficits resulting from sports-related mild TBI generally resolve within days and rarely last more than 3 months.[9,10] These findings must be placed in the context of patients who tend to be motivated and performance driven, however; these findings cannot necessarily be generalized to all subsets of patients who experience a mild TBI. Neither loss of consciousness nor posttraumatic amnesia (PTA) reliably stratifies those patients at greatest risk for cognitive deficits. In the sports medicine literature on mild TBI, cognitive impairments are most severe immediately after a closed head injury and resolve within 48 hours.[9,10] These findings support the importance of cognitive rest immediately after a mild TBI.

Behavioral/Psychiatric Disorders

Behavioral disorders

There are several behavioral manifestations associated with TBI. Clinicians must determine if the symptoms were present before an injury or are the result of the injury (ie, primary cause or exacerbant). Behavioral manifestations can also be due to a primary psychiatric disorder that becomes expressed as a result of the stress of the injury. Weak defense mechanisms, poor social support, medications, and drug use can all complicate the presentation. Symptoms complex can also be complicated by an emotional response the injury, limitations secondary to the injury, and fear of disability (**Fig. 1**).

Affective and behavioral disturbances after TBI may be expressed as personality changes appreciated by the patients or their family/caregiver. Personality changes may include aggression, impulsivity, irritability, emotional lability, or apathy.[11,12] These changes are more frequently reported after moderate and severe TBI; there is insufficient evidence linking many of these symptoms to mild TBI.[13] Impulsivity and irritability may lead to verbal and physical inappropriateness expressed as verbal outbursts or combativeness. It may be due to impaired judgment secondary to an underlying structural lesion or the exacerbation of an underlying psychiatric disorder or to an emotional response to trauma.

Depression

Major depression is one of the most frequently reported NBS of TBI; the actual prevalence varies from study to study based on methodology but seems to be approximately 25% to 50% after moderate to severe TBI versus a general population prevalence of 17%.[14–16] The degree to which a premorbid psychiatric disorder increases the risk for NBS after TBI is unclear, but studies indicate a positive correlation: Seel and colleagues[17] described fatigue (29%), distractibility (28%), anger/irritability (28%), and rumination (25%) as the most common depressive symptoms in a prospective, multicenter study of 666 nonacute moderate-severe TBI patients. Twenty-seven percent of the TBI patients met criteria for major depression, with feelings of hopelessness, worthlessness, and anhedonia differentiating depressed from nondepressed patients.

Risk factors for developing major depression after TBI fall into 2 categories: premorbid psychiatric pathology and low socioeconomic status. The relationship between rates of depression and the severity of TBI is unclear. The greatest chronicity of major depression seems to occur, however, in patients with both moderate-severe TBI and prior psychiatric illness.[2]

Studies have found a link between TBI and suicidality as well as between psychiatric comorbidity in the setting of TBI and suicidality.[18,19] In a retrospective study of 5034 patients, Silver and colleagues[18] reported that patients with a history of TBI with loss of consciousness had a 4-times greater likelihood of attempted suicide than those

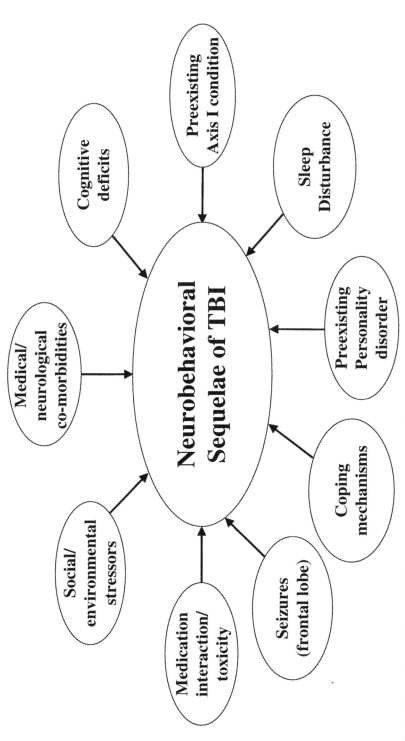

Fig. 1. Concomitant factors of NBS sequelae.

without TBI, 8.1% versus 1.9%, respectively. This risk of suicide attempt remained even after controlling for demographics, quality-of-life variables, alcohol abuse, and any comorbid psychiatric disorders. In a systematic review of the literature, Hesdorffer and colleagues[13] found insufficient evidence linking mild TBI and completed suicide.

Anxiety disorders/posttraumatic stress disorder

Anxiety disorders are reported after mild TBI, most commonly in individuals who also have a limb injury.[13,16] Increased age, a history of posttraumatic stress disorder (PTSD), and an avoidant coping style increases risk of acute stress symptoms after TBI.[20,21] An acute stress disorder predisposes to the development of PTSD after TBI: PTSD has been associated primarily with mild TBI in the military population whereas there is insufficient evidence linking it to mild TBI in the civilian population.[21]

Recall of the traumatic event has been identified as a predictor of developing PTSD.[22,23] Turnbull and colleagues[23] in a study of 55 patients reported that having traumatic memories of the injury were associated with increased psychological distress. Amnesia for event, although not protective against PTSD, was related to a decreased severity of symptoms. Other predictors of the development of PTSD, as well as its severity, include avoidant coping style, behavioral coping style (vs cognitive coping style), and prior unemployment (an indicator of premorbid level of functioning).[24] There is ongoing controversy regarding the relationship between PTSD and PTA, the point being the likelihood of having the disorder if a patient does not recall the traumatic event. The primary question is how patients can have PTSD if they cannot re-experience the actual trauma via intrusive thoughts or nightmares. The proposed counterargument to the controversy is the theory that TBI patients with PTA for the traumatic event re-experience the trauma event through the imagination from second-hand accounts or the patients' own mind[25] and that patients may also be able to re-experience fragments or islands of memory within the amnestic period, thus meeting the re-experiencing criterion of PTSD.[26]

The military experience differs from the civilian experience regarding the association of PTSD with mild TBI: Hoge and colleagues[27] studied soldiers with mild TBI and a variety of postinjury symptoms. After adjusting for PTSD and depression, mild TBI was no longer significantly associated with symptoms except headache. The investigators postulated that PTSD and depression are important mediators of the relationship between mild TBI and physical health problems.

Aggression

Aggression is a commonly reported behavioral symptom of TBI, again, most commonly associated with moderate and severe injuries. Tateno and colleagues[8] studied 89 consecutive inpatients with moderate to severe TBI and found that 34% exhibited aggressive behavior within the first 6 months of injury. Risk factors for aggression after TBI include frontal lobe injury, premorbid affective disorder, personality disorder, or alcohol or substance abuse.

Substance related disorders

A review of the literature by van Reekum and colleagues[15] reported a 22% prevalence of substance abuse in TBI patients versus a 15% lifetime prevalence in the general population. A review of subsequent studies by Rogers and Read[14] in 2007 showed a prevalence of 12%. Premorbid substance use has been found strongly associated with post-TBI drug use, and multiple studies have cited substance abuse as a risk factor for TBI rather than the other way around. A 30-year longitudinal study by Koponen and colleagues[28] showed that 71% of TBI patients who were using drugs currently also did so pre-TBI. A systematic review of the literature found limited evidence of an association between TBI and decreased drug and alcohol use up to 3 years postinjury.[13]

SOMATIC SYMPTOMS
Headache

Headache is the most commonly reported somatic symptom after mild TBI, with a prevalence ranging from 25% to 90%.[29–31] Post-TBI headaches may be classified as acute, beginning within 2 weeks of the injury and resolving within 2 months, or chronic, beginning within 2 weeks and persisting for more than 8 weeks. The common co-occurrence of headache with other NBS was noted by Baandrup and Jensen[30]: 53% had at least 1 other somatic complaint (fatigability, sleep disturbance, dizziness, or alcohol intolerance), 49% had at least 1 cognitive complaint (memory dysfunction or impaired concentration/attention), and 26% had at least 1 psychiatric complaint (irritability, aggressiveness, anxiety, depression, or emotional lability); 17% had all 3 types of complaints and 17% had none.

A premorbid history of headache increases the risk of posttraumatic headaches, and those with pretraumatic headache may experience a worsening of the headache after injury. The presence of posttraumatic headache has not been consistently correlated with the severity of the injury; some investigators have reported that mild TBI patients have higher rates of headache during the initial post traumatic phase than patients with more severe injury.[32] In the majority of mild TBI cases, headaches resolve within 3 months.[2]

Dizziness/Nausea

Dizziness is commonly reported after head injury although most studies do not separate the vague complaint of dizziness from that of vertigo.[33] The mechanisms of vertigo and dizziness are different and must be teased apart in the history and physical examination. Vertigo can result from a central or peripheral lesion, with central lesions potentially life-threatening. In the acute phase, the clinician must always consider a vertebral artery dissection in a TBI patient complaining of vertigo. Peripheral causes include cupulolithiasis, perilymphatic fistula, posttraumatic Meniere disease, damage to the vestibular nerve, and use of ototoxic medications. Dizziness/vertigo is reported in 24% to 78% of mild TBI patients acutely, significantly higher than the prevalence in non-TBI patients in the community.[34] As with headache, dizziness generally resolves within 3 months in patients with mild TBI whereas persistence may be more problematic in patients with moderate and severe TBI.[35] Anticholinergics (eg, meclizine) should be used judiciously, if at all, in treating patients with a complaint of dizziness; there is no good evidence to support their use and their sedative properties often make patients feel worse.

Fatigue

Fatigue is reported in up to 73% of patients post-TBI and may become a persistent and debilitating symptom.[36–38] The presence of fatigue is associated with poorer social integration, decreased level of productive activities, and decreased overall quality of life. When fatigue persists, it may present a barrier to recovery. Post-TBI fatigue is most likely the result of a combination of etiologies, including pain, sleep disorders, cognitive deficits, depression, and anxiety. Hypopituitarism, with resultant neuroendocrine abnormalities, such as growth hormone deficiency and cortisol deficiency, may also be associated with post-TBI fatigue.[39] Other possible contributing factors include vertigo, diplopia, and iatrogenic causes, such as psychotropic or analgesic medications.

Sleep Disturbance

Sleep disturbances are frequent after a TBI although the etiology is complex. These disturbances span the spectrum of sleep disorders and are reported in up to 73% of post-TBI patients.[40] Key to managing sleep disorders is identifying the factors contributing to the presentation.[41]

Seizures

Posttraumatic seizures can be focal or generalized; focal seizures can be simple or complex based on the lack (simple) or presence (complex) of loss of awareness or consciousness. Both simple and complex partial seizures can evolve into a secondary generalized seizure with tonic-clonic activity and postictal confusion. Due to the high incidence of TBI to the frontal or temporal lobe, the focus of posttraumatic seizures is often in these areas. Seizures of frontal lobe origin can be difficult to diagnose because they can present with a wide variety of clinical manifestations, frequently mimicking psychiatric disorders, yet can have a normal electroencephalogram (EEG).[1]

Seizures of frontal origin are often characterized by bizarre clinical manifestations, such as RMA, simple or complex automatisms (trashing, kicking, tapping, running, or agitation), and/or nonspecific auras, including dizziness or lightheadedness.[1] The bizarreness of frontal lobe seizures, without associated tonic-clonic activity or loss of consciousness, results in the diagnosis frequently overlooked. To compound this issue, much of the frontal lobe is inaccessible to standard scalp EEG recording; consequently, an EEG can be normal even during an ictal episode, which can result in the false exclusion of a seizure disorder when too much reliance is placed on a single diagnostic test. Standard EEG in any type of focal epilepsy detects interictal epileptiform abnormalities in only 29% to 55% of patients and several series have reported no ictal EEG change in 33% to 36% of patients.[42] Some series have reported that only 14% of patients with frontal lobe seizures have localized frontal lobe discharges.[1]

Table 1 reviews some of the clinical characteristics of frontal lobe origin. When agitation, brief outbursts of rage and aggression, and/or new-onset bizarre behavior occurs in association with a TBI, a detailed history and careful characterization of

Table 1
Clinical characteristics of frontal lobe seizures

Presentation	Frontal Lobe Seizure
Stereotypicity	Yes
RMA	Yes
Aura	Nonspecific
Duration	Brief
Abrupt onset	Yes
Abrupt ending	Yes
Postictal phase	Possible
Frequency	Often in clusters
Nocturnal	Possible
Situational	No
Goal-directed aggression	No

the events is warranted. If the episodes are periodic, stereotypic, and brief in duration with a variable postictal phase, then the possibility of a frontal lobe seizure should be entertained.

Approach to the Patient with Neurobehavioral Complaints after a TBI

Evaluating the NBS of TBI requires a deep understanding of a patient's neurologic, psychiatric, and primary illness both pre- and postinjury. At times, it can be difficult to differentiate NBS after a TBI from similar symptomatology secondary to a preexistent psychiatric disorder. To complicate matters, affective symptoms can be the first clinical presentation of frontal lobe dysfunction independent of its etiology and/or of a dementing process possibly secondary to past TBIs (ie, chronic traumatic encephalopathy).

NBS are easier to put in context in patients with moderate or severe TBI who have demonstrable lesions on neuroimaging. The mild TBI group is more of a challenge and although the literature suggests the majority of patients make a complete recovery, there is a subset who do not.[2] Several studies have been performed trying to delineate the etiology and establish the existence of NBS in mild TBI; findings have been controversial and inconclusive.[2]

As discussed previously, the literature reports a high incidence of depression, anxiety, sleep disturbances, headaches/pain syndrome, fatigue, and dizziness in TBI patients: many of these studies, however, are underpowered, retrospective, or flawed by bias. In addition, most of the studies included patients of all TBI severities and included patients with a prior psychiatric and substance abuse histories.[16] Studies on patients with pain and non-TBI related injures report a surprisingly high incidence of neurobehavioral complaints. A correlation between pain and NBS has been reported, and pain has been associated with the persistence of symptoms.[43–45] Occurrence of cognitive complaints in non-TBI chronic pain patients has been demonstrated, questioning the relationship between TBI per se and NBS.[45] Iverson and McCracken have reported that non-TBI patients have a similar incidence of NBS to those patients with a TBI.[43] They reported disturbed sleep, fatigue, and/or irritability in 81% of patients and 1 or more cognitive problems in 42% of patients.

Depression can be used as an example to demonstrate the difficulty linking NBS symptoms with TBI. To meet criteria for depression, 5 symptoms need to be present during a 2-week period: depressed mood and/or lack of interest plus insomnia, hypersomnia, fatigue or loss of energy, diminished ability to think or concentrate, and other symptoms. Some of these symptoms are commonly reported as NBS, however: depression due to TBI might be differentiated from a premorbid depression based on the onset of the symptoms, associated presence of feeling worthlessness or hopelessness, significant weight changes, excessive guilt, or suicidal ideation. Bombardier and colleagues[16] studied a cohort of 559 TBI patients and reported that 53.1% of the patients were depressed at some time within the 12 months after a TBI. The diagnosis was made after telephone interview. Patients with prior history of depression or depression at injury were included. The study was conducted at a single level 1 trauma center and a high number of participants were Medicaid recipients. All of these factors might potentially have skewed the results. They did not discuss that depressed mood can be an NBS of TBI in the absence of other criteria. The same is true of fatigue, decrease in energy, decreased concentration, and sleep disturbances. All of these symptoms need to be considered in the setting of the injury, the individual response, past and present comorbidities, and concomitant pharmacotherapy.

In adjustment disorder, the development of emotional or behavioral symptoms occurs in response to an identifiable stressor. Predominant symptoms are depressed and anxious mood, which can occur individually or can be mixed, depending on the subtype. Disturbance of conduct, which is manifested by behavioral changes, can also be present, in which case both the affective and the behavioral components can be misinterpreted with NBS. Symptoms usually occur within 3 months of the onset of head trauma, which is similar to what happens in NBS.

The major question confronting clinicians is whether or not outcomes change when patients are treated with antidepressants for depressed mood or anxious mood even if these symptoms are not secondary to major depression but are in the context of the psychosocial stressors often encountered after a TBI. There is insufficient evidence to answer this question and future studies must try to determine the relative contributions of central nervous system lesions, physical disabilities, and environmental stressors on the manifestation of NBS. The importance of answering this question is obvious: there are risks of pharmacotherapy especially when a patient is cognitively compromised after a TBI. Antidepressants can interfere with cognitive function, especially with attention and memory, and can cause sleep disturbances. Also, headaches and extrapyramidal movements can be associated with antidepressant therapy and potentially interfere with motor function, especially in the elderly or in patients in whom motor function is already compromised from the injury.

Creating a differential diagnosis and management plan

Determining etiology of a neurobehavioral complaint requires a systematic and comprehensive evaluation. NBS of TBI are nonspecific and clinicians must be careful to not draw a false conclusion before a proper assessment has been made. For example, a TBI patient with a depressed mood may have a major depressive disorder but could also have an adjustment disorder, a lesion in the mesial frontal region, injury to the basal ganglia, or hypothyroidism. An adjustment disorder might not require pharmacotherapy whereas a major depression disorder does; depression from a mesial frontal lesion would have questionable benefit from antidepressants. Depression from a basal ganglia lesion could potentially get worse with antidepressants due to the possibility of secondary extrapyrimadal symptoms with bradykinesia mimicking psychomotor retardation. Not only must the etiology of the depression be determined but also the clinician must remember the possibly the depression may be an expression of an existing condition and not directly due to the TBI.

Cognitive deficit of attention plays a major role in NBS and recognizing them may be the key to a successful management plan. The differential diagnosis of dysfunction of attention includes a structural lesion, an underlying medical problem, a primary psychiatric disorder, or drug side effect (in particular, compounds with high anticholinergic properties or antihistaminergic properties). Sleep disturbances and pain syndromes can also interfere with attention. Attention can be affected by a lesion in the orbitofrontal region, resulting in high distractibility, or due to a lesion in the dorsolateral region, resulting in an inability to switch mindset or to multitask (**Box 2**). Mood disorder, anxiety disorder, psychotic disorder, and/or personality disorder can also interfere with attention, as can fatigue secondary to the injury or to a medical problem.

Bizarre or unusual behavior after TBI can be the result of structural lesions, psychiatric disorders, drug toxicity, metabolic disorders, or frontal lobe seizures. Frontal lobe seizures deserve special mention because their clinical presentation can be characterized by bizarre behavior (eg, RMA) or automatisms, such as repetitive tapping, kicking, running, or trashing. These episodes can be associated with or without loss of awareness, no loss of consciousness, nonspecific auras, and variable postictal confusion (see **Table 1**). Findings can appear psychiatric in origin and presentation can be associated with a normal interictal or ictal EEG.[1]

> **Box 2**
> **Frontal lobe lesions and its clinical presentations**
>
> Dorsolateral frontal region: injury may be expressed as difficulties in switching parameters or planning; a certain mental inflexibility can be noted, which can ultimately result in irritability, slowness in performance, and/or low frustration tolerance with potential social and performance repercussion.
>
> Orbitofrontal region: injury can manifest clinically with agitation, disinhibition, and/or poor impulse control.
>
> Medial frontal region: injury can manifest itself with apathy, which can be misdiagnosed with major depression.

Complaints of NBS after TBI are best addressed by a multidisciplinary team. Family involvement is important to promote an understanding and support system needed for successful management. The literature on mild TBI demonstrates that education can decrease the severity and duration of NBS, partially by normalizing the situation and providing the reassurance needed to patiently allow recovery to occur.[5] Ponsford and colleagues[4] studied 202 mild TBI patients and reported that patients given an information booklet on mild TBI and coping strategies for symptoms were significantly less symptomatic at 3 months than those who were not provided education. An extensive review of articles on early intervention after mild TBI by Borg and colleagues[46] showed that early educational information reduces long-term complaints.

SUMMARY

The development of NBS after TBI is associated with several factors making the identification of etiology and the prognosis challenging. The severity of symptoms has some relation to the severity of injury. The NBS after mild TBI are the most difficult to diagnose and treat because neuroimaging and physical examination are often normal. When present, NBS after mild TBI generally resolve within 3 months and when they become more persistent, a search for contributing factors beyond the initial injury should be done. To accomplish this, a systematic and comprehensive evaluation should be performed and the presenting complaint must be placed in the context of a patient's premorbid state. Neuroimaging is generally nondiagnostic in mild TBI patients with NBS; thus, additional assessment may require neurophysiologic and neuropsychological testing. Treatment of TBI patients with NBS cannot be accomplished without a clear understanding of the underlying etiology and placed within patients' social and functional framework. Normalizing the experience through education to patients and their family facilitates recovery.

REFERENCES

1. Riggio S, Harner RN. Repetitive motor activity in frontal lobe epilepsy. In: Jasper HH, Riggio S, Goldman-Rakic PS, editors. Epilepsy and the functional anatomy of the frontal lobe. New York (NY): Raven Press; 1995. p. 153–66.
2. Carroll LJ, Cassidy JD, Peloso PM, et al. Prognosis for mild traumatic brain injury: results of the WHO Collaborating Centre Task Force on mild traumatic brain injury. J Rehabil Med 2004;(Suppl 43):84–105.
3. Alves W, Macciocchi S, Barth J. Postconcussive symptoms after uncomplicated mild head injury. J Head Trauma Rehabil 1993;8:48–59.

4. Ponsford J, Willmott C, Rothwell A. Impact of early intervention on outcome following mild head injury in adults. J Neurol Neurosurg Psychiatry 2002;73: 330–2.
5. Ruff RM, Camenzuli L, Mueller J. Miserable minority: emotional risk factors that influence the outcome of a mild traumatic brain injury. Brain Inj 1996;8:61–5.
6. Lundin A, de Boussard C, Edman G, et al. Symptoms and disability until 3 months after mild TBI. Brain Inj 2006;20:799–806.
7. Meares S, Shores EA, Taylor AJ, et al. Mild traumatic brain injury does not predict acute postconcussion syndrome. J Neurol Neurosurg Psych 2008;79:300–6.
8. Dikmen S, Corrigan J, Levin H, et al. Cognitive outcome following traumatic brain injury. J Head Trauma Rehabil 2009;24:430–8.
9. Bleiberg J, Cernich AN, Cameron K, et al. Duration of cognitive impairment after sports concussion. Neurosurgery 2004;54:1073–80.
10. McCrea M, Guskiewicz KM, Marshall SW, et al. Acute effects and recovery time following concussion in collegiate football players: the NCAA concussion study. JAMA 2003;290:2556–63.
11. Tateno A, Jorge RE, Robinson RG. Clinical correlates of aggressive behavior after traumatic brain injury. J Neuropsychiatry Clin Neurosci 2003;15:155–60.
12. Greve KW, Sherwin E, Stanford MS, et al. Personality and neurocognitive correlates of impulsive aggression in long-term survivors of severe traumatic brain injury. Brain Inj 2001;15:255–62.
13. Hesdorffer D, Rauch S, Tamminga C. Long term psychiatric outcomes following traumatic brain injury: a review of the literature. J Head Trauma Rehabil 2009; 24:452–9.
14. Rogers JM, Read CA. Psychiatric comorbidity following traumatic brain injury. Brain Inj 2007;21:1321–33.
15. van Reekum R, Cohen T, Wong J. Can traumatic brain injury cause psychiatric disorders? J Neuropsychiatry Clin Neurosci 2000;12:316–27.
16. Bombardier CH, Fann JR, Dikmen SS, et al. Rates of major depressive disorder and clinical outcomes following traumatic brain injury. JAMA 2010;303:1938–45.
17. Seel RT, Kreutzer JS, Rosenthal M, et al. Depression after traumatic brain injury: a national institute on disability and rehabilitation research model systems multicenter investigation. Arch Phys Med Rehabil 2003;84:177–84.
18. Silver JM, Kramer R, Greenwald S, et al. The association between head injuries and psychiatric disorders: findings from the New Haven NIMH Epidemiologic Catchment Area Study. Brain Inj 2001;15:935–45.
19. Simpson G, Tate R. Suicidality in people surviving a traumatic brain injury: prevalence, risk factors and implications for clinical management. Brain Inj 2007;21: 1335–51.
20. Bryant RA. Posttraumatic stress disorder and traumatic brain injury: can they co-exist? Clin Psychol Rev 2001;21:931–45.
21. Harvey AG, Bryant RA. Predictors of acute stress following mild traumatic brain injury. Brain Inj 1998;12:147–54.
22. Gil S, Caspi Y, Ben-Ari IZ, et al. Does memory of a traumatic event increase the risk of posttraumatic stress disorder in patients with traumatic brain injury? A prospective study. Am J Psychiatry 2005;162:963–9.
23. Turnbull SJ, Campbell EA, Swann IJ. Post-traumatic stress disorder symptoms following a head injury: does amnesia for the event influence the development of symptoms? Brain Inj 2001;15:775–85.
24. Bryant RA, Marosszeky JE, Crooks J, et al. Coping style and post-traumatic stress disorder following severe traumatic brain injury. Brain Inj 1999;14:175–80.

25. Bryant RA, Harvey AG. Relationship between acute stress disorder and posttraumatic stress disorder following mild traumatic brain injury. Am J Psych 1998;155:625–9.
26. King NS. Post-traumatic stress disorder and head injury as a dual diagnosis: "Islands" of memory as a mechanism. J Neurol Neurosurg Psych 1997;62:82–4.
27. Hoge CW, McGurk D, Thomas JL, et al. Mild traumatic brain injury in soldiers returning from Iraq. N Engl J Med 2008;358:453–63.
28. Koponen S, Taiminen T, Portin R. Axis I and II psychiatric disorders after traumatic brain injury: a 30-year follow-up study. Am J Psychiatry 2002;159:1315–21.
29. Uomoto JM, Esselman PC. Traumatic brain injury and chronic pain: differential types and rates by head injury severity. Arch Phys Med Rehabil 1993;74:61–4.
30. Baandrup L, Jensen R. Chronic post-traumatic headache—a clinical analysis in relation to the international headache classification 2nd edition. Cephalalgia 2005;25:132–8.
31. Paniak C, Reynolds S, Phillips K, et al. Patient complaints within 1 month of mild traumatic brain injury: a controlled study. Arch Clin Neuropsychol 2002;17:319.
32. Couch JR, Bearss C. Chronic daily headache in the posttrauma syndrome: relation to the extent of head injury. Headache 2001;41:559.
33. Chamelian L, Feinstein A. Outcome after mild to moderate traumatic brain injury: the role of dizziness. Arch Phys Med Rehabil 2004;85:1662–6.
34. Anstey KJ, Butterworth P, Jorm AF, et al. A population survey found an association between self-reports of traumatic brain injury and increased psychiatric symptoms. J Clin Epidemiol 2004;57:1202–9.
35. Masson F, Maurette P, Salmi LR, et al. Prevalence of impairments 5 years after a head injury, and their relationship with disabilities and outcome. Brain Inj 1996;10:487–97.
36. Bushnik T, Englander J, Wright J. The experience of fatigue in the first 2 years after moderate-to-severe traumatic brain injury: a preliminary report. J Head Trauma Rehab 2008;23:17–24.
37. Cantor JB, Ashman T, Gordon W, et al. Fatigue after traumatic brain injury and its impact on participation and quality of life. J Head Trauma Rehabil 2008;23:41–51.
38. Ashman TA, Cantor JB, Gordon WA, et al. Objective measurement of fatigue following traumatic brain injury. J Head Trauma Rehabil 2008;23:33–40.
39. Popovic V. Growth hormone deficiency as the most common pituitary defect after TBI: clinical implications. Pituitary 2005;8:239–43.
40. Rao V, Rollings P. Sleep disturbances following traumatic brain injury. Curr Treat Options Neurol 2002;4:77–87.
41. Clinchot DM, Bogner J, Mysiw WJ, et al. Defining sleep disturbance after brain injury. Am J Phys Med Rehabil 1998;77:291–5.
42. Quesney LF. Seizures of frontal lobe origin. In: Pedley T, Meldrum B, editors. Recent advances in epilepsy, vol. 3. London: Churchill Livingstone; 1986. p. 81–100.
43. Iverson GL, McCracken LM. 'Postconcussive' symptoms in persons with chronic pain. Brain Inj 1997;11:783–90.
44. Hart RP, Martelli MF, Zasler ND. Chronic pain and neuropsychological functioning. Neuropsychol Rev 2000;10:131–49.
45. McCracken LM, Iverson GL. Predicting complaints of impaired cognitive functioning in patients with chronic pain. J Pain Symptom Manage 2001;21:392–6.
46. Borg J, Holm L, Peloso PM, et al. Non-surgical intervention and cost for mild traumatic brain injury: results of the WHO Collaborating Centre Task Force on Mild Traumatic Brain Injury. J Rehabil Med 2004;(Suppl 43):76–83.

Neuropsychiatry of Aggression

Scott D. Lane, PhD, Kimberly L. Kjome, MD,
F. Gerard Moeller, MD*

KEYWORDS

• Aggression • Pharmacotherapy • Diagnosis • Neurobiology

Aggressive behavior is prevalent in most species, and aggressive behavior patterns may serve an adaptive function. In humans, extreme and persistent forms of aggression often indicate psychopathology,[1] especially when they persist across the lifetime.[2,3]

Although several definitions have been proposed, in this article human aggression is operationally defined as (1) a social behavior that involves the interaction at least 2 people; (2) behavior that is intended to harm another person; who (3) finds this harm aversive and would act to avoid it.[4,5] This definition includes the requirement of a social context (ie, verbal and nonverbal interaction). Thus, aggression directed toward self (ie, self-injury, suicide) is outside the scope of this issue. Provocation and retaliation are known to be critical determinants of aggression, and these factors necessarily require a social context.[6]

BRAIN REGIONS ASSOCIATED WITH PATHOLOGIC AGGRESSION

In general, both human and nonhuman studies find that subcortical brain regions, particularly the limbic system and specifically the amygdala, are associated with the processing of emotionally salient events, including aggression.[7] The limbic system consists of several components that interact and project to areas of autonomic and somatomotor emotional control.[8] The amygdala has repeatedly been shown to mediate fear, defensive reactions, emotional learning, and motivation.[7] The amygdala and hypothalamus interact in the emotions of anger and fear.[9] Patients with damage to the amygdala show impairment in the recognition of fearful facial expressions,[10] and the amygdala is active in many human social conditioning and fear paradigms.[11]

In addition to subcortical regions, several cortical brain regions have been associated with emotions. The dorsolateral prefrontal cortex (DLPFC) and the orbitofrontal

Financial support: Supported by R01AA016965 (SDL) and P50DA009262 (FGM).
Financial Disclosures: The authors have nothing to disclose.
Department of Psychiatry and Behavioral Sciences, University of Texas Health Science Center at Houston, 1941 East Road Houston, TX 77054, USA
* Corresponding author.
E-mail address: Frederick.g.moeller@uth.tmc.edu

cortex (OFC) receive limbic inputs from the amygdala and other medial temporal areas as well as sensory inputs, and thus may integrate sensory information with affective signals.[12] Damage to limbic and prefrontal cortex (PFC) regions negatively affects cognition, memory, and emotional processes.[13] Several theories propose that (1) it is the interconnected network between the limbic (amygdala), OFC, and DLPFC regions that primarily subserves the processing of emotional and goal-driven behavior (eg, hedonic function), and (2) damage or dysfunction in any of these areas or this network results in problems with the regulation of emotion and subsequent difficulties with inhibitory and aggressive behavior.[14]

There is considerable evidence that the limbic-dorsolateral prefrontal and orbital frontal network facilitates the activation and inhibition of aggressive behavior. Patients with brain lesions in OFC have higher aggression/violence scores compared with normal controls and patients with lesions in other brain regions.[15] Following frontal lobe damage, particularly injury to the ventromedial prefrontal cortex, subjects who exhibited sociopathic behavior showed decreased autonomic skin conductance responses to emotional visual stimuli.[13] Patients with Alzheimer disease presenting problems with behavioral disinhibition showed decrements in OFC, DLPFC, and anterior cingulate metabolic activity that were not present in patients with Alzheimer dementia without such problems.[16] In patients with organic mental syndromes and violent behavior, lesions in the amygdala-hippocampal region were found in brain imaging scans that were not present in nonviolent organic patients.[17] These studies concluded that widespread damage to the amygdala (as opposed to pinpoint surgical lesions) produces behavioral disinhibition and violent behavior.

The connection between neuropsychiatric abnormalities and violent criminal behavior has been noted, in that "orbitofrontal injury is specifically associated with aggression" and "focal frontal lobe dysfunction is associated with aggressive dyscontrol and increased risk of violence."[18] Similarly, for the neurobiology of personality disorders, impulsive aggression is characterized by abnormal functioning in the amygdala, OFC, DLPFC, and anterior cingulate cortex (ACC).[19] Psychiatric patients with a history of repetitive purposeless violent behavior showed lower resting temporal and prefrontal metabolic activity compared with normal controls.[20] There was a significant inverse correlation between life history of aggressive impulse difficulties and OFC regional metabolic activity.[21] Subjects who committed unplanned impulsive murders were found to have lower PFC and higher subcortical (eg, amygdala, hippocampus) metabolic activity compared with controls.[22] Patients with *Diagnostic and statistical manual version IV* (DSM-IV) personality disorders and clinically significant impulsive aggression showed an absence of activation in OFC and ACC in response to the serotonin agonist drug m-CPP.[23] Individuals with a criminal history of domestic violence who also met alcohol dependence criteria had lower metabolic activity in hypothalamus, thalamus, and OFC than both nonviolent alcoholics and healthy controls.[24] Neuroimaging studies that experimentally induced anger in humans showed increased activation in the DLPFC and OFC.[25] In nonhuman primates, OFC and DLPFC lesions reliably produce increased aggressive behavior.[26]

The brain neuronal circuitry underlying aggressive behavior seems extensive and complex. Studies in humans suggest that increased aggressive behavior may be associated with decreased functioning in orbital and dorsolateral prefrontal cortical areas, and increased functioning in medial temporal (especially amygdala) brain regions. The relative balance of activity between dorsolateral prefrontal, orbital frontal, and limbic brain regions may be important in predisposing to violence and abnormal processing of emotional stimuli.[18]

SEIZURES AND AGGRESSION

There have been medical legal cases in which epilepsy has been used as a defense against charges of violence. However, recent studies provide evidence that acts of aggression during seizures are simple and unsustained; they are not planned or performed in an organized fashion, nor are they purposeful or directed. When aggression occurs in the setting of a seizure, the onset is usually sudden, duration is short, and the act is generally in response to being held down or as part of a defensive motion. Seizure-related aggression is usually part of an automatism that is characteristically unsustained, short lived, or fragmentary.[27]

To better understand the relation between aggression and epilepsy, an international task force from 16 epilepsy programs selected 19 patients who were believed to have aggressive behavior during their seizure. This sample of patients was selected from a group of 5400 patients with epilepsy. The events were recorded by video-monitoring electroencephalography (EEG) and analyzed. After reviewing the clinical characteristics and their correlation with EEG discharges, the task force made recommendations to guide the determination of causation of aggression in patients with epilepsy[28]: (1) the diagnosis of epilepsy should be established by a neurologist with special training in epilepsy; (2) the presence of epileptic automatisms should be documented by history, closed-circuit television monitoring, and EEG biotelemetry; (3) presence of aggression during epileptic automatisms should be verified by videotaped seizures and correlated with EEG ictal epileptiform discharges; (4) the aggressive or violent episode should be characteristic of the patient's habitual seizures, at which point (5) a clinical judgment should be made by the neurologist who will then attest whether, in his or her opinion, the act and/or alleged crime was part of the seizures.[28]

A complete history, including clinical characteristics, medical, psychiatric comorbidities, social history, and other concomitant factors and circumstances, is essential before making a diagnosis and before designing the necessary treatment.

DEMENTIA AND AGGRESSION

Patients with dementia can present with aggression and/or agitation. Symptoms can be caused by a superimposed delirium, and/or by the nature and severity of the underlying degenerative or structural disorder. Identifying and treating the underlying cause is key to maximizing outcome. As reviewed by Ballard and colleagues,[29] agitation and aggression are frequent symptoms in patients with dementia, which is distressing to family members and can lead to significant morbidity. In a retrospective review conducted by Jost and Grossberg[30] of patients who were diagnosed with Alzheimer disease, symptoms were defined in 3 groups to include agitation, mood symptoms, and psychotic symptoms. The investigators found that agitation occurred in the first year after the diagnosis, psychotic symptoms at the time of the diagnosis, and mood symptoms preceded the diagnosis on average by 2 years. A comprehensive approach to these patients should include basic testing of cognitive functions because it might lead to an early accurate diagnosis with all the necessary implications.

AGGRESSION AND PSYCHIATRIC DIAGNOSIS
Intermittent Explosive Disorder

DSM-IV text revision (DSM-IV-TR) diagnostic criteria for intermittent explosive disorder (IED) are: "A. Several discrete episodes of failure to resist aggressive impulses that result in serious assaultive acts or destruction of property. B. The degree of aggressiveness expressed during the episodes is grossly out of proportion to any precipitating psychosocial stressors. C. The aggressive episodes are not better accounted for by another mental disorder and are not due to the direct physiologic effects of a substance (eg, a drug of abuse, a medication) or a general medical condition (eg, head trauma, Alzheimer's disease)." In these criteria, aggression is a key feature of the diagnosis.[31] An additional key feature of the diagnosis of IED is that it is a diagnosis of exclusion; if the aggression is believed to be better accounted for by another psychiatric or nonpsychiatric medical condition, the diagnosis of IED cannot be made. However, the determination of whether the aggression is better accounted for by another condition is left to the clinician, with little guidance on how this determination is to be made. In some cases the determination is simple. In a situation in which a patient who has no history of aggression before a head injury suddenly develops aggression after the injury, the diagnosis of aggression related to the brain injury would be made to the exclusion of IED. However, in many cases the diagnosis is less clear. Many patients with aggressive behavior have minor head trauma and substance abuse, and the causal relationship between these factors and the aggression can be difficult to ascertain. Obtaining information from friends and family of the patient regarding the association between aggression and other potential factors such as substance abuse or head trauma is critical in the determination of the causal relationship. As with the general evaluation of aggression, regardless of the cause, a thorough history, physical examination, and neurologic examination are also important. Factors such as rapid onset of symptoms, association with neurologic findings on physical examination, or frontal release signs (described in detail later) can be reasons for additional tests, such as neuropsychological testing and brain magnetic resonance imaging (MRI). From a treatment perspective, unless the aggression is clearly better accounted for by another psychiatric diagnosis or nonpsychiatric medical condition, the critical question is whether the aggression is primarily impulsive or planned. Impulsive aggression has been shown to respond to treatment with pharmacotherapy, whereas planned or premeditated aggression has not.

Aggression and Psychosis

The relationship between aggression and psychotic disorders, in particular schizophrenia, is controversial.[32] One potential reason for the conflicting results on the association between psychosis and aggression is that past history of aggressive behavior related to antisocial personality disorder and substance abuse are independently associated with aggression, and thus need to be taken into account in the study of psychosis and violence. Taking these factors into account, there is some evidence that psychosis accompanied by depression or distress is associated with an increased risk of violence.[32]

Aggression and Substance Abuse

Alcohol

The epidemiologic evidence linking alcohol to aggressive behavior is overwhelming. Alcohol intoxication, abuse, and dependence are highly associated with violent criminal activity.[33,34] The non–health-related costs of alcohol abuse to society (ie, those resulting from criminal behavior) are estimated at $13 billion annually.[35] A substantial proportion of these crimes are of a violent nature; alcohol may be involved in 40% to 50% of all violent crimes, including homicide and assault.[36] This pattern is present in adolescents and young adults.[37] There is a positive correlation between the quantity of ethanol consumed and the frequency of a wide variety of acts of violence including sexual assault, child abuse, and homicide.[38] Individuals who engage in aggressive behavior report a greater amount of ethanol consumption than those without such a history.[39] In addition, alcohol consumption is greater in individuals who are more likely to commit violence, such as individuals with antisocial personality disorders.[1]

There is an extensive history of laboratory investigation regarding alcohol effects on aggression.[40,41] Reviews of laboratory-based studies have consistently concluded that alcohol increases aggressive responding.[38,41] More than any other drug, alcohol is known to increase the probability of aggression in laboratory conditions.[41]

Other abused drugs

Historically, several benzodiazepines have been used effectively to manage aggression in psychiatric patient populations.[42] However, previous reports have noted an association between benzodiazepine use and aggressive/violent behavior.[43] Past reviews have documented increased risk of criminal behavior following extended use,[44] and violence and loss of self-control in patient populations prescribed benzodiazepines.[45] From the extant data, it is unknown whether these increases were observed primarily in individuals with a history of violent behavior or underlying personality disorder.

Recreational use of flunitrazepam (Rohypnol) increased the odds of involvement in physical assault, sexual assault, and motor vehicle accidents.[46] A survey of drug users in Mexico City found an association between flunitrazepam abuse and street fights, robbery, and rape.[47] In forensic studies, psychiatric patients and juvenile offenders who abused flunitrazepam were more commonly involved in offenses involving robbery, weapons, drugs,[48] acts of impulsive violence, and serious violent criminal offenses.[49] Thus, like alcohol, abuse of certain benzodiazepines may be related to aggression. This association may be caused by shared pharmacologic mechanisms of action at γ-aminobutyric acid receptors, and concomitant loss of inhibitory control. However, because benzodiazepines have also been shown to be clinically effective in mitigating agitation and aggressive behavior, it seems likely that there is a subset of individuals for whom heavy use or abuse of benzodiazepines may facilitate aggressive behavior. History of criminal violence and/or personality disorders may be contributing factors.

One previous literature review concluded that there was little evidence suggesting that marijuana use was directly associated with aggressive behavior.[50] However, more recent data suggest that marijuana use may be related to increased likelihood of violence, particularly with use during adolescence. Studies show increased likelihood of weapons offenses and attempted homicide in inner city youth of low socioeconomic status[51]; a link between marijuana use during early adolescence and violent experiences in later adolescence in Columbian youth[52]; heavy use and abuse of marijuana was predictive of violent crimes (vs property crimes) in delinquent adolescents[53]; and violent behavior during adolescence was associated with marijuana use and dependence in early adulthood.[54] The complexity of this relationship cannot be overemphasized. Developmental factors and comorbid conduct/behavior disorders highlight the difficulty of understanding direction and causality in the relationship between marijuana use and aggression. Further complexity is added by studies suggesting that aggressive behavior may increase during periods of marijuana withdrawal.[55]

Several studies suggest a relationship between aggressive behavior and the use of central nervous system (CNS) stimulants. Day-to-day substance use in men was related to violence toward female partners, with cocaine and/or alcohol use associated with increases in physical aggression.[56] Denison and colleagues[57] reported that violent behavior increased during periods of cocaine and/or cocaine-alcohol use, and that the severity of violence was altered once cocaine use escalated into cocaine dependence. Dysregulation of the limbic system following chronic use has been suggested as a mechanism by which cocaine use may lead to heightened aggression.[58,59] In support of this, Moeller and colleagues[60] found that, compared with controls, cocaine-dependent subjects were more aggressive than control subjects on both psychometric and laboratory measures of aggression, and showed a significant correlation between measures of aggression and growth hormone response to a buspirone challenge, which was not observed in controls. However, a subsequent study by Moeller and colleagues[61] suggested that the relationship between cocaine-use variables (eg, craving, withdrawal) and aggression is mediated primarily by the presence of antisocial personality disorder. In addition to cocaine, aggressive behavior patterns may be associated with the abuse of other CNS stimulants including methamphetamine[62] and 3,4-methylenedioxy-methamphetamine (MDMA or ecstasy).[63]

Epidemiologic data indicate that, generally, the presence of a psychiatric disorder increases risk for violent behavior, but this risk is greatly increased by the presence of substance abuse symptoms.[64] Most prominent is the finding that comorbid substance use disorders and axis-II personality disorders (particularly conduct, antisocial personality, and borderline personality disorders) increase the risk for violent behavior more than either disorder alone; by one account on the order 15:1 to 20:1 compared with community-matched base rates.[64] Adolescent drug users were more prone to fighting and assault than non–drug users, and were more likely to be victims of violent behavior.[65] At least in natural settings, the collective implication of such data is that, rather than a direct pharmacologic effect of abused drugs on aggressive behavior, there are important interactions with concomitant factors, such as history of aggressive behavior and presence of psychiatric disorders, that must be understood.

DIAGNOSTIC EVALUATION OF AGGRESSION
History and Presentation

Aggression is a behavioral finding of many causes, necessitating a detailed history and physical examination in establishing the cause and potential treatments. A comprehensive approach to include premorbid function, prior psychiatric and medical comorbidities, history of alcohol and/or substance abuse, concomitant medications, presence of absence of social support, and coping mechanisms is imperative because identifying and treating the underlying cause is key to maximizing the outcome.

Specific questions in the history about aggression may help characterize illness and inform clinicians about the potential for future aggressive acts. Legal history (including reason for, number, and length of incarcerations; history of abuse toward spouse, child, or other person or animals) should be obtained as well as ownership and carrying pattern of firearms. Developmental components relating to patterns of abuse and childhood environment, as well as developmental delays, childhood legal history, diagnosis with conduct disorder or oppositional defiant disorder, may also help to further characterize presentation of aggression.

Physical Examination

In general, a basic evaluation for aggressive behavior should include a complete medical, neurologic, and psychiatric evaluation. Laboratory tests should include a complete blood count, metabolic panel, thyroid functions, urine drug screen, and urinalysis. In addition, although of lower yield, B12 and folate levels may be helpful. Brain imaging and EEG may be indicated based on the history and physical examination findings, as described later.

Physical findings in individuals with aggressive behavior of psychiatric origin, although generally nonspecific, may be helpful in understanding underlying causes of aggression. Likewise, as mentioned previously, a diagnosis of IED is made by exclusion of nonpsychiatric medical causes of aggression. Hence, this diagnosis can only be made after a thorough medical evaluation.

Abnormal vital signs and/or acute change in mental status may suggest delirium and should be investigated. In institutionalized patients with dementia, urinalysis and chest radiographs may be particularly helpful in determining the cause of delirium.

Sudden changes in behavior or focal neurologic findings suggest focal brain abnormality that should be evaluated by MRI or computed tomography scans. Gradual decline in cognitive functioning concomitant with aggression suggests dementia, which would necessitate a thorough workup for causes of dementia, including brain imaging, neuropsychological testing, and EEG.

Additional findings on physical examination may include signs of past physical altercations, including healed signs of fracture, contusion, laceration, gunshot wound, and other signs of violence. Frontal release signs may direct the history and evaluations toward a diagnosis of dementia; skull injuries may suggest a traumatic cause.

TREATMENT OF AGGRESSION

Pharmacotherapy for aggression can be separated into acute and chronic phases. The goal for the treatment of acute aggressive behavior, which is generally initiated in the emergency department or in an inpatient unit, is elimination of the aggressive behavior for the safety of the patient and staff. In pharmacotherapy for acute aggression, sedation is accepted and even sought after, although it is considered an unacceptable side effect in the treatment of chronic aggression. With these factors in mind, medications used for the treatment of acute aggression tend not to have specific effects on aggression but to have substantial sedative effects. A common practice is the use of injectable benzodiazepines and antipsychotic medication, alone or in combination. In a recent Cochrane meta-analysis of studies on the use of benzodiazepines for the treatment of acute aggression, Gillies and colleagues[66] concluded that the benzodiazepine lorazepam reduced excitement after 24 hours compared with placebo and produced similar sedation to antipsychotic medication. When comparing benzodiazepines plus antipsychotic medication with antipsychotic medication alone, there was no difference in the need for additional medication to achieve sedation between the 2 treatments, but there was a higher rate of extrapyramidal symptoms in the group that received antipsychotic medication alone.[66] The finding that patients treated with antipsychotic medication alone had higher rates of extrapyramidal side effects is consistent with the study of Huf and colleagues,[67] who showed that, in a group of 316 patients who received intramuscular medication for sedation for aggression, subjects who received haloperidol alone had more extrapyramidal symptoms than subjects who received haloperidol plus promethazine.

Antipsychotic medications vary in their extrapyramidal side effects based on potency of dopamine receptor antagonism and affinity for other receptors, such as the muscarinic cholinergic receptor, with lower-potency antipsychotic medications generally having fewer extrapyramidal side effects than higher-potency antipsychotic medications. There is a growing body of evidence that newer-generation antipsychotic medications other than clozapine do not have a specific reduction in extrapyramidal side effects beyond the potency and inherent anticholinergic effects.[68] However, few controlled trials have compared older-generation with newer-generation antipsychotic medications for acute aggression.

Pharmacotherapy for Chronic Aggression

As mentioned earlier, the goal of pharmacotherapy for chronic aggressive behavior is elimination or reduction of aggression without producing general sedation or other intolerable side effects. Although there are a large number of case reports and open-label trials of various medications for aggression,[69] there are few double-blind, placebo-controlled trials of medication for chronic aggressive behavior. Because there is a substantial placebo effect in the treatment of aggression (similar to virtually every other psychiatric and nonpsychiatric medical disorder), it is difficult to assess the efficacy of pharmacotherapy from open-label trials and case reports should be evaluated with skepticism. The most commonly used classes of medications for chronic treatment of aggression are discussed later, along with the evidence supporting their use for this indication and potential drawbacks.

ANTIPSYCHOTIC MEDICATION

As described earlier, antipsychotic medication is used routinely alone or in combination with benzodiazepines or promethazine for the treatment of acute aggression. However, for the treatment of chronic aggressive behavior, for which sedation is not an acceptable side effect, there is little evidence to support the use of first-generation antipsychotic medication. However, there are some data to support a specific antiaggressive effect for at least some of the second-generation antipsychotic medications.

In children with mental retardation and autism, and adults with dementia, there are data to support a specific antiaggressive effect that seems to be separate from the sedative effect of risperidone, at least at lower doses.[29] In a meta-analysis by Ballard and Howard[70] in 2006, the conclusions were that risperidone at 1 and 2 mg daily produced a significant improvement in aggression in patients with dementia. In patients with schizophrenia, there is evidence that risperidone may reduce aggression to a greater degree than first-generation antipsychotic medication.[71] The main drawbacks with risperidone are related to side effects of extrapyramidal symptoms, orthostasis, and sedation. As mentioned earlier, there is a growing body of evidence that newer-generation antipsychotic medications do not have lower extrapyramidal side effects than older-generation antipsychotic medications.[68] In addition, the US Food and Drug Administration (FDA) has added a black box warning to risperidone and other antipsychotic medications regarding the increased mortality in elderly patients with dementia treated with antipsychotic medication, largely related to cardiovascular or infectious causes.[29] Other second-generation antipsychotic medications have also been studied for chronic aggression in patients with dementia. In the meta-analysis by Ballard and Howard[70] in 2006, in addition to risperidone, olanzapine produced a significant improvement in aggression in patients with dementia at a dose of 5 to 10 mg per day. Fewer data are available for other second-generation antipsychotic medications. One study of quetiapine found a significant worsening of agitation, possibly related to the effect of quetiapine on muscarinic receptors or brain-derived neurotrophic factor,[72] but one study of aripiprazole did indicate improvement in agitation.[73] Similar to findings in patients with dementia, there is some evidence from small-scale and open-label studies that other second-generation antipsychotic medications reduce aggression in patients with conduct disorder, but these conclusions need to be replicated in larger controlled studies.[74]

Clozapine is a second-generation antipsychotic for which there is some additional evidence that it reduces aggression independently of sedative effects.[75] Most of the evidence supporting a specific antiaggressive effect of clozapine comes from studies of patients with psychosis.[76] In addition to the drawbacks of other second-generation antipsychotic medications, clozapine also has a risk of a potentially lethal reduction in white blood cell count, which limits its use in patients who are refractory to other medications.

LITHIUM

One of the earliest placebo-controlled trials of a medication for chronic aggressive behavior was performed by Sheard and colleagues,[77] in which 66 male prisoners (age 16–24 years) without a history of treatment of a psychiatric disorder were treated with lithium or placebo in a double-blind fashion for up to 3 months. Results of the study showed that the subjects treated with lithium had a significant reduction in aggressive behavior compared with the subjects treated with placebo.

Since the study by Sheard and colleagues, several other studies have examined lithium as a treatment of chronic aggression, showing similar results in a variety of patient groups including patients with mental retardation and children with conduct disorder.[78,79] As with anticonvulsants (described in detail later), there is some evidence that lithium is most effective in patients with affective or impulsive aggression, as opposed to premeditated aggression.[80] The main drawbacks with lithium as a treatment of chronic aggression are the side effects and need for blood level monitoring. Lithium has a narrow therapeutic window, with a potential for substantial toxicity if blood levels exceed recommended levels of 0.6 to 1.2 mEq/L. Even if blood levels are maintained in this range, lithium has side effects that include tremor, sedation, nausea, and polyuria; there is some evidence that patients with head trauma may be at greater risk for neurotoxicity, especially if these patients are also taking antipsychotic medication.[81]

ANTICONVULSANTS

Anticonvulsants are probably the most widely studied class of medications for treatment of chronic aggression. One of the first double-blind placebo-controlled trials of anticonvulsants for aggression was performed by Barratt and colleagues,[82] who compared phenytoin with placebo in inmates with violent behavior. In that study, subjects were treated with 300 mg of phenytoin daily in divided doses. Inmates who had impulsive aggression showed a significant reduction in aggressive behavior compared with placebo, but no change in premeditated aggression. Subjects with a known history of seizures were excluded from the study, suggesting that effects of anticonvulsants on aggression are independent of effects on seizures. A second study by Stanford and colleagues[83] supported the earlier results of Barratt and colleagues[82] of reduced impulsive aggression in patients treated with phenytoin, and a third study showed that effects of phenytoin on impulsive aggression were similar to effects of valproate.[84] Phenytoin was well tolerated at the dose used in these studies, which produced blood levels that were, on average, lower than those used to treat epilepsy.

Valproate/divalproex has also been studied for aggression in several clinical trials. Donovan[85] reported a greater number of children and adolescents with disruptive behavior disorders responding to divalproex compared with placebo for explosive temper and mood lability in a small-scale study. Similar results were found in a small-scale study comparing valproate with phenytoin and carbamazepine.[84]

However, another small-scale study in patients with pervasive developmental disorders did not find a significant difference between subjects treated with valproate and those treated with placebo.[86] A multicenter placebo-controlled trial of divalproex for impulsive aggression also did not find a significant reduction in aggression in patients overall, but there was a significantly greater response in the subset of patients with cluster B personality disorders.[87] Based on studies to date, a recent Cochrane database meta-analysis concluded that, although there is some evidence supporting valproate/divalproex for aggression, further research is warranted.[88]

Studies of other anticonvulsants have also reported mixed results in the treatment of aggression. A study by Cueva and colleagues[89] of patients with conduct disorder did not find a difference in response between carbamazepine and placebo, but a small-scale study comparing carbamazepine with valproate and phenytoin found that carbamazepine did reduce impulsive aggression, although the onset of action of carbamazepine was slower than the other 2 drugs.[84] Similarly, a small-scale trial in patients with borderline personality disorder showed decreased behavioral dyscontrol in patients treated with carbamazepine compared with patients treated with placebo.[90]

Though research is less extensive, newer anticonvulsants have been reported to reduce aggression in acute laboratory models and in controlled trials. Using a laboratory model of human impulsive aggression, aggressive behavior was diminished following acute doses of gabapentin,[91] tiagabine,[92] and topirimate.[93] In one clinical trial, topiramate reduced aggression as measured by the Stait Trait Anger Expression Inventory in patients with borderline personality disorder.[94] Similarly, oxcarbazepine has been reported to be more efficacious in reducing impulsive aggression in an outpatient trial.[95] A few controlled studies have also reported negative results. One trial reported that levetiracetam showed no difference from placebo in reducing impulsive aggression.[96]

SELECTIVE SEROTONIN REUPTAKE INHIBITORS

Although selective serotonin reuptake inhibitors (SSRIs) are widely used clinically for the treatment of aggression, few controlled trials have been published on the efficacy of SSRIs for aggression. Fluoxetine is the most widely studied of the SSRIs for aggression. Two studies reported decreased anger[97] and verbal aggression[98] in patients with personality disorders. Another study using fluvoxamine showed a reduction in mood shifts in patients with borderline personality disorder compared with placebo but no significant difference in aggression scores.[99] A more recent study reported that citalopram produced a significant reduction in anger and hostile affect in patients with high hostility scores but who were otherwise healthy.[100] The same study reported a reduction in aggression, but this only occurred in the female subjects.

There are also some data on effects of SSRIs on aggression in patients with dementia. A study comparing citalopram with risperidone showed that both treatments reduced agitation symptoms and psychotic symptoms but citalopram was associated with fewer side effects.[101] Another study of citalopram, perphenazine, and placebo in patients with dementia showed that only citalopram was associated with improvement in agitated aggression.[102]

β-BLOCKERS

Although there are few controlled trials with β-adrenergic agonists, these drugs have been most extensively studied in patients with a history of traumatic brain injury. A recent Cochrane meta-analysis of the randomized clinical trials for aggression and agitation following brain injury concluded that the best evidence of effectiveness in the management of aggression and agitation in patients with brain injury was for β-blockers.[103] However, several caveats were noted in this evidence, including that the studies of β-blockers for aggression in patients with brain injury were small scale, used large doses of β-blockers, and did not assess global outcomes or long-term follow-up. The 2 β-blockers that have been studied in controlled trials are propranolol[104] and pindolol,[105] with neither drug being clearly superior based on the studies to date.

SUMMARY

Aggression is a serious medical problem in several neurologic and psychiatric patient groups. It can be a sign of an underlying nonpsychiatric medical disorder, or a symptom of a psychiatric or substance use problem. When faced with a patient who has aggressive behavior, the most important actions include ensuring safety of the patient and staff, followed closely by an evaluation of the cause of the aggression. In acute aggression, physical restraints may be needed for a short period until the physical examination and clinical assessment have been made. Pharmacotherapy for acute aggression involves sedating medications, which have risks in themselves and can make diagnosis difficult. A goal of pharmacotherapy for chronic aggression is to reduce aggression without producing significant sedation and other side effects. Although there are several controlled trials showing efficacy of several different classes of medications for treatment of chronic aggressive behavior, these studies have small sample sizes and none of these medications are approved by the FDA for this indication. All medications have side effects and a recent consensus statement supported the use of pharmacotherapy for aggression and agitation only after nonpharmacologic interventions had failed in patients with dementia because of the risk of side effects.[106] Thus, nonpharmacologic interventions, such as reducing pain, improving sleep, and enhancing unit structure, should be applied before pharmacotherapy.

REFERENCES

1. American Psychiatric Association. Diagnostic and statistical manual of mental disorders (DSM-IV). 4th edition. Washington, DC: APA Press; 1994.
2. Archer J. The nature of human aggression. Int J Law Psychiatry 2009;32(4): 202–8.
3. Moffitt TE. Adolescence-limited and life-course-persistent antisocial behavior: a developmental taxonomy. Psychol Rev 1993;100:674–701.
4. Baron RA, Richardson DR. Human aggression. New York: Plenum Press; 1994.
5. Cherek DR, Tcheremissine OV, Lane SD. Psychopharmacology of aggression. In: Nelson RJ, editor. Biology of aggression. Oxford (UK): Oxford University Press; 2006. p. 424–46.
6. Cherek DR, Steinberg JL. Psychopharmacology of aggression in humans - laboratory studies. Aggress Behav 1988;14(2):137.
7. Cardinal RN, Parkinson JA, Hall J, et al. Emotion and motivation: the role of the amygdala, ventral striatum, and prefrontal cortex. Neurosci Biobehav Rev 2002; 26(3):321–52.
8. Kringelbach ML. The human orbitofrontal cortex: linking reward to hedonic experience. Nat Rev Neurosci 2005;6(9):691–702.
9. Davis M. Are different parts of the extended amygdala involved in fear versus anxiety? Biol Psychiatry 1998;44(12):1239–47.
10. Adolphs R, Tranel D, Damasio H, et al. Impaired recognition of emotion in facial expressions following bilateral damage to the human amygdala. Nature 1994; 372(6507):669–72.

11. Davis M, Whalen PJ. The amygdala: vigilance and emotion. Mol Psychiatry 2001;6(1):13–34.
12. Schoenbaum G, Setlow B, Saddoris MP, et al. Encoding predicted outcome and acquired value in orbitofrontal cortex during cue sampling depends upon input from basolateral amygdala. Neuron 2003;39(5):855–67.
13. Damasio AR. The somatic marker hypothesis and the possible functions of the prefrontal cortex. Philos Trans R Soc Lond B Biol Sci 1996;351(1346):1413–20.
14. Bechara A, Van Der Linden M. Decision-making and impulse control after frontal lobe injuries. Curr Opin Neurol 2005;18(6):734–9.
15. Grafman J, Schwab K, Warden D, et al. Frontal lobe injuries, violence, and aggression: a report of the Vietnam Head Injury Study. Neurology 1996;46(5): 1231–8.
16. Kumar A, Schapiro MB, Haxby JV, et al. Cerebral metabolic and cognitive studies in dementia with frontal lobe behavioral features. J Psychiatr Res 1990;24(2):97–109.
17. Tonkonogy JM. Violence and temporal lobe lesion: head CT and MRI data. J Neuropsychiatry Clin Neurosci 1991;3:189–96.
18. Brower MC, Price BH. Neuropsychiatry of frontal lobe dysfunction in violent and criminal behaviour: a critical review. J Neurol Neurosurg Psychiatry 2001;71(6): 720–6.
19. Goodman M, New A, Siever L. Trauma, genes, and the neurobiology of person-ality disorders. Ann N Y Acad Sci 2004;1032:104–16.
20. Volkow ND, Tancredi L. Neural substrates of violent behaviour. A preliminary study with positron emission tomography. Br J Psychiatry 1987;151:668–73.
21. Goyer PF, Andreason PJ, Semple WE, et al. Positron-emission tomography and personality disorders. Neuropsychopharmacology 1994;10(1):21–8.
22. Yang Y, Glenn AL, Raine A. Brain abnormalities in antisocial individuals: implica-tions for the law. Behav Sci Law 2008;26(1):65–83.
23. New AS, Hazlett EA, Buchsbaum MS, et al. Blunted prefrontal cortical 18fluoro-deoxyglucose positron emission tomography response to meta-chlorophenylpi-perazine in impulsive aggression. Arch Gen Psychiatry 2002;59(7):621–9.
24. George DT, Rawlings RR, Williams WA, et al. A select group of perpetrators of domestic violence: evidence of decreased metabolism in the right hypothal-amus and reduced relationships between cortical/subcortical brain structures in position emission tomography. Psychiatry Res 2004;130(1):11–25.
25. Dougherty DD, Shin LM, Alpert NM, et al. Anger in healthy men: a PET study using script-driven imagery. Biol Psychiatry 1999;46(4):466–72.
26. Raleigh MJ, Steklis HD, Ervin FR, et al. The effects of orbitofrontal lesions on the aggressive behavior of vervet monkeys (Cercopithecus aethiops sabaeus). Exp Neurol 1979;66(1):158–68.
27. Marcangelo MJ, Ovsiew F. Psychiatric aspects of epilepsy. Psychiatr Clin North Am 2007;30(4):781–802.
28. Delgado-Escueta AV, Mattson RH, King L, et al. The nature of aggression during epileptic seizures. Epilepsy Behav 2002;3(6):550–6.
29. Ballard CG, Gauthier S, Cummings JL, et al. Management of agitation and aggres-sion associated with Alzheimer disease. Nat Rev Neurol 2009;5(5):245–55.
30. Jost BC, Grossberg GT. The evolution of psychiatric symptoms in Alzheimer's disease: a natural history study. J Am Geriatr Soc 1996;44(9):1078–81.
31. American Psychiatric Association. Diagnostic and statistical manual of mental disorders DSM-IV-TR fourth edition (text revision). Washington, DC: American Psychiatric Publishing; 2000.

32. Hodgins S. Violent behaviour among people with schizophrenia: a framework for investigations of causes, and effective treatment, and prevention. Philos Trans R Soc Lond B Biol Sci 2008;363(1503):2505–18.
33. Ensor T, Godfrey C. Modelling the interactions between alcohol, crime and the criminal justice system. Addiction 1993;88:477–87.
34. Lanza-Kaduce L, Bishop DM, Winner L. Risk/benefit calculations, moral evaluations, and alcohol use: exploring the alcohol-crime connection. Crime Delinq 1997;43:222–39.
35. Martin SE. The links between alcohol, crime and the criminal justice system: explanations, evidence and interventions. Am J Addict 2001;10(2):136–58.
36. Murdoch D, Pihl RO, Ross D. Alcohol and crimes of violence: present issues. Int J Addict 1990;25(9):1065–81.
37. Galanter M. Recent developments in alcoholism. Alcohol and violence: epidemiology, neurobiology, psychology, family issues. New York: Plenum Press; 1997.
38. Bushman BJ. Effects of alcohol on human aggression. Validity of proposed explanations. Recent Dev Alcohol 1997;13:227–43.
39. Collins JJ, Messerschmidt PM. Epidemiology of alcohol-related violence. Alcohol Health Res World 1993;17:93–100.
40. Chermack ST, Giancola PR. The relationship between alcohol and aggression: An integrated biopsychosocial conceptualization. Clin Psychol Rev 1997;17:621–49.
41. Giancola PR, White HR, Berman ME, et al. Diverse research on alcohol and aggression in humans: in memory of John A. Carpenter. Alcohol Clin Exp Res 2003;27(2):198–208.
42. Zeller SL, Rhoades RW. Systematic reviews of assessment measures and pharmacologic treatments for agitation. Clin Ther 2010;32(3):403–25.
43. Pihl RO, Peterson J. Drugs and aggression - correlations, crime, and some proposed mechanisms. J Psychiatry Neurosci 1995;20(2):141–9.
44. Berry M. Criminal behavior following drug treatment for psychiatric disorders - medicolegal and ethical issues. CNS Drugs 1994;2(4):301–12.
45. Bond AJ, Curran HV, Bruce MS, et al. Behavioural aggression in panic disorder after 8 weeks' treatment with alprazolam. J Affect Disord 1995;35(3):117–23.
46. Calhoun SR, Wesson DR, Galloway GP, et al. Abuse of flunitrazepam (Rohypnol) and other benzodiazepines in Austin and south Texas. J Psychoactive Drugs 1996;28(2):183–9.
47. Galvan J, Unikel C, Rodriguez EM, et al. General perspective of flunitrazepam (Rohypnol) abuse in a sample of drug users of Mexico City. Salud Mental (Mex) 2000;23(1):1–7.
48. Daderman AM, Edman G. Flunitrazepam abuse and personality characteristics in male forensic psychiatric patients. Psychiatry Res 2001;103(1):27–42.
49. Daderman AM, Lidberg L. Flunitrazepam (Rohypnol) abuse in combination with alcohol causes premeditated, grievous violence in male juvenile offenders. J Am Acad Psychiatry Law 1999;27(1):83–99.
50. Abel EL. The relationship between cannabis and violence: a review. Psychol Bull 1977;84(2):193–211.
51. Friedman AS, Glassman K, Terras A. Violent behavior as related to use of marijuana and other drugs. J Addict Dis 2001;20(1):49–72.
52. Brook JS, Brook DW, Rosen Z, et al. Earlier marijuana use and later problem behavior in Colombian youths. J Am Acad Child Adolesc Psychiatry 2003; 42(4):485–92.
53. Simonds JF, Kashani J. Specific drug use and violence in delinquent boys. Am J Drug Alcohol Abuse 1980;7(3–4):305–22.

54. Poulton R. Cannabis use in young New Zealanders. N Z Med J 1997;110(1048): 279.

55. Hoaken PNS, Stewart SH. Drugs of abuse and the elicitation of human aggressive behavior. Addict Behav 2003;28(9):1533–54.

56. Fals-Stewart W, Golden J, Schumacher JA. Intimate partner violence and substance use: a longitudinal day-to-day examination. Addict Behav 2003; 28(9):1555–74.

57. Denison ME, Paredes A, Booth JB. Alcohol and cocaine interactions and aggressive behaviors. Recent Dev Alcohol 1997;13:283–303.

58. Davis WM. Psychopharmacologic violence associated with cocaine abuse: kindling of a limbic dyscontrol syndrome? Prog Neuropsychopharmacol Biol Psychiatry 1996;20(8):1273–300.

59. Miller NS, Gold MS, Mahler JC. Violent behaviors associated with cocaine use: possible pharmacological mechanisms. Int J Addict 1991;26(10):1077–88.

60. Moeller FG, Steinberg JL, Petty F, et al. Serotonin and impulsive/aggressive behavior in cocaine-dependent subjects. Prog Neuropsychopharmacol Biol Psychiatry 1994;18(6):1027–35.

61. Moeller FG, Dougherty DM, Rustin T, et al. Antisocial personality disorder and aggression in recently abstinent cocaine dependent subjects. Drug Alcohol Depend 1997;44(2–3):175–82.

62. Darke S, Torok M, Kaye S, et al. Comparative rates of violent crime among regular methamphetamine and opioid users: offending and victimization. Addiction 2010;105(5):916–9.

63. Bond AJ, Verheyden SL, Wingrove J, et al. Angry cognitive bias, trait aggression and impulsivity in substance users. Psychopharmacology 2004;171(3):331–9.

64. Steadman HJ, Mulvey EP, Monahan J, et al. Violence by people discharged from acute psychiatric inpatient facilities and by others in the same neighborhoods. Arch Gen Psychiatry 1998;55(5):393–401.

65. Kingery PM, Pruitt BE, Hurley RS. Violence and illegal drug use among adolescents: evidence from the U.S. National Adolescent Student Health Survey. Int J Addict 1992;27(12):1445–64.

66. Gillies D, Beck A, McCloud A, et al. Benzodiazepines alone or in combination with antipsychotic drugs for acute psychosis. Cochrane Database Syst Rev 2005;4:CD003079.

67. Huf G, Coutinho ES, Adams CE. Rapid tranquillisation in psychiatric emergency settings in Brazil: pragmatic randomised controlled trial of intramuscular haloperidol versus intramuscular haloperidol plus promethazine. BMJ 2007; 335(7625):869.

68. Miller DD, Caroff SN, Davis SM, et al. Extrapyramidal side-effects of antipsychotics in a randomised trial. Br J Psychiatry 2008;193(4):279–88.

69. Verhoeven WM, Tuinier S. The effect of buspirone on challenging behaviour in mentally retarded patients: an open prospective multiple-case study. J Intellect Disabil Res 1996;40(Pt 6):502–8.

70. Ballard C, Howard R. Neuroleptic drugs in dementia: benefits and harm. Nat Rev Neurosci 2006;7(6):492–500.

71. Aleman A, Kahn RS. Effects of the atypical antipsychotic risperidone on hostility and aggression in schizophrenia: a meta-analysis of controlled trials. Eur Neuropsychopharmacol 2001;11(4):289–93.

72. Ballard C, Margallo-Lana M, Juszczak E, et al. Quetiapine and rivastigmine and cognitive decline in Alzheimer's disease: randomised double blind placebo controlled trial. BMJ 2005;330(7496):874.

73. De Deyn P, Jeste DV, Swanink R, et al. Aripiprazole for the treatment of psychosis in patients with Alzheimer's disease: a randomized, placebo-controlled study. J Clin Psychopharmacol 2005;25(5):463–7.
74. Findling RL. Atypical antipsychotic treatment of disruptive behavior disorders in children and adolescents. J Clin Psychiatry 2008;69(Suppl 4):9–14.
75. Fava M. Psychopharmacologic treatment of pathologic aggression. Psychiatr Clin North Am 1997;20(2):427–51.
76. Buckley P, Bartell J, Donenwirth K, et al. Violence and schizophrenia: clozapine as a specific antiaggressive agent. Bull Am Acad Psychiatry Law 1995;23(4): 607–11.
77. Sheard MH, Marini JL, Bridges CI, et al. The effect of lithium on impulsive aggressive behavior in man. Am J Psychiatry 1976;133(12):1409–13.
78. Malone RP, Delaney MA, Luebbert JF, et al. A double-blind placebo-controlled study of lithium in hospitalized aggressive children and adolescents with conduct disorder. Arch Gen Psychiatry 2000;57(7):649–54.
79. Craft M, Ismail IA, Krishnamurti D, et al. Lithium in the treatment of aggression in mentally handicapped patients. A double-blind trial. Br J Psychiatry 1987;150: 685–9.
80. Malone RP, Bennett DS, Luebbert JF, et al. Aggression classification and treatment response. Psychopharmacol Bull 1998;34(1):41–5.
81. Glenn MB, Wroblewski B, Parziale J, et al. Lithium carbonate for aggressive behavior or affective instability in ten brain-injured patients. Am J Phys Med Rehabil 1989;68(5):221–6.
82. Barratt ES, Stanford MS, Felthous AR, et al. The effects of phenytoin on impulsive and premeditated aggression: a controlled study. J Clin Psychopharmacol 1997;17(5):341–9.
83. Stanford MS, Houston RJ, Mathias CW, et al. A double-blind placebo-controlled crossover study of phenytoin in individuals with impulsive aggression. Psychiatry Res 2001;103(2–3):193–203.
84. Stanford MS, Helfritz LE, Conklin SM, et al. A comparison of anticonvulsants in the treatment of impulsive aggression. Exp Clin Psychopharmacol 2005;13(1): 72–7.
85. Donovan SJ, Stewart JW, Nunes EV, et al. Divalproex treatment for youth with explosive temper and mood lability: a double-blind, placebo-controlled crossover design. Am J Psychiatry 2000;157(5):818–20.
86. Hellings JA, Weckbaugh M, Nickel EJ, et al. A double-blind, placebo-controlled study of valproate for aggression in youth with pervasive developmental disorders. J Child Adolesc Psychopharmacol 2005;15(4):682–92.
87. Hollander E, Tracy KA, Swann AC, et al. Divalproex in the treatment of impulsive aggression: efficacy in cluster B personality disorders. Neuropsychopharmacology 2003;28(6):1186–97.
88. Huband N, Ferriter M, Nathan R, et al. Antiepileptics for aggression and associated impulsivity. Cochrane Database Syst Rev 2010;2:CD003499.
89. Cueva JE, Overall JE, Small AM, et al. Carbamazepine in aggressive children with conduct disorder: a double-blind and placebo-controlled study. J Am Acad Child Adolesc Psychiatry 1996;35(4):480–90.
90. Gardner DL, Cowdry RW. Positive effects of carbamazepine on behavioral dyscontrol in borderline personality disorder. Am J Psychiatry 1986;143(4): 519–22.
91. Cherek DR, Tcheremissine OV, Lane SD, et al. Acute effects of gabapentin on laboratory measures of aggressive and escape responses of adult parolees

with and without a history of conduct disorder. Psychopharmacology (Berl) 2004;171(4):405–12.

92. Lieving LM, Cherek DR, Lane SD, et al. Effects of acute tiagabine administration on aggressive responses of adult male parolees. J Psychopharmacol 2008; 22(2):144–52.

93. Lane SD, Gowin JL, Green CE, et al. Acute topiramate differentially affects human aggressive responding at low vs. moderate doses in subjects with histories of substance abuse and antisocial behavior. Pharmacol Biochem Behav 2009;92(2):357–62.

94. Nickel MK, Nickel C, Kaplan P, et al. Treatment of aggression with topiramate in male borderline patients: a double-blind, placebo-controlled study. Biol Psychiatry 2005;57(5):495–9.

95. Mattes JA. Oxcarbazepine in patients with impulsive aggression: a double-blind, placebo-controlled trial. J Clin Psychopharmacol 2005;25(6):575–9.

96. Mattes JA. Levetiracetam in patients with impulsive aggression: a double-blind, placebo-controlled trial. J Clin Psychiatry 2008;69(2):310–5.

97. Salzman C, Wolfson AN, Schatzberg A, et al. Effect of fluoxetine on anger in symptomatic volunteers with borderline personality disorder. J Clin Psychopharmacol 1995;15(1):23–9.

98. Coccaro EF, Kavoussi RJ. Fluoxetine and impulsive aggressive behavior in personality-disordered subjects. Arch Gen Psychiatry 1997;54(12):1081–8.

99. Rinne T, van den Brink W, Wouters L, et al. SSRI treatment of borderline personality disorder: a randomized, placebo-controlled clinical trial for female patients with borderline personality disorder. Am J Psychiatry 2002;159(12):2048–54.

100. Kamarck TW, Haskett RF, Muldoon M, et al. Citalopram intervention for hostility: results of a randomized clinical trial. J Consult Clin Psychol 2009;77(1):174–88.

101. Pollock BG, Mulsant BH, Rosen J, et al. A double-blind comparison of citalopram and risperidone for the treatment of behavioral and psychotic symptoms associated with dementia. Am J Geriatr Psychiatry 2007;15(11):942–52.

102. Pollock BG, Mulsant BH, Rosen J, et al. Comparison of citalopram, perphenazine, and placebo for the acute treatment of psychosis and behavioral disturbances in hospitalized, demented patients. Am J Psychiatry 2002;159(3):460–5.

103. Fleminger S, Greenwood RJ, Oliver DL. Pharmacological management for agitation and aggression in people with acquired brain injury. Cochrane Database Syst Rev 2006;4:CD003299.

104. Brooke MM, Patterson DR, Questad KA, et al. The treatment of agitation during initial hospitalization after traumatic brain injury. Arch Phys Med Rehabil 1992; 73(10):917–21.

105. Greendyke RM, Kanter DR. Therapeutic effects of pindolol on behavioral disturbances associated with organic brain disease: a double-blind study. J Clin Psychiatry 1986;47(8):423–6.

106. Salzman C, Jeste DV, Meyer RE, et al. Elderly patients with dementia-related symptoms of severe agitation and aggression: consensus statement on treatment options, clinical trials methodology, and policy. J Clin Psychiatry 2008; 69(6):889–98.

Headaches: Psychiatric Aspects

Mark W. Green, MD

KEYWORDS

• Headaches • Migraines • Treatment • Psychiatric disorders

Headache is a common malady occurring in 90% of the population. Psychiatric disorders are common as well, and as a result, the 2 categories of conditions are likely to coexist in the same individuals. However, there is frequently a more complex interaction. Often the mutual progression of headache syndromes and psychiatric comorbidities interact to affect overall quality of life.

Many psychiatric syndromes and migraine (migraine being the most commonly disabling form of episodic headache) occur together in some individuals. There are numerous shared components, including family history and autonomic and sympathomimetic symptom complexes, as well as shared treatment with similar medications and behavioral regimens. Understanding the biologic connections and pathogenesis of these associated conditions should lead to improved diagnosis, treatment, and outcome in patient populations.

Characterization of headache types has been an active arena in clinical research. The International Headache Society lists several hundred headache types.[1] However, most are phenotypes of conditions that often have complex and poorly understood genetic underpinnings.

Tension-type headache is the most prevalent form of head pain, but, by definition, is rarely disabling and is generally untreated or self-treated. Consequently, these individuals rarely come to medical attention. Migraine is the most common headache that presents to health care professionals. Twelve percent of the population in the United States is afflicted with migraine.[2] Much of the burden of migraine is through the attendant psychiatric disorders.

Migraine is generally described as a condition of recurrent headaches, often unilateral and pulsatile, and often associated with photophobia, phonophobia, and nausea and exacerbated by movement. However, there are many variations of migraine. Up to 30% of migraines do not have pulsatile pain and the attacks are frequently bilateral, often leading to the misdiagnosis of tension-type headache.

The term migraine is often used in a general way to describe the state of a lowered threshold for the development of head pain. Many migraineurs have prodromal

Department of Neurology, Mount Sinai School of Medicine, 5 East 98th Street, 7th Floor, Box 1139, New York, NY 10029, USA
E-mail address: mark.green@mssm.edu

Neurol Clin 29 (2011) 65–80
doi:10.1016/j.ncl.2010.10.004   **neurologic.theclinics.com**
0733-8619/11/$ – see front matter © 2011 Elsevier Inc. All rights reserved.

symptoms occurring up to a day before the headache begins. These symptoms can include cold hands and feet, food cravings (for example, for chocolate), yawning, and a variety of mood changes, including depression or euphoria. Twenty percent of migraineurs experience focal neurologic complaints of an aura. The symptoms are often visual, but can be a sensory, language, motor, or a brainstem abnormality lasting up to an hour. A sequence of auras is common. An example would be a visual aura, followed by cheiro-oral tingling, followed by numbness. This situation is likely because of activation followed by a metabolic depression involving the primary visual cortex, the primary somatosensory cortex, and the primary motor cortex. The aura symptoms commonly, but not invariably, precede the headache. Migraine headaches characteristically last 4 to 72 hours and are often followed by postdromal symptoms such as malaise and depression, which can last up to a day. During the postdromal period, migraineurs are vulnerable for a brief recurrence of the headache with exertion or a Valsalva maneuver.

Specific pathologic features are observed in the genesis of migraine attacks. Migraineurs seem to have a hyperexcitable cerebral cortex. This characteristic has been shown in various ways. Transcranial magnetic stimulation of the occiput produces phosphenes in all individuals, but a lower intensity is needed to produce this effect in migraineurs.[3]

Cortical spreading depression (CSD) might be the common denominator for various migraine causes. Although this wave can be seen in other conditions, it is convincingly seen in migraine with aura. Less clear is the frequency of occurrence in migraine without aura, because it is difficult to study asymptomatic migraines in the earliest stages of attacks. CSD was originally identified by Leão after stimulating the cortex of rabbits. A wave spreading 3 to 6 mm/min spread across the cortex, posteriorly to anteriorly, first activating, and then depressing neuronal activity.[4] Lashley,[5] observing his own migraine auras, calculated that the observed symptoms during the aura correlated with a slow march of cortical activity at a rate of 3 mm/min. Positron emission tomography studies in spontaneous migraine attacks showed a spreading bilateral oligemia. Unlike in the older vascular theory, it has been observed that the headache in a migraine attack begins at a time of continued reduction in cerebral blood flow, making cerebral vasodilation an unlikely source of the head pain.[6] The vascular changes in aura seem to be after neuronal changes.[7] A wave of CSD or other factors occurring during a migraine activates trigeminal nociceptors in the meninges, leading to localized vasodilation, meningeal inflammation, and pain transmission.[8] The vascular changes, long believed to be the fundamental cause of aura, are therefore likely secondary to the neuronal changes brought on by this wave, first exciting, then depressing neuronal activity.

Plasma protein extravasation also occurs in the dura. Because migraine pain follows meningeal inflammation and activation of nociceptors in the meninges, it is not surprising how similar the symptoms of meningitis are to a severe migraine. The trigeminal nerve innervates the pia and the meningeal arteries, and CSD activates trigeminal afferents. Therefore, the pain of migraine is typically referred to the trigeminal nerve distribution, commonly its first division, notably the eye and the temple. The presynaptic terminal of the trigeminal nerve contains vasoactive neuropeptides including neurokinin A, substance P (SP), and calcitonin gene-related peptide (CGRP). Activation of the trigeminal sensory C fibers in this region causes release of the neuropeptides, leading to vasodilatation and plasma protein extravasation.

It is possible that the predilection of a brain to develop CSD and its fundamentally hyperexcitable state relate to the psychiatric comorbidities that accompany migraine. Later in an attack that has not been terminated, abnormalities of central processing occur as second-order trigeminal neurons are activated.[9] This situation leads to cutaneous allodynia, in which the stimuli, which are not normally painful, cause a painful reaction, and migraineurs find it uncomfortable to brush their hair, loosen their ties, and remove their jewelry. Because sensory fibers converge centrally, the pain becomes generalized in the migraineurs' head and less pulsatile. The cervical region becomes involved and they are often misdiagnosed as having tension-type headaches. This central sensitization is caused by involvement of wide dynamic range neurons in the trigeminal nucleus caudalis, which receive C fibers from the trigeminal ganglion. Increased amounts of glutamate, serotonin, nitric oxide, CGRP, and SP amplify the input received from $A\beta$ fibers.

A genetically driven vulnerability for these attacks likely underlies the disorder of recurrent migraine attacks. This situation likely involves multiple genes interacting with environmental triggers over time. Studies of migraine family trees provide evidence for this genetic basis. First-degree family members experiencing migraine with and without aura have a higher than expected prevalence of the same type of migraine.[10,11] Monozygotic twins have a higher concordance for migraine, when compared with dizygotic twins.[12] This finding suggests that although there is a significant genetic component to migraine, it cannot entirely explain its prevalence and severity. Only in familial hemiplegic migraine have genes been convincingly identified; these are associated with ion channelopathies.

PSYCHIATRIC COMORBIDITIES WITH MIGRAINE

Comorbidity means that 2 conditions occur in the same individual more often than expected by chance. Psychiatric comorbidities are a common presentation in sufferers of migraine headache.

Migraine and Depression

Depression is the most common psychiatric comorbidity with migraine and often poses a challenge in the treatment of both disorders.[13] Those with migraine have an odds ratio for depression of 2.5.[14] This risk is more highly associated with women than men.[15] In addition, the incidence of depressive symptoms is higher in those with a longer history of headaches and with a higher attack frequency.[15] Those with tension-type headaches do not suffer from this increased risk of depression when compared with controls.[13] There is no proof that migraine frequency is increased because of the presence of anxiety or depression.

Migraine and depression share a bidirectional comorbidity, suggesting that there is some shared component to the cause of both disorders.[16] There is also a bidirectional risk for suicidality in migraineurs and depressed patients.[17] It has recently been shown that the inheritability of migraine decreased in those individuals who are depressed.[18] There are no significant qualitative differences in the migraines seen in mildly compared with severely depressed individuals.[19]

When migraine becomes chronic and transformed from its episodic form, there is an even higher likelihood of a comorbid psychiatric condition. One study showed 78% of these individuals with chronic migraine have psychiatric disorders. These disorders were major depression in 57% of cases, dysthymia in 11% of cases, panic disorder in 30% of cases, and generalized anxiety in 8% of cases. Depression and anxiety disorders were more frequently encountered in female migraineurs. However, there was no increased risk of generalized anxiety disorder in this group.[20]

In chronic daily headache (subtypes not defined), the risk of major depression and panic disorder is 1.5 to 2 times more likely in women, compared with the general population.[21]

There may be sex-related differences in the variety of comorbid conditions. One study suggested that only migrainous women, and not migrainous men, suffered from an increased risk of anxiety, depression, somatic complaints, and hysteria.[22]

The relationship of affective disorders and migraine is unclear. Does migraine trigger affective disorder in some whereas affective disorder triggers migraine attacks in others? In general, affective disorders present before migraine symptoms.[11] It is possible that depressed individuals have a lower threshold for pain and these patients may experience a greater number of headaches. However, no genetic link to both migraine and depression has been identified.

Treating both migraine and comorbid depression is challenging. Not all antidepressant medications are effective for migraine therapy. The serotonin reuptake inhibitors, which are widely used in the treatment of depression, are generally not useful in the prevention of migraine. Amitriptyline has level-A evidence for the treatment of migraine, but is commonly not used in sufficient amounts to treat major depression, should that be comorbid. Other tricyclic antidepressants, notably doxepin, nortriptyline, and protriptyline, have level-C evidence for efficacy in migraine. Venlafaxine is more potent in its ability to inhibit serotonin reuptake compared with norepinephrine. It seems that 75 to 150 mg can treat migraine.[23,24] Mirtazapine, known to enhance serotonergic and noradrenergic neurotransmission, might be helpful in the treatment of both conditions.[25]

Bipolar disorder is another significant psychiatric condition comorbid with migraine. There is a lifetime prevalence of migraine in these individuals of 40% (44% in women and 31% in men). This relationship is particularly prominent with individuals with bipolar II disorder, who have a migraine prevalence of 65% (75% in women and 40% in men).[26] There are some differences in their psychiatric presentation as well. Depression, rather than mania, is the reason for a medical consultation, followed by a flip of depression into mania after treatment with antidepressant medication.

Migraine and Anxiety

Just as migraine is comorbid with depression, it is also comorbid with generalized anxiety disorder, with 11% of migraineurs having an anxiety disorder as opposed to 2% of the general population.[27]

Migraineurs with depression and anxiety tend to suffer more severe migraine attacks and respond poorly to their headache treatment. In addition, they are more likely to overuse their acute migraine agents.[28] This situation could contribute to an increased chance of developing the syndrome of medication-overuse headache (MOH), a chronic condition.

Migraine and Panic

A significant relationship of migraine to panic disorders has long been identified.[29] Migraineurs are 12 times more likely to have panic attacks compared with the general population.[30] There is a crossover of symptom complexes in these disorders. Some migraine attacks can be accompanied by panic symptoms such as anxiety, palpitations, feelings of cold extremities, and fear of imminent death.[31]

Autonomic symptoms such as nausea, vomiting, and dizziness are commonly reported in both disorders.[29] It is possible that those with a panic disorder and migraine sufferers share a fundamental abnormality of autonomic regulation. Because those with panic disorder tend to somatize, it is also possible that the symptoms, which lead to the diagnosis of a panic disorder, are exaggerated, and more often reported by patients and health care professionals.

Social phobias and migraine are also associated comorbid conditions. The stresses and daily hassles that complicate migraine are also reported in these syndromes.

Migraine and Stress

Three-quarters of migraineurs report that there were triggers of their attacks, with 80% stating that stress is a major trigger.[32] The concept of stress is often ambiguous. The inability to reach a goal, whether the cause is internal or external, can be a significant stressor to individuals. The stress of the headache disorder itself is often significant. Often the headache occurs, not at the height of the stress, but when the stressor is withdrawn. Stress is often protective for the development of attacks. There is evidence that stress can produce analgesia.[33,34]

The sympathetic nervous system and the hypothalamic-pituitary-adrenal axis are activated acutely during a stressful situation. Corticotrophin-releasing hormone (CRH) is released as part of this response, leading to cortisol release from the hypothalamus, leading to epinephrine release. Subsequently there is activation of the β-endorphin and dopaminergic systems. However, should this response be long-term, pronociceptive and immunosuppressive systems become activated.[35] This factor, along with others, can lead to activation of N-methyl-D-aspartic acid and μ opioid receptors.[36] Proinflammatory mediators such as interleukin β (IL-β), tumor necrosis factor α, IL-6, and nitric oxide are also subsequently activated. Stress also affects mast cells located in the dura. CRH, released during stressful situations, activates and degranulates mast cells, which are located near the trigeminal afferents in the meninges and dura.[37] These events could easily trigger a migraine attack.

Adolescents have reported stress to be the major trigger of headaches in 40% of individuals.[38] Cognitive coping strategies can be used and reduce the likelihood of the stressor triggering a headache attack. In an adolescent diary study, these strategies reduced the incidence of attacks occurring the day after the stressor, but not the day of the event.[39] The severity of such hassles of daily life is correlated with the frequency and intensity of headaches.[40] These daily events may be more important to the perpetuation of chronic headaches than specific life events.

Posttraumatic stress disorder (PTSD) has always been pervasive, but of even more recent concern given the large number of soldiers recently returning from war. Of those soldiers returning from the Iraq war who have been diagnosed as having PTSD, 32% list headaches as a significant complaint.[41]

Confounding the high prevalence of headache in soldiers is the fact that mild head trauma is seen in half of these individuals who seek care for headaches. This situation could cause a new headache or enhance a preexisting primary headache disorder. Mild head trauma, as opposed to severe trauma, is more likely to trigger headaches.[42,43]

Orofacial pain, often associated with headache, is also rendered more disabling in those with a history of traumatic life events. A total of 42% of individuals with both orofacial pain and headaches reported traumatic life events and their Migraine Disability Assessment Scores of headache disability were significantly higher than those not reporting such events.[44]

PTSD is associated with an enhanced activation of the amygdala and limbic system when confronted with threats. This activation is associated chemically with an increased sympathetic drive and activation of the hypothalamic-pituitary axis.[45,46]

A history of violence is not commonly shared with a treating physician. One study reported that this information was discussed with only 15% of patients.[46] This percentage may be increased by specifically inquiring about these past events when obtaining a patient history. Despite this reduced reporting, a history of physical, and particularly sexual, abuse is commonly reported in sufferers of chronic daily headache.[47,48] Up to 29% of those with chronic daily headaches report a history of physical abuse and up to 31% report a history of sexual abuse. Among migraine syndromes, the prevalence is even higher, with physical or sexual abuse reported in 42%. In those with PTSD and migraine, 65% report a history of physical or sexual abuse.

An association of migraine with a history of physical child abuse has been identified.[49] The occurrence of child abuse nearly doubled the risk of the development of migraine in individual patients.

The treatment of comorbid headache and PTSD is unclear. Selective serotonin reuptake inhibitors (SSRIs), used widely to treat PTSD, are commonly ineffective, or may even enhance migraines. Tricyclic antidepressants and venlafaxine may have a positive effect on both conditions.[50] Some alternatives might be mirtazapine, venlafaxine, or nefazodone, which might have a positive effect in the treatment of both conditions. Atypical antipsychotics, such as olanzapine, quetiapine, and rispirdone, may also be efficacious in the treatment of both conditions.[51]

Certain psychiatric syndromes may be seen in younger patients. Adolescents with tension-type headaches have not been found to have any more psychopathic symptoms when compared with headache-free individuals. However, adolescents with migraine exhibit 3 times the number of conduct problems, hyperactivity, inattention, and emotional symptoms when compared with headache-free adolescents.[52]

Migraine and Borderline Personality Disorder

The incidence of borderline personality disorder in the general population is 2%, but in the headache population, particularly in those with comorbid psychopathology and medication overuse, the incidence is higher.[53,54] This situation makes headache management particularly challenging. Treatment recommendations and pitfalls of management in this particular population are reviewed by Saper.[55] Pharmacotherapy, psychotherapy, good communication between treating practitioners to avoid splitting, treatment contracts, and heightened awareness by the practitioner about countertransference issues are emphasized.

Migraine and Psychosis

Psychotic disorders are also comorbid with headache syndromes. Schizophrenia has been associated with a low incidence of headache, as well as other pain disorders.[56,57] Such individuals often have an impaired awareness of somatic events in general as well as a blunted affective response to pain. However, Kuritzky and colleagues[58] and Ayata and colleagues[59] have disputed this and reported that schizophrenics had more complaints of more frequent headaches and headaches of longer duration than controls.

Migraineurs are genetically predisposed to a great many psychiatric comorbidities. It seems that psychiatric syndromes can shape the experience of headache attacks for sufferers and the frequency of symptom reporting. The presence of migraine may also be associated with behavioral and learning problems at school. Environmental factors such as physical and psychological trauma also play a role in severity and frequency of attacks as well as response to treatment. It is therefore important that these comorbid disorders be identified and their treatment included in a comprehensive migraine management plan.

THE TREATMENT OF MIGRAINE

There are different treatment approaches to managing migraines depending on the frequency and severity of attacks as well as associated medical and psychiatric conditions.

Acute medications are those generally used to abort individual attacks. The triptans are said to be migraine specific, but can relieve many forms of headache. Therefore it is important not to assume that a positive response to a triptan is a diagnostic test of migraine. These agents are agonists of the 5-HT_{1B} and 5-HT_{1D} receptors. They block vasodilatation and neurogenic inflammation. Because meningeal nociceptors are activated in a migraine, the triptans also seem to block pain transmission of these nociceptors before their synapse with the trigeminal nucleus caudalis, which is where the second-order trigeminal neurons originate. There is little evidence that triptans can enter the central nervous system and whether this ability has any therapeutic implications. Once the migraine attack has advanced to the point that there is central sensitization, this class of drugs is unlikely to be effective. These medications block the peripheral activation but not the self-sustaining central effects of the migraine attack.

Since the triptan era, the US Food and Drug Administration (FDA) has mandated that current agents seeking approval for the acute treatment of migraine reduce not only pain but also light and sound sensitivity and nausea. Unlike ergotamine tartrate and current formulations of dihydroergotamine, which often enhance nausea, triptans reduce this symptom.

Butalbital-containing agents are frequently prescribed in the treatment of migraine, but few data exist to support their efficacy in this setting. Butalbital is a barbiturate with a plasma half-life of 35 hours, but a clinical duration of action of only 4 to 6 hours. This quality means that even modestly frequent redosing can lead to drug accumulation. Butalbital-containing agents have been associated with an alarming risk for the development of MOH.

Nonsteroidal antiinflammatory agents are important agents for treating acute migraine attacks. Advantages of this class of medications in the treatment of migraine include that they rarely lead to the syndrome of medication-overuse headache, and they lack the psychoactive features that can lead to this syndrome. However, the frequent use of these agents can lead to renal or hepatic disease and gastric ulceration, and increase the risk of vascular disease.

Not all classes of medications used commonly for headache treatment have been proved to be helpful. Opioids should rarely be used in the treatment of migraine. Their efficacy in migraine is low for a variety of reasons. Opioid receptors are poorly represented in trigeminovascular neurons, which conduct head pain. Opioids can be proinflammatory, degranulating mast cells, which can enhance the inflammation in the meninges. CSD can be triggered by the presence of the most powerful excitatory amino acid, glutamate. The glutamate transporter enzyme, which is the enzyme that normally transports this acid back into the neuron, is blocked by opioids. If used frequently, these agents easily lead to the syndrome of MOH. Dysphoric individuals often self-treat their attacks with opioids to obtain relief of the dysphoria.

Preventive medications are generally used when frequency is greater than 1 or 2 attacks per week or when infrequent headaches are severe or long-lasting. Only 4 agents are approved by the FDA for prophylaxis of migraine: propranolol, timolol, divalproex, and topiramate. Methysergide, previously approved by the FDA for the prevention of migraine, is no longer on the market in the United States, although it is still used in other countries.

The mechanism of action of preventive antimigraine agents is unknown, although topiramate, valproate, propranolol, amitriptyline, and methysergide have all been shown to reduce CSD.[59] Should this site of action prove to be predictive of antimigraine prophylaxis, this greatly assists in the development of these agents in the future. Previously, all currently used preventive drugs were found to reduce migraines when prescribed for other purposes.

There are important issues to consider when using antidepressants as preventive agents in migraine with bipolar and major depressive disorders.

Several agents used in the treatment of depression can be useful in the treatment of migraine. Although low doses of tricyclic antidepressants often suffice to suppress migraines, they would not be expected to adequately treat migraine with major depression. Of equal concern is that many with depression have bipolar disorder, which may be unrecognized by the clinician. Bipolar patients may become manic when exposed to antidepressants. It has been suggested that this effect is particularly prominent in migraineurs.[26]

It is often recommended to use tricyclic antidepressants in migraineurs who experience difficulty in falling asleep and in maintaining sleep. However, the architecture of sleep that occurs with the use of these agents is abnormal.[60]

SSRIs, which are better tolerated than tricyclic antidepressants, have not been convincingly shown to be effective in the prophylaxis of migraine. Some selective serotonin/norepinephrine reuptake inhibitors have some data, albeit limited, supporting their use in the treatment in a migraineur with comorbid depression.

β-Blockers have been useful in migraine prophylaxis. Several of these agents have been shown to be effective in the prevention of migraine, notably propranolol, atenolol, nadolol, nebivolol, and timolol. Because there is a high comorbidity of migraine and depression, and β-blockers have been said to cause depression, there is often concern about using such agents in migraineurs. Because of methodological and selection issues in the studies that originally led to this notion, it is not clear whether β-blockers can trigger depression.

Valproic acid has been shown to be an effective agent for the prophylaxis of migraine and is, in addition, a mood stabilizer. It is one of the preventive treatments for migraine approved by the FDA. This situation makes this agent a logical choice for a migraine preventive agent in a bipolar individual. Weight gain and risk of teratogenicity with pregnancy often limit its use.

Topiramate is also an effective agent for the prevention of migraine. The mood-stabilization studies for this agent have been largely negative. This agent also has FDA approval for migraine prophylaxis. Weight loss induced by the use of this drug is a nearly unique feature with migraine prophylactic agents. Paresthesias and taste perversions are troublesome but benign. Cognitive abnormalities, in particular difficulty with word retrieval, can be problematic.

Nonmedication treatments are also available in the treatment of migraine and can be effective when used in combination with medication therapy. Cognitive behavioral therapy and biofeedback both have level-A evidence for efficacy in the prevention of migraine.

A meta-analysis of 23 randomized controlled trials concerning the use of cognitive behavior therapy, relaxation, and biofeedback in children and adolescents with migraine and tension-type headache has documented their efficacy. A statistically and clinically significant reduction in headaches, associated with long-term improvement, was documented.[61]

Medication interactions arise when psychiatric and headache syndromes are treated concurrently. Given the high comorbidity of migraine and depression, and the widespread use of triptans in the acute treatment of migraine, the serotonin syndrome has been of great concern. This interaction has been reported with SSRIs, serotonin- and norepinephrine-inhibiting antidepressants, and monoamine oxidase inhibitors, all capable of increasing serotonin levels. The prevalence of this interaction is low. It seems that activation of the 5-HT_{2a} receptor causes a serious serotonin syndrome, and triptans normally have no affinity for this receptor, being largely

5-HT$_{1b}$ and 5-HT$_{1d}$ agonists.[62] Nonetheless, the FDA alert suggests that a fatal sero-tonin syndrome is possible when triptans are coadministered with some antidepres-sants.[63] No convincing cases of the serotonin syndrome have been reported with the use of ergots, including bromocriptine.

TENSION-TYPE HEADACHES

Tension-type headaches are a commonly misunderstood variety of headache, although the most prevalent. However, because these headaches are rarely disabling, those individuals often do not seek professional care, and adequately self-treat. Orig-inally named tension headache, it was ambiguous whether this term was referring to muscle tension or psychic tension. The term was later changed to muscle-contraction headache until it was recognized that muscle contraction was not an adequate marker of the presence or severity of these headaches. It is not clear that the current nomen-clature of tension-type headache clarifies these issues.

The episodic form of tension-type headache is diagnosed by attacks lasting 30 minutes to 7 days. At least 2 of the following characteristics need to be associated with the pain: bilateral location; pressing, tightening, and nonpulsatile; mild or moderate in severity; and not aggravated by routine physical activity. In addition there cannot be nausea or vomiting, and photophobia or phonophobia can be present, but not both. Frequently when attacks are more severe and do not fulfill these criteria, they are termed migraines. If the attacks occur more than 15 times monthly, they are classified as chronic tension-type headaches. Chronic tension-type headache, as opposed to the episodic form, is disabling because of its chronicity. Many of these individuals, like those with chronic migraine, overuse acute medications, which are responsible for the transformation and perpetuation of the chronic pain.

It remains unclear whether the pain of tension-type headache is centrally located or emanates from extracranial skeletal muscles. Most likely, the brief episodes have a peripheral mechanism and the more continuous pain is centrally located. The elec-tromyograms (EMGs) of peripheral muscles reveal some increase in activity in the chronic form, but not in the episodic form.[64] The degree of physical hardness of the muscle and the degree of pain are not always correlated.

Emotional stress remains the most common trigger of these attacks.[65,66] As in chronic migraine, the high numbers of daily hassles correlate with the number of head-aches.[67] Although there is not a clear correlation of chronic tension-type headache and depression, some depressive scales can be increased.[68] Despite the high comor-bidity of migraine with depression and panic attacks, this comorbidity has not been identified in those with tension-type headaches and headache-free individuals.[13,21]

The medical treatment of episodic tension-type headaches generally involves simple analgesics such as nonsteroidal antiinflammatory medications. Ibuprofen and nap-roxen are most commonly used. The preventive treatment of chronic tension-type headache is more challenging. Most practitioners advocate the use of amitriptyline, which was found in a study to be effective as opposed to citalopram.[69] One positive study in chronic tension-type headache also showed that there was no correlation between headache improvement and improvement in pericranial muscle tension or temporal muscle exteroceptive suppression of voluntary activity (ES2).[70] In general, the doses of tricyclic antidepressants used are lower than those used for depressive syndromes. There is no evidence to support the use of benzodiazepines or botulinum toxin. There is weak evidence to support the use of tizanidine.[71] Mirtazapine might also have some efficacy in chronic tension headaches.[72] A recent meta-analysis of preventive drugs for tension-type headache concluded that none was effective.[73]

EMG biofeedback has good evidence for efficacy in the treatment of chronic tension-type headache and should always be used, if available. This treatment, combined with relaxation training, can reduce headaches by 50%.[74] It is unclear whether physical therapy, chiropractic therapy, occipital nerve stimulation, or acupuncture are efficacious.

CHRONIC HEADACHE AND ITS TREATMENT

Approximately 3% of sufferers from episodic migraine transform their attacks to a chronic form within a 1-year period.[75] Several risk factors are known to be associated with this transformation, including medication overuse, the frequency of headaches at baseline, obesity, caffeine consumption, stressful life events, and depression.[76–78] Major life events, particularly in those older than 40 years, often occur within 2 years of the transformation of episodic into chronic headaches. This association does not prove causality, because the major life event could lead to the overuse of psychoactive medications, leading to chronic daily headache.

MOH can occur in migrainous individuals who use large amounts of acute medications. It occurs in 1% to 2% of the population and affects 3 times more women than men. One-quarter of those with chronic daily headache can trace the cause to the overuse of acute medications.[79–81] Over time, medication overuse can transform an episodic headache into chronic head pain with superimposed exacerbations. Migrainous individuals return to their pain-free state in between paroxysms, but there is a baseline pain in those with medication overuse.

MOH is more prevalent in migraineurs when compared with sufferers of neck or low back pain.[82] Those with pain syndromes, but without migraine, do not develop headaches de novo and then progress in frequency and chronicity. This finding has been shown with several conditions, including arthritis, in which migraineurs taking analgesics for their joint pains developed chronic headaches.[83] The prognosis for untreated MOH is poor and there may a point at which it is untreatable.

In those with MOH, there is an increased risk of depression.[15] Other comorbidities seen in migraineurs with medication overuse include panic disorder, anxiety, and social phobias.[84]

There are various reasons why those with psychiatric disorders are often those overusing medication. It is suspected that many individuals with medication overuse are self-treating a comorbid disorder. Anxious individuals might be attracted to barbiturates for their anxiolytic properties. Butalbital, a short-acting barbiturate with a long biologic half-life, is present in many preparations used to treat headache. Dysphoric individuals might be attracted to the use of opioids. Those with hypersomnia for a variety of reasons, including depression and various sleep disorders, might overuse caffeine in their diet and in medications. There are additional reasons why these individuals can increase their acute medications. Undertreating or delaying treatment of an acute attack commonly leads to incomplete relief. Often redosing follows. Fear of a headache (with little confidence that the pain can be terminated without using the acute agent), obsessional drug-taking behavior, and anticipatory anxiety all lead to this state.

The psychological profiles of those with MOH and the episodic form differed in some respects. The patients with MOH reported more hypochondriasis and health concerns on the MMPI-2 (Minnesota Multiphasic Personality Inventory, second edition).[85]

Triptans and nonsteroidal antiinflammatory agents, also used in the treatment of migraine, had little likelihood of inducing and perpetuating headaches in a recent study. This finding is in contradistinction to opioid, butalbital combination, and over-the-counter products with caffeine.[86] These agents are generally devoid of psychoactive properties.

The treatment of MOH involves withdrawal of the overused agent, if present. This action is initially associated with a worsening of symptoms, generally followed by improvement. Regardless of treatment, the prognosis is poor with chronic MOH. There are many studies addressing this prognosis, and a representative study revealed that at 4 years following treatment, only one-third of these individuals remained off the offending medications.[87] Preventive medications for chronic headache have not been well studied in the past, with most prevention studies excluding individuals with headache for more than 15 days monthly. Recent studies involving onabotulinumtoxin A in the chronic migraine have suggested modest efficacy.[88] It seems that chronic migraines, even in the presence of medication overuse, can respond to this therapy. Topiramate prevention with the use of triptans for acute treatment was effective in converting chronic migraine into the episodic form.[89] Fluoxetine, used in the treatment of depression and obsessive-compulsive behavior, did increase headache-free days and caused a mood improvement, including those without depression.[90]

MALINGERING AND DRUG SEEKING

Accusations of malingering and drug seeking are common in patients with headache, particularly in the emergency department setting, in which the practitioners often are unfamiliar with the individual and in which parenteral opioids are available and often used. Pain is a subjective and immeasurable experience. Malingering individuals intentionally feign or exaggerate painful symptoms with the hope of fooling the treating practitioner into prescribing an agent of their choice, often an opioid. Feigning illness in the emergency department setting is common and was discovered in 13% of emergency department patients in one study.[91]

Malingerers typically have some external gain, which drives their behavior, although that factor may be elusive to the treating physician. These factors include using or selling narcotics and avoiding responsibilities. Many are antisocial and therefore have a history of additional antisocial behaviors other than drug seeking. Those with persistent malingering have little interest in a therapeutic outcome. However, even obvious malingering does not preclude the coexistence of a serious psychosocial or medical disorder that requires management.

Malingerers tend to dramatically present their complaints and, if any physical findings are noted, they are usually out of proportion to the purported pain. Skepticism by the physician is commonly met with hostility. Although the practitioner is obligated to share their concerns with the patient, this should be done in a nonjudgmental way, with the hope of breaking the repetitious pattern of medical office and emergency room visits.

Factitious pain is motivated by the desire of the individual to occupy the role of a suffering individual. This motivation is different from that of the malingerer. Those with Munchausen syndrome often self-inflict injury and try to produce a convincing medical syndrome.

COGNITIVE DECLINE

A transient cognitive disorder is associated with spells of migraine and cluster attacks.[92] Does decreasing cognitive function result from recurrent migraine attacks? Deep white-matter lesion changes can be seen with frequent headaches, in particular in women. The nature of these changes, whether they represent ischemic areas or abnormalities in the blood-brain barrier, is unknown. However, there is no evidence that migraine is associated with a cognitive decline.[93]

SUMMARY

Headache, and in particular, migraine, is often associated with comorbid psychiatric illness. The complex relationships between these disorders are slowly becoming understood. Successful management requires an integrated approach of neurologic and psychiatric management.

REFERENCES

1. Headache Classification Subcommittee of the International Headache Society. The International Classification of Headache Disorders: 2nd edition. Cephalalgia 2004;24(Suppl 1):1–160.
2. Stewart WF, Lipton RB, Celentano DD, et al. Prevalence of migraine headache in the United States: relation to age, income, race, and other socioeconomic factors. JAMA 1992;267:64–9.
3. Aurora SK, Welch KM. Brain excitability in migraine: evidence from transcranial magnetic stimulation studies. Curr Opin Neurol 1998;11(3):205–9.
4. Leão AAP. Spreading depression of activity in cerebral cortex. J Neurophysiol 1944;7:359–90.
5. Lashley KS. Patterns of cerebral integration indicated by the scotomas of migraine. Arch Neurol Psychiatry 1941;46:331–9.
6. Woods RP, Iacoboni M, Mazziotta JC. Brief report: bilateral spreading cerebral hypoperfusion during spontaneous migraine headache. N Engl J Med 1994; 331(25):1689–92.
7. Hadjikhani N, Sanchez Del Rio M, Wu O, et al. Mechanisms of migraine aura revealed by functional MRI in human visual cortex. Proc Natl Acad Sci U S A 2001; 98(8):4687–92.
8. Strassman AM, Levy D. Response properties of dural nociceptors in relation to headache. J Neurophysiol 2006;95:1298–306.
9. Burstein R, Cutrer MF, Yarnitsky D. The development of cutaneous allodynia during a migraine attack: clinical evidence for the sequential recruitment of supraspinal nociceptive neurons in migraine. Brain 2000;123(Pt 8):1703–9.
10. Russell MB, Iselius L, Olesen J. Inheritance of migraine investigated by complex segregation analysis. Hum Genet 1995;96:726–30.
11. Russell MB, Olesen J. Increased familial risk and evidence of genetic factor in migraine. BMJ 1995;311:541–4.
12. Gervil M, Ulrich V, Kyvik KO, et al. Migraine without aura: a population based twin study. Ann Neurol 1999;46:606–11.
13. Merikangas KR, Merikangas JR, Angst J. Headache syndromes and psychiatric disorders: association and familial transmission. J Psychiatr Res 1993;27: 197–210.
14. Passchier J, Schouten J, van der Donk J, et al. The association of frequent headaches with personality and life events. Headache 1991;31:116–21.
15. Mitsikostas DD, Thomas AM. Comorbidity of headache and depressive disorders. Cephalalgia 1999;19:211–7.
16. Breslau N, Lipton RB, Stewart WF, et al. Comorbidity of migraine and depression: investigating potential etiology and prognosis. Neurology 2003;60:1308–12.

17. Breslau N, Davis GC. Migraine, physical health and psychiatric disorder: a prospective epidemiologic study in young adults. J Psychiatr Res 1993;27: 211–21.
18. Ligthart L, Nyholt D, Penninx B, et al. The shared genetics of migraine and anxious depression. Headache 2010;50(10):1549–60.
19. Ligthart L, Penninx B, Nyholt D, et al. Migraine symptomatology and major depressive disorder. Cephalalgia 2010;30:1073–81.
20. Juang K, Wang S, Fuh J, et al. Comorbidity of depressive and anxiety disorder I chronic daily headache and its subtypes. Headache 2000;40:818–23.
21. Merikangas KR, Stevens DE, Angst J. Headache and personality: results of a community sample of young adults. J Psychiatr Res 1993;27:187–96.
22. Crisp AH, Kalucy RS, MacGuinnes B, et al. Some clinical, social and psychological characteristics of migraine subjects in the general population. Postgrad Med J 1977;53:691–7.
23. Adelman LC, Adelman JU, Von Seggern R, et al. Venlafaxine extended release (XR) for the prophylaxis of migraine and tension-type headache: a retrospective study in a clinical setting. Headache 2000;40:572–80.
24. Suleyman SN, Talu GK, Kiziltan E, et al. The efficacy and safety of venlafaxine in the prophylaxis of migraine. Headache 2005;45:144–52.
25. Levy E, Margolese HC. Migraine headache prophylaxis and treatment with low-dose mirtazapine. Int Clin Psychopharmacol 2003;18:301–3.
26. Low N, Galbaud du Fort G, Cervantes P. Prevalence, clinical correlates, and treatment of migraine in bipolar disorder. Headache 2003;43:940–9.
27. Breslau N, Davis GC, Andreski P. Migraine, psychiatric disorders, and suicide attempts: an epidemiologic study of young adults. Psychol Res 1991;37:11–23.
28. Rains J, Mekies C, Geraud G, et al. Anxiety, stress and coping behaviors in primary care migraine patients: results of the SMILE study. Cephalalgia 2008; 28:1115–25.
29. Stewart W, Linet M, Celentano D. Migraine headaches and panic attacks. Psychosom Med 1989;51:559–69.
30. Breslau N, Davis GC. Migraine, major depression and panic disorder: a prospective epidemiologic study of young adults. Cephalalgia 1992;12:85–90.
31. Ossipova VV, Kolosova OA, Vein AM. Migraine associated with panic attacks. Cephalalgia 1999;19:728–31.
32. Kelman L. The triggers or precipitants of the acute migraine attack. Cephalalgia 2007;27:394–402.
33. Bodner RJ. Neuropharmacological and neuroendocrine substrates of stress-induced analgesia. Ann N Y Acad Sci 1986;467:345–60.
34. Terman CW, Liebeskind JC. Relation of stress-induced analgesia to stimulation-produced analgesia. Ann N Y Acad Sci 1986;467:345–60.
35. Maier SF. Bi-directional immune-brain communication: implications for understanding stress, pain, and cognition. Brain Behav Immun 2003;17:69–85.
36. Imbe H, Iwai-Liao Y, Senba E. Stress-induced hyperalgesia: animal models and putative mechanisms. Front Biosci 2006;11:2179–92.
37. Strassman AM, Raymond SA, Burstein R. Sensitization of meningeal sensory neurons and the origin of headaches. Nature 1996;384:560–4.
38. Passchier J, Orlebeke JF. Headaches and stress in schoolchildren: an epidemiological study. Cephalalgia 1985;5:167–76.
39. Massey E, Garnefsky N, Gebhardt W, et al. Daily frustration, cognitive coping and coping efficacy in adolescent headache: a daily diary study. Headache 2009;49: 1198–205.

40. Fernandez EW, Sheffield J. Relative contributions of life events versus daily hassles to the frequency and intensity of headaches. Headache 1996;36:595–602.
41. Hoge CW, Terhakopian A, Castro CA, et al. Association of posttraumatic stress disorder with somatic symptoms, health care visits, and absenteeism among Iraq war veterans. Am J Psychiatry 2007;164:150–3.
42. Wilkinson M, Gilchrist E. Post traumatic headache. Ups J Med Sci Suppl 1980;31: 48–51.
43. Theeler B, Erickson C. Mild head trauma and chronic headaches in returning US soldiers. Headache 2009;49:529–34.
44. Branch M. Headache disability in orofacial pain patients is related to traumatic life events. Headache 2009;49:535–40.
45. Hopper JW, Frewen PA, van der Kolk BA, et al. Neural correlates of reexperiencing, avoidance, and dissociation in PTSD: symptom dimensions and emotion dysregulation in responses to script-driven trauma imagery. J Trauma Stress 2007;20:713–25.
46. Kelso EB, Haber J. Selections from the current literature: clinical detection of abuse. Fam Pract 1996;13:408–11.
47. Tietjien GE, Brandes JL, Digre KB, et al. The influence of abuse on headache, mood, and somatic symptoms in women. Headache 2005;45:772.
48. Peterlin BL, Ward TW, Lidicker J, et al. A retrospective, comparative study on the frequency of abuse in migraine and chronic daily headache. Headache 2007;47: 397–401.
49. Fuller-Thomson E, Baker T, Brennenstuhl S. Investigating the association between childhood physical abuse and migraine. Headache 2010;50:749–60.
50. Griffith JL, Razavi M. Pharmacological management of mood and anxiety disorders in headache patients. Headache 2006;46(Suppl 3):S133–41.
51. Adetunji B, Mathews M, Williams A, et al. Use of antipsychotics in the treatment of post-traumatic stress disorder. Psychiatry 2005;2:43–7.
52. Milde-Busch A, Boneberger A, Heinrich S, et al. Higher prevalence of psycho-pathological symptoms in adolescents with headache. A population-based cross-sectional study. Headache 2010;50:738–48.
53. Swartz M, Blazer D, George L, et al. Estimating the prevalence of borderline personality disorder in the community. J Pers Disord 1990;4:257–72.
54. Widiger T, Weissman M. Epidemiology of borderline personality disorder. Hosp Community Psychiatry 1991;42:257–72.
55. Saper J, Lake A. Borderline personality disorder and the chronic headache patient: review and management recommendations. Headache 2002;42:663–74.
56. Mehta D, Wooden H, Mehta S. Migraine and schizophrenia [letter]. Am J Psychiatry 1980;137:1126.
57. Dworkin RH. Pain insensitivity in schizophrenia: a neglected phenomenon and some implications. Schizophr Bull 1994;20:235–48.
58. Kuritzky A, Mazeh D, Levi A. Headache in schizophrenic patients: a controlled study. Cephalalgia 1999;19:725–7.
59. Ayata C, Jin H, Kudo C, et al. Suppression of cortical spreading depression in migraine prophylaxis. Ann Neurol 2006;59:652–61.
60. Carette S, Oakson G, Guimont C, et al. Sleep electroencephalography and the clinical response to amitriptyline in patients with fibromyalgia. Arthritis Rheum 1995;38:1211–7.
61. Trautmann E, Lackschewitz H, Kroner-Herwig B. Psychological treatment of recurrent headache in children and adolescents–a meta-analysis. Cephalalgia 2006;26:1411–26.

62. Gillman PK. Triptans, serotonin agonists, and serotonin syndrome (serotonin toxicity): a review. Headache 2010;50:264–72.
63. US Food and Drug Administration (FDA public health advisory). Combined use of 5-hydroxytriptamine receptor agonists (triptans), selective serotonin reuptake inhibitors (SSRIs) or selective serotonin/norepinephrine reuptake inhibitors (SNRIs) may result in life-threatening serotonin syndrome. 2007. Available at: http://fda.gov/cder/drug/advisory/SSRI_SS200607.htm. Accessed October 18, 2010.
64. Schoenen J, Gerard P, De Pasqua V, et al. Multiple clinical and paraclinical analyses of chronic tension-type headache associated or unassociated with disorder of pericranial muscles. Cephalalgia 1991;11:135–9.
65. Spierings EL, Ranke AH, Honkoop PC. Precipitating and aggravation factors of migraine versus tension-type headache. Headache 2001;41:554–8.
66. Rasmussen BK. Migraine and tension-type headache in a general population: precipitating factors, female hormones, sleep pattern and relation to lifestyle. Pain 1993;53:65–72.
67. DeBenedittis G, Lorenzetti A. The role of stressful life events in the persistence of primary headache: major life events vs. daily hassles. Pain 1992;51:35–42.
68. Yücel B, Kora K, Özyalcin S, et al. Depression, automatic thoughts, alexithymia, and assertiveness in patients with tension-type headache. Headache 2002;42:194–9.
69. Bendtsen L, Jensen R, Olesen J. A non-selective (amitriptyline), but not a selective (citalopram), serotonin reuptake inhibitor is effective in the prophylactic treatment of chronic tension-type headache. J Neurol Neurosurg Psychiatry 1996;61:285–90.
70. Gobel H, Hamouz V, Hansen C, et al. Amitriptyline reduces clinical headache-duration and experimental pain sensitivity but does not alter pericranial muscle activity readings. Pain 1994;59:241–9.
71. Fogelholm R, Murros K. Tizanidine in chronic tension-type headache: a placebo controlled double-blind cross over study. Headache 1992;32:509–13.
72. Bentsen L, Jensen R. Mirtazapine is effective in the prophylactic treatment of chronic tension-type headache. Neurology 2004;62:1706–11.
73. Verhagen A, Damen L, Berger MY, et al. Lack of benefit for prophylactic drugs of tension-type headache in adults: a systematic review. Fam Pract 2010;27(2):151–65.
74. Holroyd KA, Penzien DB. Client variables and behavioral treatment of recurrent tension headaches: a meta-analytic review. J Behav Med 1986;9:515–36.
75. Scher A, Stewart WF, Liberman J, et al. Prevalence of frequent headache in a population sample. Headache 1998;38:497–506.
76. Bigal ME, Lipton RB. Modifiable risk factors for migraine progression. Headache 2006;46:1334–43.
77. Scher AL, Stewart WF, Buse D, et al. Major life changes before and after the onset of chronic daily headache: a population-based study. Cephalalgia 2008;28:868–76.
78. Scher AI, Stewart WF, Ricci JA, et al. Factors associated with the onset and remission of chronic daily headache in a population based study. Pain 2003;106:81–9.
79. Zwart JA, Dyb G, Hagen K, et al. Analgesic overuse among subjects with headache, neck, and low-back pain. Neurology 2003;62:1540–4.
80. Pascal J, Colas R, Castillo J. Epidemiology of chronic daily headache. Curr Pain Headache Rep 2001;5:529–36.
81. Colas R, Munoz P, Temprano R, et al. Chronic daily headache with analgesic overuse: epidemiology and impact on quality of life. Neurology 2004;62:1338–42.

82. Katsavara Z, Schneeweiss S, Kurth T, et al. Incidence and predictors for chronicity of headache in patients with episodic migraine. Neurology 2004;62: 788–90.
83. Bahra A, Walsh M, Menon S, et al. Does chronic daily headache arise de novo in association with regular use of analgesics? Headache 2003;43:179–90.
84. Radat F, Sakh D, Lutz G, et al. Psychiatric comorbidity is related to headache induced by chronic substance use in migraineurs. Headache 1999;39:477–80.
85. Sances G, Galli F, Anastasi S, et al. Medication-overuse headache and personality: a controlled study by means of the MMPI-2. Headache 2009;50: 198–209.
86. Scher AI, Lipton RB, Stewart WF, et al. Patterns of medication use by chronic and episodic headache sufferers in the general population: results from the frequent headache epidemiology study. Cephalalgia 2010;30:321–8.
87. Pini LA, Cicero AF, Sandrini M. Long-term follow-up of patients treated for chronic headache with analgesic overuse. Cephalalgia 2001;21:878–83.
88. Dodick D, Turkel C, DeGryse R, et al. Onabotulinumtoxin A for treatment of chronic migraine: pooled results from the double-blind, randomized, placebo-controlled phases of the PREEMPT clinical program. Headache 2010; 50:921–36.
89. Mei D, Ferraro D, Zelano G, et al. Topiramate and triptans revert chronic migraine with medication overuse to episodic migraine. Clin Neuropharmacol 2006;29: 269–75.
90. Saper J, Silberstein SD, Lake AE, et al. Double-blind trial of fluoxetine: chronic daily headache and migraine. Headache 1994;34:497–502.
91. Yates BD, Nordquist CR, Schultz-Ross RA. Feigned psychiatric symptoms in the emergency room. Psychiatr Serv 1996;47:998–1000.
92. Meyer JS, Thornby J, Crawford K, et al. Reversible cognitive decline accompanies migraine and cluster headaches. Headache 2000;40:638–46.
93. Baars M, van Boxtel M, Jolles J. Migraine does not affect cognitive decline: results from the Maastricht aging study. Headache 2009;50:176–84.

White Matter: Beyond Focal Disconnection

Christopher M. Filley, MD[a,b,*]

KEYWORDS

- Disconnection • Neural networks • Diffusion tensor imaging
- White matter dementia • Depression • Schizophrenia

The myelinated fibers of white matter interact with the neuronal cell bodies and synapses of gray matter to support all operations of the brain. Long understood as critical for sensory and motor function, the cerebral white matter has also steadily gained attention as essential for the higher functions.[1–6] White matter lesions are well known, for example, to produce focal neurobehavioral deficits such as aphasia, apraxia, and agnosia, and a variety of disconnection syndromes have provided a foundation for modern behavioral neurology.[1]

In recent years, the contributions of white matter to other aspects of cognition and emotion have been increasingly recognized. As a cognitive syndrome, white matter dementia has been described as a sequel of diffuse or multifocal white matter dysfunction.[2,6] Much interest has also been generated by the role of white matter connectivity in emotion[2,4] and the hypothesis that white matter dysfunction may underlie a wide range of idiopathic neuropsychiatric disorders that have thus far defied understanding.[7–9]

This review considers the cognitive and emotional relevance of white matter beyond focal disconnection. White matter dementia is presented as a common but underappreciated cognitive syndrome associated with the widespread cerebral neuropathology of most white matter disorders. A focused account follows of the psychiatric syndromes that may occur in patients with known white matter disorders, and lastly, the emerging investigation of white matter dysfunction in the pathogenesis of a variety of psychiatric disorders is briefly described. White matter dementia reflects network disconnection with prominent frontal lobe manifestations,[2,6] whereas neuropsychiatric disorders implicate disconnection within frontotemporal networks subserving normal emotion.[10–14] While much remains unknown, the evidence that white matter neuropathology

The author has no disclosures.

[a] Behavioral Neurology Section, University of Colorado School of Medicine, 12631 East 17th Avenue, MS B185, Aurora, CO 80045, USA
[b] Denver Veterans Affairs Medical Center, 1055 Clermont Street, Denver, CO 80220, USA
* Behavioral Neurology Section, University of Colorado School of Medicine, 12631 East 17th Avenue, MS B185, Aurora, CO 80045.
E-mail address: christopher.filley@ucdenver.edu

Neurol Clin 29 (2011) 81–97
doi:10.1016/j.ncl.2010.10.003   **neurologic.theclinics.com**
0733-8619/11/$ – see front matter © 2011 Elsevier Inc. All rights reserved.

contributes to a wide range of cognitive and behavioral dysfunction introduces a host of intriguing clinical and research implications.

AN OVERVIEW OF BRAIN WHITE MATTER
Anatomy

White matter comprises roughly half the volume of the adult brain,[15] and some 135,000 km of myelinated fibers course within the cerebrum.[16] At the macroscopic level, white matter consists of millions of myelinated axons joined in tracts, fascicles, bundles, and peduncles; in the brain, neuroanatomists have usefully distinguished between projection, association, and commissural fiber systems.[17] Association and commissural tracts are most important for neurobehavioral function, as they link cortical and subcortical gray matter regions into neural networks.[2,13,18] Not to be neglected are small white matter fascicles that also course within the cerebral cortex and deep gray matter of the basal ganglia and thalamus.[19] White matter neuroanatomy continues to evolve with modern investigation, and the finer details of cerebral macroconnectivity are becoming clearer.[20] The microscopic structure of white matter is dominated by myelin, a complex mixture of 70% lipid and 30% protein that encircles the length of axons except for the nodes of Ranvier, and oligodendrocytes, the myelin-forming glial cells of the central nervous system.[21,22]

Physiology

The defining feature of white matter function is the increase of axonal conduction velocity conferred by myelination. Exploiting the saltatory conduction enabled by the nodes of Ranvier, myelinated axons conduct action potentials far more rapidly than unmyelinated fibers, and the efficiency of widely distributed neural networks is markedly enhanced.[17] The common-sense assumption that slowed neural transmission will manifest as slowed cognition is in fact proving to be accurate; recent evidence indicates that cognitive speed is indeed dependent on the integrity of white matter tracts,[23,24] confirming that information transfer in the brain is facilitated by myelinated systems. This capacity of white matter permits the seamless and highly integrated operations of large-scale neural networks distributed within and between the hemispheres, linking the gray matter of the cerebral cortex with other cortical regions and numerous subcortical nuclei.[25] Distributed neural networks are thought to subserve arousal, attention, executive function, memory, language, praxis, visuospatial ability, recognition, and a range of emotional domains including motivation, comportment, social cognition, and others less well defined.[2,13,25] In all these networks, a distinction emerges between the microconnectivity of gray matter, in which synaptic function subserves information processing, and the macroconnectivity of white matter, whereby remote gray matter areas are unified into functionally coherent neural ensembles.[19,26]

Development and Aging

White matter structure displays a unique trajectory in the brain over the entirety of development and aging.[2] Recent evidence has consistently supported an inverted "U" or quadratic depiction of cerebral white matter over the life span, such that peak white matter volume in the brain is reached at about 50 years of age, with accumulation before then and loss thereafter.[27] While gray matter structure and function must also be considered in the origin of normal behaviors that appear over the life span, changes in white matter are increasingly implicated. In development, for example, it is evident that the acquisition of normal maturity temporally coincides with the myelination of the frontal lobes in young adulthood.[9] In aging, a special vulnerability of white matter has been noted, particularly in anterior cerebral regions, where volume loss may underlie the cognitive changes of normal aging.[28] These age-related alterations imply that white matter is in a continual process of volumetric change that has neurobehavioral consequences. Thus, white matter lesions of any kind noted by clinicians on computed tomography (CT)—and even better on magnetic resonance imaging (MRI)—should be seen as superimposed on normal age-related variations in white matter that may influence their clinical impact.

Evolutionary Significance

The size of the human brain, in particular the frontal lobes, has increased dramatically over the course of evolution, and expansion of the cerebral cortex has been assumed to drive this enlargement. However, while the size of the cerebral cortex has increased, the cerebral white matter has expanded to an even greater degree.[29] Moreover, in the prefrontal regions, white matter is disproportionately larger in humans than in other primates.[29] These observations suggest a special role of white matter in the organization of human capacities such as executive function and social cognition. Indeed, differences in white matter structure correlate with measured intelligence and a range of cognitive and emotional skills,[4] so that myelinated systems can be seen as complementing gray matter in the mediation of higher functions. Another neurobiological feature with adaptive value, usually associated with cortical synapses but now also evident in myelin, is plasticity.[4] In essence, experience changes white matter structure; activity-dependent myelination has been shown in several animal models, and in studies of piano players who develop increased white matter tract organization in proportion to the number of hours practiced.[4] White matter is also increasingly recognized to have at least some capacity to restore itself after injury; the study of remyelination has long been pursued and continues to attract attention, and the recent discovery of endogenous stem cells in the subventricular zone raises intriguing questions about the potential for white matter to respond to structural damage by gliogenesis or neurogenesis.[30]

WHITE MATTER DEMENTIA

Dementia is an increasing threat to medicine and society, and Alzheimer disease (AD) by itself poses a major challenge, but dementia can also occur in well over 100 other disorders in which cerebral white matter is prominently or exclusively affected.[2] These disorders fall into the categories of genetic, demyelinative, infectious, inflammatory, toxic, metabolic, vascular, traumatic, neoplastic, and hydrocephalic.[2,19,31] **Table 1** lists these categories and relatively well-studied examples of each[32–41]; many other disorders can also be found in each of these categories.[2,19,31] The obvious exception to this list is the neurodegenerative diseases, in which white matter damage is generally considered secondary to gray matter neuropathology; even this assumption may be premature, however, as one current model posits that the earliest neuropathology of AD may in fact be found within cerebral white matter.[5]

  The prevalence of dementia in the white matter disorders as a whole is not known, but the problem is likely underestimated. Neurobehavioral manifestations in patients with these disorders often escape detection because of reduced access to health care (as can burden many people with toluene abuse), the relative insensitivity of cognitive screening tests such as the Mini-Mental State Examination (MMSE[42]) to cognitive impairment from white matter pathology,[2] or overriding clinical emphasis on elemental sensory and motor problems such as visual loss, hemiparesis, ataxia, and incontinence

Table 1
Categories of white matter disorders and representative examples

Genetic	Metachromatic leukodystrophy[32]
Demyelinative	Multiple sclerosis[33]
Infectious	Progressive multifocal leukoencephalopathy[34]
Inflammatory	Systemic lupus erythematosus[35]
Toxic	Toluene leukoencephalopathy[36]
Metabolic	Cobalamin (B_{12}) deficiency[37]
Vascular	Binswanger disease[38]
Traumatic	Traumatic brain injury[39]
Neoplastic	Gliomatosis cerebri[40]
Hydrocephalic	Normal pressure hydrocephalus[41]

in patients with white matter disorders. When carefully sought, cognitive dysfunction in white matter disorders is far more common than is often assumed. In multiple sclerosis (MS), for example, the reported prevalence of cognitive dysfunction rose from about 5%[43] to 43% after well-designed neuropsychological studies were conducted,[33] and one study found 23% of MS patients to be demented.[44] Similarly, many millions of older people around the world harbor substantial white matter ischemic disease that is now thought to either produce or contribute to the onset of dementia.[2] The term white matter dementia was introduced in 1988[6] to highlight the often neglected cognitive loss experienced by patients with white matter disorders, often progressing to dementia, that may be completely reversible if recognized early.[2]

The clinical profile of white matter dementia reflects the usual diffuse or multifocal neuropathology of white matter disorders.[2] Focal white matter disconnection syndromes are relatively uncommon because single white matter lesions are unusual, and a more likely cognitive sequel of white matter neuropathology is white matter dementia or a precursor cognitive impairment syndrome. **Box 1** presents the clinical features of white matter dementia.[2,6,13,19] Slowing of cognitive processing is typical, and this pervasive deficit in turn contributes to impaired executive function and sustained attention, deficits often described in terms of the closely related concept of working memory. Simultaneously, memory retrieval deficits in declarative memory are present while memory encoding is largely spared. Visuospatial skills are compromised, often reflecting

Box 1
The clinical profile of white matter dementia

Cognitive slowing

Executive dysfunction

Sustained attention deficit

Memory retrieval deficit

Visuospatial impairment

Psychiatric disorder

Relatively preserved language

Normal extrapyramidal function

Normal procedural memory

combined constructional and motor disturbances. Psychiatric dysfunction is common and may take many forms. Important areas of spared function are language, extrapyramidal function, and procedural memory.[2,19,31]

The specific features of white matter dementia can best be explained in the context of the distinction between cortical and subcortical dementia.[2,19,31] Although this distinction has been criticized because of much overlap between the 2 categories,[45] a neuroanatomically based classification of dementia has merit in investigating cognition just as focal cerebral lesions can help elucidate brain-behavior relationships. White matter dementia differs from both cortical (eg, AD) and subcortical dementia (including Huntington disease [HD] and Parkinson disease [HD]), as its unique neuroanatomical basis would suggest.[2,19,31] Amnesia and aphasia are not typical of white matter dementia, in keeping with the sparing of cerebral cortical regions devoted to declarative memory and language, whereas cognitive slowing and impaired sustained attention are common. Thus, in contrast to AD, which manifests worse declarative memory encoding and verbal function, white matter dementia is characterized by slower processing speed and more impaired sustained attention.[46] White matter dementia is similar to classic subcortical dementia, as both manifest prominent cognitive slowing, executive dysfunction, impaired sustained attention, and declarative memory retrieval deficits,[2,6,13,19] but in sharp contrast to subcortical dementia, white matter dementia does not feature prominent extrapyramidal dysfunction[47,48] and procedural memory is normal.[49–52]

One of the most convincing examples of white matter dementia is toluene leukoencephalopathy.[36,53–58] This drug abuse syndrome, far less recognized than abuse syndromes related to alcohol, stimulants, and opiates, results from the intentional inhalation of toluene vapors, typically from spray paint or other readily available commercial products, and severe dementia may ensue with the clinical features described above.[54,56] MRI detects diffuse white matter involvement,[55,56] and the severity of dementia correlates with the degree of white matter involvement as well as the duration of toluene abuse.[56] Autopsy of toluene leukoencephalopathy patients discloses selective white matter loss with sparing of the cerebral cortex, subcortical gray matter, and even cerebral axons until very late in the clinical course.[36,57] Despite other forms of drug abuse receiving more attention, toluene abuse is a widespread problem in the United States and around the world, and reported use of solvent vapor among young people—as high as 22%—indicates the potential magnitude of this problem.[36,58] Because most white matter disorders involve some component of gray matter neuropathology, either cortical or subcortical, the profound dementia that occurs in many cases of toluene leukoencephalopathy provides a compelling example of how selective white matter damage may produce devastating cognitive consequences.

White matter dementia has mainly been documented in the parallel literature describing cognitive deficits in all categories of white matter disorder.[2,19,31] Perusal of this literature does indeed reveal striking commonalities in the clinical features of dementia,[2,19,31] shown in **Box 1**, demonstrating a fundamental principle of behavioral neurology that the location of neuropathology is more important than its specific type in producing clinical phenomenology. Experimental evidence adds additional support to the concept. A clinical study compared dementia patients with 25% or more of the white matter affected by various disorders disclosed by conventional MRI with age-matched AD patients, and found that the former group had more cognitive slowing, attentional dysfunction, and memory retrieval impairment.[59] These findings showed that white matter dementia clearly differs from AD using a Neurobehavior Clinic sample with many different white matter disorders, and supported the neurobehavioral profile shown in **Box 1**. Animal models have also been supportive. In traumatic brain injury

(TBI), for example, the degree of diffuse axonal injury in the cerebral white matter has been strongly correlated with duration of coma and neurologic outcome in monkeys subjected to rotational head injury.[60] Studies of vascular disease in mice induced by bilateral carotid artery stenosis have shown that ischemic cerebral white matter lesions, sparing both hippocampus and cortex, produce selective deficits in working memory while leaving intact the memory function subserved by the hippocampus.[61] Models such as these permit controlled experimental investigation of the cognitive effects of selective cerebral white matter damage.

PSYCHIATRIC SYNDROMES IN WHITE MATTER DISORDERS

Neurologists have long described psychiatric syndromes in patients with neurologic disorders. These descriptions often derive from patients who have a prominent degree of cerebral white matter neuropathology.[2,19,31] MRI has proven invaluable in detecting white matter abnormalities, and the advent of diffusion tensor imaging (DTI) in the last decade has begun to add more information by virtue of its capacity to provide detailed depiction of myelinated tracts.[62] DTI is based on the diffusion of water molecules, which normally occurs in the direction of white matter tracts, a property known as anisotropy; when a tract is damaged, water diffusion becomes more random as the directionality of the tract is reduced, and isotropy results. Measures such as fractional anisotropy (FA) and mean diffusivity (MD) are used to quantitate white matter integrity, and DTI also enables tractography, the mapping of white matter pathways. Although some technical issues remain to be resolved with further study, DTI has powerfully expanded white matter neuroimaging by moving past the macrostructural lesions seen on CT and conventional MRI to the microstructure of myelin and axons. **Box 2** lists several prominent syndromes that have often been observed in patients with disorders that prominently affect the cerebral white matter. While not exhaustive, this list highlights the range of psychiatric syndromes that may occur in patients with white matter disorders, and suggests that myelinated tracts play an important role in the organization of emotion. Selected examples of specific disorders that illustrate key points are discussed.

Depression

Among all the white matter disorders, depression appears to be the most common psychiatric syndrome.[2] MS, systemic lupus erythematosus (SLE), and TBI are known to be strongly associated with depression, and in older people with leukoaraoisis (LA) on CT or MRI, depression is increasingly appreciated.[2,63–65] Ischemic white matter disease contributes directly to depression in older people,[63] whether visible as LA[64]

Box 2
Psychiatric syndromes in white matter disorders

Depression

Mania

Psychosis

Disinhibition

Euphoria

Pathologic laughter and crying

Apathy

or detectable as altered white matter integrity on DTI.[65] Thus depression can occur earlier in life with white matter involvement from a range of insults, but may be particularly common in old age when cerebrovascular disease is superimposed on white matter already undergoing age-related changes.[28] The presence of LA implies a more refractory form of depression with a less favorable outcome, and considerable evidence suggests the possibility that white matter ischemia may predispose to AD as well as play a role in depression.[5,63]

Mania

Neurologic diseases can produce manic behavior, a phenomenon known as secondary mania.[66] A range of disorders have been associated with secondary mania, including stroke, MS, neurosyphilis, Creutzfeldt-Jakob disease, postinfectious demyelination, SLE, TBI, benign and malignant neoplasms, and frontotemporal dementia,[66] and many affected patients have lesions specifically involving cerebral white matter.[2] A common localization for focal lesions associated with secondary mania is within the right anterior temporal and orbitofrontal regions, and selective white matter involvement of these areas has been reported.[67,68]

Psychosis

A variety of white matter disorders have been observed to produce schizophrenia-like psychosis.[69] The leukodystrophies are the best studied of this group, in particular metachromatic leukodystrophy (MLD), in which psychosis regularly precedes dementia in late-onset cases.[69-71] Demyelinative disorders including MS, SLE, and white matter tumors including astrocytoma and oligodendroglioma may also present with psychosis.[12,40,69,70] Schizophrenia-like psychosis appears most likely to develop, however, in individuals with diseases disrupting the formation of normal myelin, often termed dysmyelinative diseases.[69] The location of white matter neuropathology producing psychosis is typically in the frontal and temporal regions.[12,40,69,70]

Disinhibition

The erosion of comportment can be a devastating neurobehavioral disorder with a host of medical, psychiatric, social, and legal consequences.[72] The clinical descriptor for this condition is disinhibition, and orbitofrontal involvement is typical in these cases.[72] A tendency for disinhibition to be particularly associated with right anterior cerebral lesions has been noted,[73] and both gray and white matter may be implicated. Although qualitatively distinct, disinhibition nevertheless has much in common with mania, and the shared cerebral localization of these syndromes likely reflects a similar pathogenesis. Neuropathology from dysmyelination, stroke, TBI, or a neoplasm involving white matter of the orbitofrontal regions is often responsible for disinhibition.[2]

Euphoria

Persistent cheerfulness in the absence of the motor overactivity typical of mania has been termed euphoria, and this striking syndrome has been classically observed in MS patients, of whom about 10% are affected.[74] Euphoria in MS is strongly associated with cognitive decline and widespread white matter disease burden, and is thought to reflect primarily frontal lobe demyelination.[74] Loss of insight and impaired judgment are prominent neurobehavioral deficits contributing to euphoria.

Pathologic Laughter and Crying

This syndrome, often called pseudobulbar affect and sometimes emotional lability or emotional incontinence, refers to episodic laughter or crying that is inconsistent with the clinical context and without commensurate feelings.[75] Classically considered the result of corticobulbar tract involvement, recent localization analysis has found basis pontis lesions to be most closely associated with the syndrome, with internal capsule and cerebral peduncle lesions also implicated in many cases.[75] As pathologic laughter and crying is common in patients with cerebrovascular disease, MS, and TBI, all of which feature long tract involvement, the importance of white matter disruption in this syndrome seems clear.

Apathy

The amotivational state of apathy can be distinguished from the mood disorder of depression, and apathy is typical of many patients with medial frontal involvement, particularly in the region of the anterior cingulate gyrus.[76] Focal white matter lesions in this area can produce apathy,[2] as can diffuse white matter changes from disorders such as the toxic leukoencephalopathies.[36,53–58] Apathy is also prominent with white matter changes in dementias of older people, as demonstrated in a study of patients with AD, vascular dementia, and mild cognitive impairment.[77] Apathy in the setting of white matter changes is closely related to the cognitive slowing that occurs as part of the profile of white matter dementia.[2,6,19,31]

PSYCHIATRIC DISEASES WITH WHITE MATTER ABNORMALITIES

The etiology and pathogenesis of several major psychiatric diseases remain poorly understood despite advances in treatment over the last half century. Standard neuro-pathological investigation has been applied with little success to the investigation of schizophrenia, depression, and other debilitating psychiatric illnesses. In recent years, largely stimulated by advances in structural and functional neuroimaging, the study of psychiatric diseases has focused more on putative network dysfunction and away from lesion-based models of pathogenesis. This emphasis has naturally implicated the cerebral white matter as a tissue of much interest regarding disconnection of neural networks subserving normal emotion. This altered connectivity can be generally estimated with CT and MRI when LA or lacunar stroke damages the macrostructure of white matter, but detection of microstructural changes, implying less obvious neuro-pathology in myelin and glial cells, requires more sensitive technologies. Among newer structural neuroimaging methods, which include magnetic resonance spectroscopy and magnetization transfer imaging, DTI has been most often applied to the micro-structure of white matter,[78] and is most useful in direct investigation of white matter tracts in idiopathic psychiatric disorders beyond the resolution of conventional neuro-imaging. A list of common psychiatric diseases being investigated for the potential contribution of white matter neuropathology is shown in **Box 3**.

Schizophrenia

Schizophrenia continues to perplex neuroscientists because of a paucity of distinctive neuropathological findings, despite much evidence that the disease has a neurobio-logical basis.[10,14,79] Whereas gray matter changes have been found that are consis-tent with synaptic pathology, functional imaging data suggest a more diffuse disorder of frontal and temporal neural networks,[79] and the strong association of neurologic white matter disorders and psychosis[69] had led investigators to focus on white matter in the investigation of schizophrenia.[8] Structural brain imaging with conventional MRI has been conducted, with many studies showing white matter volume reduction in the frontal lobes and corpus callosum, although concurrent changes in gray matter are evident.[8,14] Reduced numbers of oligodendrocytes in white

Box 3
Psychiatric diseases with white matter abnormalities
Schizophrenia
Depression
Bipolar disorder
Obsessive-compulsive disorder
Posttraumatic stress disorder
Autism
Attention deficit/hyperactivity disorder (ADHD)

matter have also been observed.[8] DTI has been pursued and, in general, abnormalities have been found in frontal and temporal lobe white matter and the corpus callosum[78]; the most often reported measure is FA, which is decreased in most but not all studies of cerebral white matter in schizophrenia.[8] Down-regulation of oligodendrocyte and myelin genes has also been noted, although it is unclear whether these genes are susceptibility genes or only represent epiphenomena of a more pervasive neurodevelopmental process that may also lead to mood disorders.[8]

Depression

Whereas schizophrenia has been called the graveyard of neuropathology, the mood disorders, including depression and bipolar disorder, have been likened to an uncharted wilderness.[80] However, neuropathological and neuroimaging evidence is accumulating to suggest the occurrence of gray and white matter abnormalities, microscopic and macroscopic, in the mood disorders.[80] The microscopic neuropathology of depression is most evident in frontal cortices, where abnormalities of synapses and glial cells are found, and the neuropathology of white matter has not been as revealing.[80] However, the impact of vascular white matter disease seen on neuroimaging has garnered much attention, particularly in view of the frequent observation that depression is accompanied by cognitive loss that may also be caused by these macroscopic lesions. The consistent association of depression with LA in older people has been described,[2,63–65] leading to the concept of vascular depression,[64] although a genetic contribution to late-onset depression also has support. Longitudinal study of older people without cerebrovascular disease using conventional MRI has disclosed an association between depressive symptoms and left frontal white matter volume loss, but this study could not determine whether the white matter changes were a cause or a result of depressive symptoms.[81] DTI is also being explored for evidence of microscopic white matter changes, and a majority of studies of affective disorder, conducted in childhood through old age, have found reduced anisotropy in the frontal and temporal white matter.[78,82]

Bipolar Disorder

Bipolar disorder has been found to feature neuropathological findings in the cerebral cortex similar to those of depression, but white matter has not been subjected to such detailed study.[80] As in depression, however, a strong association of LA, commonly in the frontal lobes, with bipolar disorder has been observed using conventional MRI, suggesting the concept of vascular mania.[83] A genetic contribution to bipolar disorder also has considerable support; similar to recent findings in schizophrenia, reduced numbers of oligodendrocytes and decreased white matter volume have been found, and genetic evidence exists for altered expression of oligodendrocyte and myelin genes in bipolar disorder.[83] Moreover, white but not gray matter volume reduction has been observed in first-episode bipolar disorder patients.[84] DTI has also been employed to probe microscopic white matter neuropathology in bipolar disorder, and available information suggests abnormalities in the frontal lobes.[78]

Obsessive-Compulsive Disorder

This form of anxiety disorder has recently been viewed as involving a disturbance of frontal-subcortical circuits, including areas of the frontal cortices, basal ganglia (most notably the caudate), and the thalamus. White matter tracts within this circuit have attracted attention, as they establish the connectivity of the various component regions. While conventional MRI studies have found areas of gray matter volume loss in frontal cortical regions, bilaterally decreased prefrontal white matter volume has also been noted.[85] DTI studies of this disorder have been conducted, and changes have been found in the cingulum.[78,86]

Posttraumatic Stress Disorder

Posttraumatic stress disorder is an anxiety disorder receiving renewed attention in the United States as current military conflicts have produced many more affected individuals. The most compelling recent evidence for brain abnormalities exists for changes in the amygdala and hippocampus, limbic structures for which evidence has been gathered to suggest that severe stress may produce structural damage leading to a range of anxiety disorders.[87,88] However, white matter changes have also been noted in this condition, as in a recent DTI study reporting that frontal and limbic tracts are primarily affected.[89] Consistent with the theme of network disconnection, microstructural white matter abnormalities may occur in networks dedicated to the regulation of anxiety that include medial temporal gray matter structures, the frontal lobes, and associated white matter tracts.[89]

Autism

While a substantially increased prevalence of autism has been observed in recent years, its neurobiology remains obscure. In contrast to schizophrenia, which is often shown to manifest reduced white matter, autism has been noted in most studies to display an increase in white matter volume, with a concomitant increase in head size.[90–92] The frontal lobes may show the largest expansion of white matter, but temporal and parietal lobe expansion has also been reported. DTI studies generally show white matter abnormalities in frontal, temporal, and parietal white matter as well as the corpus callosum.[78] The pathogenesis of autism has been speculated to involve altered connectivity that interferes with the processing of complex information requiring multiple neural networks.[91] Whereas white matter changes have been frequently detected, autism often involves clinical features suggesting cortical involvement such as language impairment and seizures, and indeed, abnormal synaptic function in the cortex may occur in parallel with white matter changes.[91]

Attention Deficit/Hyperactivity Disorder

This disorder has long defied understanding despite the availability of effective medications, suggesting a neurobiological pathogenesis. Recent structural and functional neuroimaging studies have led to the hypothesis that white matter neuropathology may result in disrupted connectivity in distributed networks underlying attention and working memory.[93] Conventional MRI has shown a reduction in white matter volume compared with controls.[94] DTI studies have shown alterations in frontal-parietal networks subserving attention and executive function, either bilaterally distributed[95] or more prominent on the right.[96] These frontal-parietal white matter changes suggest delayed brain maturation of networks that should be developing normally, and it is noteworthy that adults with a history of childhood ADHD may show an increase of white matter volume that could represent a compensatory response to reduced neural network efficiency.[93]

DISCUSSION

The evidence from both the neurologic and psychiatric disorders reviewed here strongly suggests that white matter plays a major role in cognitive and emotional function. Disruption of myelinated systems in the brain can produce white matter dementia, and may help explain a range of puzzling neuropsychiatric disorders. Implicit in these observations is the notion of multiple neural network disturbance, meaning that the clinical phenomenology of these complex disorders has its basis in widespread cerebral dysfunction that simultaneously compromises several neurobehavioral domains. By contrast, the classic disconnection syndromes of behavioral neurology can be more securely localized to one network because a solitary lesion disrupts a specific cognitive domain. Thus, the many deficits of white matter dementia and idiopathic psychiatric diseases such as schizophrenia, depression, and autism—involving many aspects of behavior including cognitive speed, attention, executive function, social cognition, comportment, memory, motivation, and mood—imply dysfunction of multiple networks, whereas a classic disconnection syndrome such as conduction aphasia, for example, indicates a single lesion isolated within the language network.

With this background, white matter dysfunction clearly merits continued attention as a potential source of cognitive loss and neuropsychiatric illness. For this assertion to have any meaning, however, an appreciation of how tract dysfunction interrupts neural network function is necessary. As white matter is organized to transmit information efficiently between gray matter regions, impaired axonal transmission is a key concept.[2,4,7] The slowing of conduction velocity produced by white matter dysfunction may lead to asynchronous, temporally degraded integration of interdependent cerebral regions devoted to the generation and regulation of cognitive and emotional operations.[2,4,7] Thus the efficient, highly regulated interplay of cerebral regions critically devoted to cognitive and interpersonal relationships may be compromised, and white matter dementia or a variety of neuropsychiatric disorders may result. Myelin damage by itself can cause significant neurobehavioral disturbance, and axonal injury typically worsens the outcome[97]; in cases such as advanced MLD, progressive MS, severe Binswanger disease, or TBI with extensive diffuse axonal injury, transmission of action potentials may be completely lost, leading to more profound clinical deterioration that reflects damage to the specific networks involved.[2,19,31]

Although white matter dementia and neuropsychiatric disorders related to white matter dysfunction are too multifaceted to be localized to one tract, system, or neural network, the principle of localization still applies in this context. The clinical profile of white matter dementia, with prominent cognitive slowing, executive dysfunction, impaired sustained attention, and memory retrieval deficits, clearly implicates networks in which the frontal lobes are engaged.[2] When structural lesions produce neuropsychiatric dysfunction, both frontal and temporal lobe systems are most likely to be implicated, a generalization consistent with much clinical experience.[10–12] Taken together, these observations lead to the conclusion that tracts providing bilateral frontal and temporal lobe connectivity are crucial to the organization and maintenance of the normal human behavioral repertoire. While much remains to be learned about the neural networks mediating cognition and emotion, the frontal lobes, exerting their supervisory capacity with respect to all behavior, and the temporal lobes with their prominent limbic connections, are centrally involved. These networks depend heavily on white matter, which is highly developed in humans,[30] and most abundant in the anterior cerebrum.[2,28] The importance of white matter is further highlighted by its volumetric expansion in early life when idiopathic psychiatric disorders are most likely to present,[2,9] and its decline in late life when dementia is most prevalent.[2,27]

The further investigation of white matter may therefore yield benefits not only for patients with neurologic white matter disorders that alter cognitive and emotional function but also for many others who have primary psychiatric disease in which white matter neuropathology may be critical. Many questions stem from these ideas. An important theoretical issue is the characterization of distributed neural networks within which these syndromes are postulated to develop,[2,25,76] as more clarity is needed in defining brain regions underlying complex cognitive and emotional functions. Specific clinical questions also arise. For example, in neurologic disorders of white matter, will conventional treatment strategies such as corticosteroids or immunomodulatory treatment for MS suffice for neurobehavioral dysfunction, or are additional interventions needed? In psychiatric diseases, are white matter findings of primary pathogenic significance or only secondary to gray matter dysfunction, or is there a combined pathogenesis that disrupts both white and gray matter components of distributed neural networks? If white matter neuropathology is primary, what is the relative importance of genetic and environmental factors in etiology? And what new treatments can be devised based on the emerging understanding of white matter dysfunction? Evidence in treatment-resistant depression showing the efficacy of deep brain stimulation in the white matter adjacent to the subgenual cingulate gyrus[98] suggests that the treatment as well as pathogenesis of neuropsychiatric illness may be revealed by considering white matter.

For neuroscientists, the study of white matter continues to offer a fertile research area with the potential to add much to our understanding of brain-behavior relationships. With the emphasis in recent decades on the prominence of distributed neural networks, white matter assumes an increasingly crucial position in formulations of how the brain mediates cognitive and emotional function. Comparable to the human genome, the connectome is a recently proposed concept to designate a comprehensive structural description of the connections forming the human brain, and white matter plays a central role in the nascent study of connectomics.[99–102] This initiative, now supported by public research funding to help develop of a freely available database, will be facilitated by neuroinformatics as details of connectionist neuroanatomy are elaborated in both white and gray matter with the use of structural and functional neuroimaging. Concomitantly, the investigation of potential network causes of brain disorders affecting cognition and emotion may lead to many clinical advances.[99–102]

Much as the study of focal cerebral disconnection syndromes was invigorated 45 years ago,[1] behavioral neurology and neuropsychiatry have now begun to benefit from a consideration of widespread white matter disconnection in distributed neural networks devoted to cognition and emotion. From this approach, which has implications for a host of problematic disorders, significant new understanding of the cerebral basis of cognition, emotion, and their disturbances now seems likely.

REFERENCES

1. Geschwind N. Disconnexion syndromes in animals and man. Brain 1965;88: 237–94, 585–644.
2. Filley CM. The behavioral neurology of white matter. New York: Oxford University Press; 2001.

3. Catani M, ffytche DH. The rises and falls of disconnection syndromes. Brain 2005;128:2224–39.
4. Fields RD. White matter in learning, cognition, and psychiatric disorders. Trends Neurosci 2008;31:361–70.
5. Bartzokis G. Alzheimer's disease as homeostatic responses to age-related myelin breakdown. Neurobiol Aging 2009. [Epub ahead of print].
6. Filley CM, Franklin GM, Heaton RK, et al. White matter dementia. Clinical disorders and implications. Neuropsychiatry Neuropsychol Behav Neurol 1988;1:239–54.
7. Kumar A, Cook IA. White matter injury, neural connectivity and the pathophysiology of psychiatric disorders. Dev Neurosci 2002;24:255–61.
8. Walterfang M, Wood SJ, Velakoulis D, et al. Neuropathological, neurogenetic and neuroimaging evidence for white matter pathology in schizophrenia. Neurosci Biobehav Rev 2006;30:918–48.
9. Bartzokis G. Brain myelination in prevalent neuropsychiatric developmental disorders: primary and comorbid addiction. Adolesc Psychiatry 2005;29:55–96.
10. Post RM. Neural substrates of psychiatric syndromes. In: Mesulam M-M, editor. Principles of behavioral and cognitive neurology. 2nd edition. New York: Oxford University Press; 2000. p. 406–38.
11. Davison K. Schizophrenia-like psychoses associated with organic cerebral disorders: a review. Psychiatr Dev 1983;1:1–33.
12. Filley CM, Kleinschmidt-DeMasters BK. Neurobehavioral presentations of brain neoplasms. West J Med 1995;163:19–25.
13. Filley CM. The behavioral neurology of cerebral white matter. Neurology 1998; 50:1535–40.
14. Pearlson GD. Neurobiology of schizophrenia. Ann Neurol 2000;48:556–66.
15. Miller AK, Alston RL, Corsellis JAN. Variation with age in the volumes of grey and white matter in the cerebral hemispheres of man: measurements with an image analyzer. Neuropathol Appl Neurobiol 1980;6:119–32.
16. Saver JL. Time is brain-quantified. Stroke 2006;37:263–6.
17. Nolte J. The human brain. 5th edition. St Louis (MO): Mosby; 2002.
18. Aralasmak A, Ulmer JL, Kocak M, et al. Association, commissural, and projection pathways and their functional deficit reported in literature. J Comput Assist Tomogr 2006;30:695–715.
19. Filley CM. White matter: organization and functional relevance. Neuropsychol Rev 2010;20:158–73.
20. Schmahmann JD, Pandya DN. Fiber pathways of the brain. New York: Oxford University Press; 2006.
21. Baumann N, Pham-Dinh D. Biology of oligodendrocyte and myelin in the mammalian nervous system. Physiol Rev 2001;81:871–927.
22. Bennaroch EF. Oligodendrocytes. Susceptibility to injury and involvement in neurologic disease. Neurology 2009;72:1779–85.
23. Turken AU, Whitfield-Gabrieli S, Bammer R, et al. Cognitive speed and the structure of white matter pathways: convergent evidence from normal variation and lesion studies. Neuroimage 2008;42:1032–44.
24. Kochunov P, Coyle T, Lancaster J, et al. Processing speed is correlated with cerebral health markers in the frontal lobes quantified by neuroimaging. Neuroimage 2010;49:1190–9.
25. Mesulam M-M. Large-scale neurocognitive networks and distributed processing for attention, language, and memory. Ann Neurol 1990;28:597–613.
26. Filley CM. White matter and behavioral neurology. Ann N Y Acad Sci 2005;1064: 162–83.

27. Bartzokis G, Beckson M, Lu PH, et al. Age-related changes in frontal and temporal lobe volumes in men. Arch Gen Psychiatry 2001;58:461–5.

28. Sullivan EV, Pfefferbaum A. Diffusion tensor imaging and aging. Neurosci Biobehav Rev 2006;30:749–61.

29. Schoenemann PT, Sheehan MJ, Glotzer LD. Prefrontal white matter is disproportionately larger in humans than in other primates. Nat Neurosci 2005;8:242–52.

30. Picard-Riera N, Nait-Oumesmar B, Baron-Van Evercooren A. Endogenous adult neural stem cells: limits and potential to repair the injured central nervous system. J Neurosci Res 2004;76:223–31.

31. Schmahmann JD, Smith ED, Eichler FS, et al. Cerebral white matter. Neuroanatomy, clinical neurology, and neurobehavioral correlates. Ann N Y Acad Sci 2008;1142:266–309.

32. Shapiro EG, Lockman LA, Knopman D, et al. Characteristics of the dementia in late-onset metachromatic leukodystrophy. Neurology 1994;44:662–5.

33. Rao SM, Leo G, Bernardin L, et al. Cogntive dysfunction in multiple sclerosis. I. Frequency, patterns, and prediction. Neurology 1991;42:685–91.

34. Paul RH, Laidlaw DH, Tate DF, et al. Neuropsychological and neuroimaging outcome of HIV-associated progressive multifocal leukoencephalopathy in the era of antiretroviral therapy. J Integr Neurosci 2007;6:191–203.

35. Kozora E, Hanly JG, Lapteva L, et al. Cognitive dysfunction in systemic lupus erythematosus: past, present, and future. Arthritis Rheum 2008;58:3286–98.

36. Filley CM, Halliday W, Kleinschmidt-DeMasters BK. The effects of toluene on the central nervous system. J Neuropathol Exp Neurol 2004;63:1–12.

37. Chatterjee A, Yapundich R, Palmer CA, et al. Leukoencephalopathy associated with cobalamin deficiency. Neurology 1996;46:832–4.

38. Caplan LR. Binswanger's disease—revisited. Neurology 1995;45:626–33.

39. Alexander MP. Mild traumatic brain injury: pathophysiology, natural history, and clinical management. Neurology 1995;45:1253–60.

40. Filley CM, Kleinschmidt-DeMasters BK, Lillehei KO, et al. Gliomatosis cerebri: neurobehavioral and neuropathological observations. Cogn Behav Neurol 2003;16:149–59.

41. Shprecher D, Schwalb J, Kurlan R. Normal pressure hydrocephalus: diagnosis and treatment. Curr Neurol Neurosci Rep 2008;8:371–6.

42. Folstein MF, Folstein SE, McHugh PR. "Mini-mental state". A practical method for grading the cognitive state of patients for the clinician. J Psychiatr Res 1975;12:189–98.

43. Kurtzke JF. Neurologic impairment in multiple sclerosis and the Disability Status Scale. Acta Neurol Scand 1970;46:493–512.

44. Boerner RJ, Kapfhammer HP. Psychopathological changes and cognitive impairment in encephalomyelitis disseminata. Eur Arch Psychiatry Clin Neurosci 1999;249:96–102.

45. Whitehouse PJ. The concept of cortical and subcortical dementia: another look. Ann Neurol 1986;19:1–6.

46. Filley CM, Heaton RK, Nelson LM, et al. A comparison of dementia in Alzheimer's disease and multiple sclerosis. Arch Neurol 1989;46:157–61.

47. Tranchant C, Bhatia KP, Marsden CD. Movement disorders in multiple sclerosis. Mov Disord 1995;10:418–23.

48. Ozturk V, Idiman E, Sengun IS, et al. Multiple sclerosis and parkinsonism: a case report. Funct Neurol 2002;17:145–7.

49. Knopman D, Nissen MJ. Procedural learning is impaired in Huntington's disease: evidence from the serial reaction time task. Neuropsychologia 1991; 29:245–54.

50. Gabrieli JD, Stebbins GT, Singh J, et al. Intact mirror-tracing and impaired rotary-pursuit skill learning in patients with Huntington's disease: evidence for dissociable memory systems in skill learning. Neuropsychology 1997;11: 272–81.
51. Lafosse JM, Corboy JR, Leehey MA, et al. MS vs. HD: can white matter and subcortical gray matter pathology be distinguished neuropsychologically? J Clin Exp Neuropsychol 2007;29:142–54.
52. Dujardin K, Laurent B. Dysfunction of the human memory systems: role of the dopaminergic transmission. Curr Opin Neurol 2003;16(Suppl 2):S11–6.
53. Filley CM, Kleinschmidt-DeMasters BK. Toxic leukoencephalopathy. N Engl J Med 2001;345:425–32.
54. Hormes JT, Filley CM, Rosenberg NL. Neurologic sequelae of chronic solvent vapor abuse. Neurology 1986;36:698–702.
55. Rosenberg NL, Spitz MC, Filley CM, et al. Central nervous system effects of chronic toluene abuse – clinical, brainstem evoked response and magnetic resonance imaging studies. Neurotoxicol Teratol 1988;10:489–95.
56. Filley CM, Heaton RK, Rosenberg NL. White matter dementia in chronic toluene abuse. Neurology 1990;40:532–4.
57. Rosenberg NK, Kleinschmidt-DeMasters BK, Davis KA, et al. Toluene abuse causes diffuse central nervous system white matter changes. Ann Neurol 1988;23:611–4.
58. Yücel M, Takagi M, Walterfang M, et al. Toluene misuse and long-term harms: a systematic review of the neuropsychological and neuroimaging literature. Neurosci Biobehav Rev 2008;32:910–26.
59. Mendez MF, Perryman KM, Bornstein YL. White matter dementias: neurobehavioral aspects and etiology. J Neuropsychiatry Clin Neurosci 2000;12:133.
60. Gennarelli TA, Thibault LE, Adams JH, et al. Diffuse axonal injury and traumatic coma in the primate. Ann Neurol 1982;12:564–74.
61. Shibata M, Yamasaki N, Miyakawa T, et al. Selective impairment of working memory in a mouse model of chronic cerebral hypoperfusion. Stroke 2007;38: 2826–32.
62. Basser PJ, Jones DK. Diffusion-tensor MRI: theory, experimental design and data analysis-technical review. NMR Biomed 2002;15:457–67.
63. Thomas AJ, O'Brien JT. Depression and cognition in older adults. Curr Opin Psychiatry 2008;21:8–13.
64. Herrmann LL, Le Masurier M, Ebmeier KP. White matter hyperintensities in late life depression: a systematic review. J Neurol Neurosurg Psychiatry 2008;79: 619–24.
65. Lamar M, Charlton RA, Morris RG, et al. The impact of subcortical white matter disease on mood in euthymic older adults: a diffusion tensor imaging Study. Am J Geriatr Psychiatry 2010;18:634–42.
66. Mendez MF. Mania in neurologic disorders. Curr Psychiatry Rep 2000;2:440–5.
67. Starkstein SE, Boston JD, Robinson RG. Mechanisms of mania after brain injury. 12 case reports and review of the literature. J Nerv Ment Dis 1988;176:87–100.
68. Paskavitz JF, Anderson CA, Filley CM, et al. Acute arcuate fiber demyelinating encephalopathy following Epstein-Barr virus infection. Ann Neurol 1995;38: 127–31.
69. Walterfang M, Wood SJ, Velakoulis D, et al. Diseases of white matter and schizophrenia-like psychosis. Aust N Z J Psychiatry 2005;39:746–56.
70. Filley CM, Gross KF. Psychosis with cerebral white matter disease. Neuropsychiatry Neuropsychol Behav Neurol 1992;5:119–25.

71. Hyde TM, Ziegler JC, Weinberger DR. Psychiatric disturbances in metachromatic leukodystrophy. Insights into the neurobiology of psychosis. Arch Neurol 1992;49:401–6.
72. Mesulam M-M. Behavioral neuroanatomy: large-scale neural networks, association cortex, frontal syndromes, the limbic system, and hemispheric specializations. In: Principles of behavioral and cognitive neurology. 2nd edition. New York: Oxford University Press; 2000. p. 1–120.
73. Starkstein SE, Robinson RG. Mechanism of disinhibition after brain lesions. J Nerv Ment Dis 1997;185:108–14.
74. McDonald WI, Ron MA. Multiple sclerosis: the disease and its manifestations. Philos Trans R Soc Lond B Biol Sci 1999;354:1615–22.
75. Parvizi J, Coburn KL, Shillcutt SD, et al. Neuroanatomy of pathological laughing and crying: a report of the American Neuropsychiatric Association Committee on Research. J Neuropsychiatry Clin Neurosci 2009;21:75–87.
76. Cummings JL. Frontal-subcortical circuits and human behavior. Arch Neurol 1993;50:873–80.
77. Jonsson M, Edman A, Lind K, et al. Apathy is a prominent neuropsychiatric feature of radiological white-matter changes in patients with dementia. Int J Geriatr Psychiatry 2010;25:588–95.
78. White T, Nelson M, Lim KO. Diffusion tensor imaging in psychiatric disorders. Top Magn Reson Imaging 2008;19:97–109.
79. Harrison PJ. The neuropathology of schizophrenia. A critical review of the data and their interpretation. Brain 1999;122:593–624.
80. Harrison PJ. The neuropathology of primary mood disorder. Brain 2002;125:1428–49.
81. Dotson VM, Davitzikos C, Kraut MA, et al. Depressive symptoms and brain volumes in older adults: longitudinal magnetic resonance imaging study. J Psychiatry Neurosci 2009;34:367–75.
82. Sexton CE, Mackay CE, Ebmeier KP. A systematic study of diffusion tensor imaging in affective disorders. Biol Psychiatry 2009;66:814–23.
83. Mahon K, Burdick KE, Szeszko PR. A role for white matter abnormalities in the pathophysiology of bipolar disorder. Neurosci Biobehav Rev 2010;34:533–54.
84. Vita A, De Peri L, Sachetti E. Gray matter, white matter, brain, and intracranial volumes in first-episode bipolar disorder: a meta-analysis of magnetic resonance imaging studies. Bipolar Disord 2009;11:807–14.
85. van den Heuvel OA, Remijnse PL, Mataix-Cols D, et al. The major symptom dimensions of obsessive-compulsive disorder are mediated by partially distinct neural systems. Brain 2009;132:853–68.
86. Ha TH, Kang DH, Park JS, et al. White matter alterations in male patients with obsessive-compulsive disorder. Neuroreport 2009;20:735–9.
87. LeDoux J. The amygdala. Curr Biol 2007;17:R868–74.
88. Nemeroff CB, Bremner JD, Foa EB, et al. Posttraumatic stress disorder: a state-of-the-science review. J Psychiatr Res 2006;40:1–21.
89. Schuff N, Zhang Y, Zhan W, et al. Patterns of altered cortical perfusion and diminished subcortical integrity in posttraumatic stress disorder: a MRI Study. Neuroimage 2010. [Epub ahead of print].
90. Herbert MR, Ziegler DA, Makris N, et al. Localization of white matter volume increase in autism and developmental language disorder. Ann Neurol 2004;55:530–40.
91. Minshew NJ, Williams DL. The new neurobiology of autism: cortex, connectivity, and neuronal organization. Arch Neurol 2007;64:945–50.

92. Geschwind DH, Levitt P. Autism spectrum disorders: developmental disconnection syndromes. Curr Opin Neurobiol 2007;17:103–11.
93. Konrad K, Eickhoff SB. Is the ADHD brain wired differently? A review on structural and functional connectivity in attention deficit hyperactivity disorder. Hum Brain Mapp 2010;31:904–16.
94. Castellanos FX, Lee PP, Sharp W, et al. Developmental trajectories of brain volume abnormalities in children and adolescents with attention-deficit/hyperactivity disorder. JAMA 2002;288:1740–8.
95. Silk TJ, Vance A, Rinehart N, et al. White-matter abnormalities in attention deficit hyperactivity disorder: a diffusion tensor imaging study. Hum Brain Mapp 2009; 30:2757–65.
96. Makris N, Buka SL, Biederman J, et al. Attention and executive systems abnormalities in adults with childhood ADHD: a DT-MRI study of connections. Cereb Cortex 2008;18:1210–20.
97. Medana IM, Esiri MM. Axonal damage: a key predictor of outcome in human CNS diseases. Brain 2003;126:515–30.
98. Mayberg HS, Lozano AM, Voon V, et al. Deep brain stimulation for treatment-resistant depression. Neuron 2005;45:651–60.
99. Sporns O, Tononi G, Kötter R. The human connectome: a structural description of the human brain. PLoS Comput Biol 2005;1:e42.
100. Bohland JW, Wu C, Barbas H, et al. A proposal for a coordinated effort for the determination of brainwide neuroanatomical connectivity in model organisms at a mesoscopic scale. PLoS Comput Biol 2009;5:e1000334.
101. Williams R. The human connectome: just another 'ome? Lancet Neurol 2010;9: 238–9.
102. Kennedy DN. Making connections in the connectome era. Neuroinformatics 2010;8:61–2.

Affective Symptoms in Early-Onset Dementia

Kenneth Podell, PhD[a,b,*], Karen Torres, PsyD[c]

KEYWORDS

- Early-onset dementia • Chronic traumatic encephalopathy
- Neuropsychological deficits • Alzheimer disease • Depression
- Anxiety

Neuropsychology is a hybrid science that combines elements of psychology, neurology, and psychiatry, and that helps us improve our understanding of brain-behavior relationships. Clinical neuropsychology studies behavior, emotions, and cognitive abilities to understand the underlying (dysfunctional) neural systems involved, as well as better characterizing the disorder or disease state being studied. In essence, it takes the phenotypic expression and using other relevant data (test results and history, for example), and assists the health care provider determine an accurate diagnosis to guide treatment and other recommendations. Nowhere is this most relevant than in the differential diagnosis of psychiatric and neurologic diseases where common phenotypic expressions (ie, cognitive and emotional sequelae) can be the same but emanate from very different genotypes (or causes). For example, a common referral question could be to "rule out dementia versus pseudo-dementia" in an elderly patient with signs of depression. Here, the expression or phenotype of neuropsychological deficits of memory, organizational skills, and concentration is as easily related to depression[1] as the early stages of a neurodegenerative dementia such as Alzheimer disease (AD). Although complex and difficult to tease apart at times, it can be even more difficult in younger patients (ie, those in their 40s and 50s) when the likelihood of the neurologic disorder being present is statistically much lower than a psychiatric disorder. Moreover, these same psychiatric symptoms can be the harbinger of a neurodegenerative disorder. It is often at this stage where neuropsychological expertise can be most effective in differential diagnoses.

[a] Division of Neuropsychology, Henry Ford Health System, 1 Ford Place - 1E, Detroit , MI 48202, USA
[b] Department of Psychiatry and Behavioral Neurosciences, Wayne State University, Detroit, MI, USA
[c] Department of Psychiatry, Cambridge Health Alliance/Harvard Medical School, 1493 Cambridge Street, Cambridge, MA 02139, USA
* Corresponding author. Division of Neuropsychology, Henry Ford Health System, 1 Ford Place - 1E, Detroit, MI 48202.
E-mail address: KPODELL1@hfhs.org

Neurol Clin 29 (2011) 99–114
doi:10.1016/j.ncl.2010.10.009
0733-8619/11/$ – see front matter © 2011 Elsevier Inc. All rights reserved.

Any medical condition that affects central nervous system (CNS) function is a risk factor for developing a neurodegenerative dementia later in life. The more common and accepted disease states are diabetes, hypertension, sleep apnea, and hyperlipidemia.[2–5] However, recent evidence has implicated less obvious factors such as affective disorders (depression and anxiety) and even chronic stress as risk factors. In this article, we review some of the less common risk factors for dementia, such as stress, depression, and anxiety. A history of repetitive head injuries can be a risk factor for developing chronic traumatic encephalopathy (CTE) later in life.

STRESS AS A MARKER FOR HPA-AXIS DYSREGULATION

Stress has been widely shown by numerous studies to affect brain functioning deleteriously via disruption of the hypothalamus-pituitary-adrenal (HPA) axis.[6] The regulation of the HPA axis of the human body when confronted by stress-induced situations is pivotal in the known pathologic changes in the brain. The HPA-axis is the mediator in the most basic human physiologic reaction to stress. The main function of the HPA axis is to maintain homeostasis in the face of perceived threat. When stress is detected, the HPA axis secretes specific hormones (glucocorticoids: cortisol in humans and cortisone in rodents) that relay negative feedback back to the HPA axis. Chronic and repeated exposure to stress (eg, extended isolation, introduction of an intruder) alters the HPA axis' mechanism of maintaining homeostasis, which subsequently alters the structural integrity of the brain. Several in vivo animal models have investigated the effect of stress on cognitive functioning. Dong and colleagues[7] used a model of social isolation with mice to demonstrate that mice isolated for 6 months began to develop beta amyloid (A) plaque formation in the cortex and hippocampus with associated impaired memory functioning. Jeong and colleagues[8] found that confining mice to a stress box with restricted mobilization for an extended length of time (8 months) resulted in significant learning and memory deficits with associated increased extracellular amyloid plaque deposition, intraneuronal A, and neurodegeneration. A comprehensive review of recent experimental AD models by Rothman and Mattson[9] found that increased levels of glucocorticoids, released under conditions of chronic stress and activation of the HPA axis, are linked with impaired memory function and elevated endogenous cortisol levels in patients with AD; thus, suggesting that the dysregulation of the HPA axis may contribute to the development of AD.[10] Similarly, other research groups have supported that chronic stress is associated with a decreased number of synapses and dendritic spines in the hippocampus.[11]

DEPRESSION AS A RISK FACTOR FOR DEMENTIA

Major depression (MD) is a complex disease and is a major risk factor for developing dementia later in life. The morphologic changes associated with depression overlap and involve the same regions of interest involved in several neurodegenerative dementias. The hippocampus, amygdala, anterior cingulate, and regions of the prefrontal cortex[12] have all shown gross pathologic changes in major depressive disorder (MDD).[1] Moreover, recent research efforts on understanding the morphologic changes associated with MDD have indicated that volume in specific brain regions is related to illness duration and number of episodes. A recent meta-analysis of structural imaging demonstrated that MDD induces chronic and long-term morphologic changes of the hippocampus.[13] A systematic meta-analysis of 102,172 participants with and without a history of depression across 8 countries found that having a lifetime of depressive episodes increases the chance of developing AD later in life.[14] Other studies have found that depression is a risk factor rather than a prodromal symptom of AD[15] and an *early* onset of depressive symptoms is associated with developing AD more than depressive symptoms alone.[16] Furthermore, McKinnon and colleagues,[17] in an extensive meta-analytic review of studies that included 2000 subjects, found consistently smaller hippocampal volumes among patients who suffered from an MDD and in whom symptoms were present for longer than 2 years or who experienced more than one episode of MD. These findings were consistently found in children and middle-aged and elderly individuals. However, it was not found among young adults (posited by the authors to be attributable to the burden of illness, short chronicity of disease, and resilience of the brain at this age). The chronicity aspect of the pathologic changes is supported by recent studies showing that antidepressant treatments reversed the increase in the neurotoxic products in those patients in their first depressive episode but not in those suffering from chronic depression.[18] The support of antidepressant medications increasing hippocampal volume is less conclusive.[19] MDD's burden on the pathologic changes in the brain accounts for the demonstrated cognitive impairments. Hickie and colleagues[20] found a positive correlation between hippocampal volume reduction in patients with MD whose depression has been resistant to traditional treatment used by primary care providers and memory decrements compared with control groups after controlling for age. Brain alterations have also been attributed to increased hippocampal glucose metabolism,[21] higher levels of cortisol causing hippocampal apoptosis and neuronal death, and reduced brain-derived neurotrophic factor (BDNF) and subsequent cognitive impairments in MDD.[22–24] In particular, several studies have found decreased BDNF levels in the hippocampus and prefrontal cortex of suicide victims[25] and in the hippocampus of chronically stressed animals.[26] Patients with severe MD evidence decreased frontal lobe volumes.[12] Patients with AD and MD show some similarity in HPA dysregulation. Studies have shown that individuals with AD exhibit chronically elevated cortisol and adrenocorticotropic hormone (ACTH) levels and marked higher levels of corticotrophin-releasing hormone (CRH) in the hypothalamic paraventricular nucleus (PVN) compared with healthy controls, which is a marker of HPA axis dysregulation[27] and rapid cognitive decline.[28] Stern's[29] notion of "cognitive reserve" may be adversely affected by the HPA axis dysregulation observed in MDD. Dysregulation affects cognitive reserve that ultimately limits the brain's ability to handle subsequent AD-related degeneration like the formation of neurofibrillary tangles and amyloid plaques.

ANXIETY'S IMPACT ON THE BRAIN

Recent work has highlighted the similarities between anxiety and dementia and more specifically the deleterious effects of anxiety on brain functioning. Tsolaki and colleagues,[30] in a study of 1271 Greek elders, found that those individuals who experienced a stressful event or situation (short- or long-lasting) of significant severity were subsequently at higher risk of being diagnosed with AD; thus, indicating that significant similarities exist between posttraumatic stress disorder (PTSD) and dementia: hippocampal vulnerability, initial symptoms of memory problems, and increased glucocorticoid levels. Similarly, individuals who suffer from PTSD without histories of alcohol abuse when compared with controls demonstrated hippocampal volume loss.[31] Bremner and colleagues[32] measured the hippocampal values in 26 Vietnam-era veterans with PTSD and compared them with matched (age and gender) healthy controls and found that the veterans had a significantly smaller (8%) right hippocampal volume, which was associated with short-term verbal memory deficits as measured with the Wechsler Memory Scale. An epidemiologic relationship exists between PTSD or experiencing traumatic events and the development of dementia. A recent study by Qureshi and colleagues,[33] including 10,481 veterans, found a higher prevalence and incidence of dementia among veterans with a history of PTSD. These veterans were twice as likely to develop the neurodegenerative disorder in comparison with their counterparts without diagnosable PTSD. This study hypothesized that the cognitive changes associated with PTSD may be an early marker of dementia or the cognitive changes associated with PTSD may place veterans at an increased risk for developing dementia.

CHRONIC TRAUMATIC ENCEPHALOPATHY

CTE, although first recognized in 1928,[34] has regained prominence in the public media through some high-profile suicides in retired National Football League athletes and more rigorous research by the prominent neuropathologists Ann McKee and Bennet Omalu. Although the research characterizing the neuropathologic changes, clinical syndrome, and causes is still in its infancy, the findings have been very robust and consistent and have clearly demarcated a progressive, yet distinct tauopathy with a unique clinical syndrome and a clear environmental component of repetitive concussive and subconcussive events. The clinical syndrome, often not evident until years after the onset, sometimes even decades after retirement, is progressive, and can last for several decades.[35] Its prevalence, time to expression, and factors causing its expression are still being studied and at this point only hypothesized.

The clinical syndrome of CTE (also known as punch-drunk syndrome, dementia pugilistica, and chronic traumatic brain injury) has 3 distinct symptom patterns: psychiatric, motor, and cognitive. Psychiatric symptoms (prominent in about one-third of the cases) include an acute onset of depressive symptoms (unrelated to any prior psychiatric history), emotional lability with erratic and unpredictable behavior, irritability, violent outbursts, paranoia, disinhibition, apathy, and substance abuse. Jordan[36] noted that the behavioral manifestations of CTE are difficult to assess in the initial phases of the disease if the premorbid personality traits are unknown. Progressive parkinsonism, although typically not an early component of the syndrome, eventually presents in about 40% of confirmed cases. The more common parkinsonian features include slow, shuffling gait, possible dysarthria and dysphagia, imbalance, rigidity, ataxia, and ocular-motor problems. Impairments in attention/concentration, memory, and executive control deficits characterize the cognitive deficits in CTE.[35,37] The clinical challenge is distinguishing the aberrant patterns of behaviors related directly to psychiatric/substance abuse disorders from similar behaviors known to be among the earliest, and more functionally impairing symptoms of CTE.

The neuropathologic changes of CTE are characterized by cerebral and medial temporal lobe atrophy, ventriculomegaly, enlarged cavum septum pellucidum, and extensive tau-immunoreactive pathology throughout the neocortex, medial temporal lobe, diencephalon, brainstem, and spinal cord. McKee astutely noted in a retrospective review of 45 cases plus 3 of her own, that the extensive pathologic changes in the limbic region linked pathologic changes in "the amygdalohippocampal-septo-hypothalamic-mesencephalic continuum" and orbito-frontal cortex to the early and often significant behavioral changes in CTE. Moreover, CTE shares pathologic features with AD, including tau-immunoreactive neurofibrillary tangles, and in approximately 40% of cases, diffuse β-amyloid plaques that are immunocytochemically identical to those found in AD, linking a common pathogenesis between CTE and AD, although the pattern of distribution is different. It may be that CTE interacts additively or synergistically with AD (similar to cerebrovascular changes in AD) causing an even greater burden on the brain manifesting in an earlier onset and more severe dementia.[35] In fact, Mann and colleagues,[38] using morphologic analysis of senile plaques, found that tau deposits provoked by repetitive blows to the head accelerates Aβ toxicity that is responsible for the earlier onset of dementia. We would like to point out that the clinical presentation, pathophysiology, causes (other than trauma), and prognosis for CTE are not well understood. All of the evidence to date has been through single cases or small group studies without formal control groups or longitudinal studies used. Thus, inferences made must be considered preliminary, although compelling and highly relevant, until better controlled studies are performed. However, it would seem reasonable to say that repetitive head trauma is a risk factor for developing dementia later in life.

IDENTIFYING THE PRODROMAL SYMPTOMS OF NEURODEGENERATIVE VERSUS PSYCHIATRIC DISORDERS

Identifying the early markers of psychiatric and neurodegenerative disorders, and distinguishing between them, is key in guiding the early and appropriate treatment of these disorders in their prodromal or early stages.[39] The use of cognitive screening measures, such as the Mini Mental State Examination (MMSE),[40] the Montreal Cognitive Assessment (MoCA),[41] and the Saint Louis University Mental Status Examination (SLUMS),[42] is common practice in assessing current cognitive functioning in medical settings. However, the sensitivity of the screening measures in general, and the MMSE in particular, has been questioned based on the observed false negative (eg, ceiling effects among the highly educated[43]) and false positive (eg, lower education and increased age can lead to an overestimation of cognitive impairment[44,45]) identifications. Recent studies have investigated the validity of screening measures other than the MMSE, given its lack of sensitivity. A study by Hoops and colleagues[46] found that the MoCA had greater sensitivity than the MMSE in detecting mild cognitive impairment (MCI) and dementia in patients with Parkinson disease. A pilot study by Tariq and colleagues[42] found that in a sample of 702 veterans, the SLUMS was a more sensitive measure in detecting mild neurocognitive disorder than the MMSE.

It is beyond the scope of this article to review all neurodegenerative dementias, but we review the more common cortical-based dementias of AD, frontotemporal dementia, and Lewy body dementia. Please see **Tables 1** and **2** for a summary of these findings.

Alzheimer's Dementia

The typical neuropsychological profile of AD consists of episodic memory impairments with associated language, semantic knowledge, executive functioning, and visuospatial deficits among the first cognitive problems noticed[47,48] without significant psychiatric manifestation other than mild depressive symptomatology. Often, others notice the cognitive deficits before the patient.

Lewy Body Dementia

Lewy body dementia (LBD) is distinguishable from the neuropsychological profile in AD in that LBD is primarily associated with fluctuating arousal, parasomnias, parkinsonism, autonomic dysfunction, and deficits in attention, visuospatial, and executive functioning (which some studies suggest may be one of the earliest deficits seen in LBDs). Depression is greater in LBD than in AD, at least in the earlier stages of the disease.[49] Recent research suggests that rapid eye movement (REM) sleep behaviors, even years or decades earlier, may be a prodromal characteristic of any of the α-synuclein dementias: Parkinson disease (PD), multiple system atrophy (MSA), and LBD.[50]

Table 1
Common characteristics and patterns of dementia types

Syndrome	Initial Complaints	Neuropsychological Profile	First to Notice Changes
Depression	Memory problems, poor focus	Fluctuating attention, slow learning curve, retrieval memory deficit with intact retention and recognition, fluctuating executive functioning, psychomotor slowing	Patient
Alzheimer's dementia	Repetition, forgetfulness, confusion	Slowly progressive anterograde memory deficit with poor learning, retention, and recognition; impaired naming; and semantic fluency and executive deficits, visuospatial processing deficits, and apraxia, aphasia and agnosia in advanced illness, functional decline	Patient/family
Lewy body dementia	Good & bad days, confusion, delusions, hallucinations, parasomnias	Progressive insidious cognitive decline with pronounced attentional fluctuations and executive deficits, marked visuoperceptual errors, retrieval memory deficit initially followed by poor retention, autonomic dysfunction and falls, motor skills marked by parkinsonism, vivid, detailed visual hallucinations	Patient/Family
Parkinson dementia	Poor initiation, slowed thinking, perceptual problems	Fluctuating attention, intact learning curve, retrieval memory deficit with poor retention and intact recognition, mildly impaired naming, slow processing speed, visuospatial processing and executive deficits, psychomotor slowing	Patient/Family

	Personality/Behavioral changes		Family
Frontotemporal dementia		Executive functioning deficits (perseveration, impulsivity, impaired planning, stimulus boundedness, mental flexibility, impaired synthesis), impaired selective attention, relatively preserved memory in earlier stages	Family
Chronic traumatic encephalopathy	Cognitive changes, personality changes, substance abuse, parkinsonism	Cognitive symptoms (often 1st) often include deficits in memory, attention/concentration & executive functioning are common early and often the first set of symptoms. Psychiatric symptoms and aberrant behaviors such as depression, irritability, aggressiveness, and substance abuse can occur early in the syndrome if not by the middle stages. Increased suicidal ideation, attempts, and successful deaths have been reported. Progressive parkinsonism in 40% of cases. Indistinguishable from Alzheimer disease and frontotemporal dementia in advanced stages.	Family/Patient

Table 2
Clinical manifestations of the dementias

Mood/Behavior	DEP: vegetative symptoms
	AD: depression, anxiety, apathy
	LBD/PD: depression > AD and may present before motor symptoms, apathy, impulsive/compulsive behavior from medication side effects in PD
	FTD: marked personality/behavior changes, unawareness, disinhibition, apathy, fixations and compulsions, emotional blunting, poor hygiene, impulsivity
	CTE: abrupt depressive symptoms with erratic behavior and outbursts
Eating	DEP: increase or decrease appetite
	AD: preference for salt and sweet
	LBD and PD: difficulties swallowing in PD
	FTD: specific food preferences, overeating
	CTE: none known
Hallucinations/Delusions	DEP: can be present in severe cases
	AD: hallucinations and delusions in advanced illness
	LBD: visual hallucinations early (often people and animals)
	PD: visual hallucinations late or related to medication side effects
	FTD: rare
	CTE: not reported
Sleep	DEP: hypersomnia or insomnia
	AD: disrupted circadian rhythms
	LBD and PD: parasomnias
	FTD: disrupted circadian rhythms
	CTE: disrupted
Other	DEP: decreased libido, psychomotor retardation
	AD: motor skills mostly preserved, decreased smell/taste
	LBD: autonomic dysfunction, neuroleptic medication sensitivity, poor saccadic pursuit, bradyphrenia, bradykinesia cognitive difficulties develop before motor symptoms (within 1 year)
	PD: autonomic dysfunction in advanced illness, neuroleptic medication sensitivity, saccadic pursuit, cognitive difficulties develop at least 1 year *after* motor symptoms
	FTD: frontal release signs, slow eye movements, incontinence, increased interest in sex
	CTE: abrupt psychiatric onset (even without prior history), early substance abuse, possibly prone to suicide attempt, parkinsonism late

Abbreviations: AD, Alzheimer dementia; CTE, chronic traumatic encephalopathy; DEP, depression; FTD, frontotemporal dementia; LBD, Lewy body dementia; PD, Parkinson disease.

Frontotemporal Dementia

Frontotemporal dementia (FTD) can include behavioral (orbito-frontal lobe variant) and language-based (temporal lobe variant) symptoms.[51] The behavioral symptomatology in FTD presents first, before any neurocognitive deficits.[52] The range of behavioral changes include apathy, irritability, lack of insight, disinhibition, and loss of personal and social norms. From a neurologic standpoint, patients with FTD may demonstrate frontal release signs. The temporal lobe variant of FTD, although usually referred to as all-encompassing primary progressive aphasia (PPA), are parceled further into progressive nonfluent aphasia, semantic dementia, and logopenic progressive aphasia.[51] Early psychiatric manifestations or abrupt behavioral changes are uncommon in PPA. Although word-finding difficulties are usually associated with PPA in general, there are several key distinctions between the PPA subsets. Patients with progressive nonfluent aphasia may be dysarthric with hesitant speech patterns and spared word comprehension. Semantic dementia is associated with early deficits in naming and knowledge of word meanings. Last, logopenic progressive aphasia includes impaired naming, single word retrieval, repetition, and errors in speech sounds.

Chronic Traumatic Encephalopathy

In CTE, behavioral, motor, and cognitive symptoms present at different stages of the disease. However, a relatively consistent sequential pattern of changes appears to be emerging. Cognitive symptoms often include deficits in memory, attention/concentration, and executive functioning[53] and are common early and often the first set of symptoms. Psychiatric symptoms and aberrant behaviors such as depression, irritability, aggressiveness, and substance abuse can occur early in the syndrome, if not by the middle stages.[35] Increased suicidal ideation, and attempts and successful deaths have been reported with recent publicized cases. As CTE progresses, the diagnostic picture is similar to that of AD and FTD.[35]

Major Depressive Disorder

The neuropsychological profile of MDD must first be differentiated from what has been typically referred to as *pseudodementia*, which is reversible cognitive impairment seen among patients who suffer from an MDD that is psychiatrically based and not neurodegeneratively based.[54] MDD also has a more chronic and progressive pattern of cognitive deficits. MDD has consistently been associated with deficits in complex and sustained attention and executive functioning, whereas processing speed is implicated inconsistently. Anterograde memory deficits, although commonly cited in the literature, also has yielded mixed results. It appears that the learning aspect and not retention or recognition is the most likely impaired characteristic of anterograde memory in MDD.[1,55] Severe depressive symptomatology is the first symptom reported in MDD. There can be patient-initiated complaints of poor attention/concentration and anterograde memory problems that at first are secondary to the depressive symptoms, but over time show a waxing and waning paralleling the disease course with a progressive decline over time that is dependent on the chronicity and frequency of depressive episodes.[1] The neuropsychological profile of anxiety disorders typically consists of impairment in verbal episodic memory (learning) and executive functioning.[56]

We thought it would be useful to discuss differentiating between the behavioral expression of depression and patients with a dorso-lateral prefrontal (DPF) syndrome given the similarities in presentations, and in our opinion, the misinterpretation of the inertia in DPF syndrome as being a sign of depression. We have noted that at times referral sources have confused the two, calling a patient depressed when in fact, the patient was not depressed at all, but rather had a significant executive deficit associated with dorso-lateral prefrontal dysfunction.[57] Both depressed patients and patients with a DPF syndrome can have very similar phenotypic expression arising from very different genotypes or etiologies. However, there are very important and clear distinctions between the two that the clinician should be readily able to identify. Being able to distinguish between the two will obviously allow for more accurate diagnosis and treatment. Although both depressed patients and patients with DPF syndrome appear to have flat affect, close observation and some simple questioning can help distinguish between the two. One of the main distinctions is insight. Depressed patients have insight, are aware of their depression, and can verbalize it. Patients with DPF syndrome are typically unaware of their deficits or behavioral changes and do not verbalize symptoms of depression. In fact, they often deny having any problems and do not describe themselves as feeling sad, down, blue, irritable, or having loss of interest and enjoyment. Often the patient with a DPF syndrome will respond "Fine" when asked if they are sad or if anything is wrong. Although on the surface, both patients who are depressed and who have DPF syndrome similarly show poor motivation and lack initiation, a critical distinction can be found between them. Depressed patients display negative affect and verbalize their lack of motivation (have insight). For example, if asked to do or go somewhere, depressed patients use words and phrases such as, "I don't want to," "I don't care," or "I don't feel like it." In contrast, patients with DPF syndrome do not make such statements. Rather, when asked to do something they will agree to do it but may not initiate any activity (avolitional). Thus, one does not perceive any *negative* affect in patients with DPF syndrome. Rather, one observes the inertia and lack of initiation. It is precisely this lack of initiation and inertia that is mistaken for the depression. Patients with DPF syndrome can literally just sit and not initiate any activities, even basic needs such as eating (even when hungry) or going to the bathroom (in more severe cases). However, when told to eat, for example, and given instructions and prompts, will do so readily and eat heartily. Observationally, differences are readily discerned between patients with depression and DPF syndrome. Depressed patients look "sad," whereas patients with DPF syndrome tend to look vacuous or expressionless. Depressed patients can be restless or frigidity, whereas patients with DPF syndrome are motorically silent and inert. They tend to sit there without any signs of intent or purposeful activity. The neuropsychological profiles of patients with depression and DPF syndrome have numerous similarities in that both demonstrate executive control deficits. However, the executive deficit in patients with DPF syndrome can be qualitatively different. Often the executive deficit is more profound and pervasive across cognitive domains such as memory, language, and attention/concentration, whereas the executive deficit in depression is more subtle and usually restricted to specific measures of executive control. Moreover, depressed patients have some insight into their deficits and impaired performance and can detect the errors they make, whereas patients with DPF syndrome lack insight and awareness and do not detect their errors.

CASE PRESENTATION

Using a case presentation, we highlight an example of an early-onset dementia (Alzheimer's disease) where the early manifestation of psychiatric symptomatology was "misleading." A 60-year-old woman presented in August 2004 for neuropsychological testing. She was referred by her psychologist who was treating the patient for anxiety, depressive symptoms, and insomnia. The patient had a long-standing history of insomnia and mild anxiety, although the symptoms of anxiety worsened and depressive symptoms developed after a series of personal stressors from 2000 to 2002 that included the death of her mother, rape, and a transformer explosion while at work that exposed her to a potentially life-threatening situation of an electrical fire, raw sewage, and *Escherichia coli*. Soon after that she developed "language, attention, and memory problems" and worsening of her baseline anxiety. In August 2002, the patient first reported speech difficulties and memory problems "especially when nervous," to her primary doctor (PCP) who recommended a neuropsychological evaluation, but the patient declined because testing was not covered by her insurance. In January of 2003, she began psychiatric and psychological treatment for generalized anxiety. In mid 2004, the treating psychologist began to suspect that it was more than just anxiety, and in August 2004, a neuropsychological evaluation was first performed.

During the interview, the patient reported short-term memory and speech problems. She noted difficulty with word finding, pronunciation, and stammering affecting her ability to function at work; for example, she no longer gave presentations and feared talking on the telephone. She also reported having difficulty with comprehension, even for relatively simple directions, and to be distracted easily. She stated that she had difficulty remembering what she just said or read and remembering the beginning of a sentence when she got to the end, but was able to recall the content of a phone conversation that she had with the neuropsychologist in 2002 when she was first referred by her PCP.

The patient also reported difficulties at work and with instrumental activities of daily living (IADLs), balancing her checkbook, remembering to take her medications, and occasionally forgetting about something she was cooking. She had increased isolation and anxiety and was fearful to use the phone because of her speech problem. She reported that symptoms of anxiety, which was mostly revolved around her health and cognitive difficulties, and fears that she was exposed to a toxin at work, improved significantly after starting 20 mg of citalopram (Celexa) the month before her visit, but that her memory and attention difficulties were unchanged. She described her mood as "pretty good." She denied depression, sadness, tearfulness, poor appetite, or suicidal and or homicidal ideation. She endorsed mild hopelessness, guilt, and lack of energy. She denied auditory and visual hallucinations, mania, and had no symptoms characteristic of PTSD. She drank a glass of wine or two per day, and denied recreational drug use. Medical history was benign and noncontributory.

Medications consisted of citalopram 20 mg daily, alendronate (Fosamax) 70 mg once a week, and zolpidem (Ambien) 5 mg as needed for sleep.

Family history was positive for memory disturbance in her mother in her 50s and died in her 70s, and her maternal grandmother who developed dementia in her 60s. Past psychiatric history was noted for chronic mild generalized anxiety; however, she noted that it never interfered with her social functioning before 2000.

The patient underwent outpatient psychotherapy several times in the past for crisis management. From 2000 to 2002, she experienced several major life stressors, as described previously. During the first neuropsychological evaluation, the patient was visibly anxious. Her thought processes were generally logical and linear without evidence of paranoia or delusion. She required some repetition of instructions but was able to sustain her focus and concentration for appropriate periods. Motor skills were intact without evidence of tremor, drift, dysmetria, frontal release signs, or romberg. Neuropsychological testing showed that the patient was able to function within the average range of general intellectual abilities, which was consistent with estimates of lifelong levels of abilities. Several areas of cognitive functioning were impaired, including executive control skills, attention/concentration, working memory, and bilateral motor speed. Semantic aspects of language processing and verbal memory were within normal limits. The most salient feature of the evaluation was marked anxiety that, in our opinion, accounted for the neuropsychological deficits. A second neuropsychological evaluation occurred approximately 1 year later where she reported worsening anxiety, memory, thinking, and comprehension. Although she was still working, she reported problems completing tasks at work and even at home. She gave examples of being unable to pack successfully for a short trip, retrieving messages from her answering machine, and multitasking.

During the interview, she was pleasant and cooperative but highly anxious. Verbal expression was noted for phonemic paraphasias, stammering, and some difficulty finding words or expressing thoughts. Motor performance was rapid and smooth. She required redirection multiple times. Attention span was good. General intellectual functioning (based on a combination of current and previous performances) was still average. Verbal skills (letter fluency, vocabulary, and verbal reasoning) continued to be intact, whereas nonverbal skills showed a decline from premorbid estimates and previous testing. She demonstrated deficits (absolute and relative to previous testing) in attention/concentration and working memory, visuospatial perception and construction, auditory comprehension, visual learning and recall, and aspects of executive functioning (eg, concept formation, mental flexibility, source memory) and semantic fluency. Verbal learning and recall declined from previous testing, but was still generally intact.

As with previous testing, anxiety had a negative impact on neuropsychological performance, but at this time there was a decline in test scores and therefore a full dementia workup was recommended. We did not think the neuropsychological profile and history were indicative of any typical dementia profiles, but were willing to explore the possibility of an atypical dementia. The patient had an extensive neurologic workup over a 10-month period to include laboratory testing, all of which were within normal limits. Brain MRI revealed mild chronic ischemic periventricular white matter changes, otherwise it was within normal limits. Electroencephalograms (EEGs) during 24 hour telemetry monitoring revealed mild background slowing, bitemporal independent slowing, and frontal intermittent rhythmic delta activity. Steroid-responsive encephalopathy associated with autoimmune thyroiditis was ruled out.

The patient completed a third neuropsychological evaluation about 2 years after the first one. A collateral was able to confirm the history for the first time and reported a rapidly progressive decline over the past several years. A marked decline in neuropsychological status was evident. The patient had severe deficits in virtually all domains but especially in executive control, working memory, and anterograde memory. She could not follow simple commands, and basic skills, such as doing arithmetic, using a calendar, and healthy and safety skills, were markedly impaired.

After proper consent was obtained, a right frontal biopsy was performed about 2.5 years after the first evaluation and revealed significant amyloid plaques and neurofibrillary tangles confirming a diagnosis of AD. The patient's conditions declined steadily requiring pharmacotherapy intervention and admission to a nursing home.

AD was not initially considered in this patient given the atypical behavioral presentation and the initial atypical neuropsychological pattern, which was characterized by intact anterograde memory, executive control, and language, instead of showing the classic neuropsychological profile of AD,[48] which is typically characterized by deficits in anterograde memory, semantic aspects of language, and executive control skills. The family history of early-onset dementia was important information to know and we may have had considered dementia earlier in the course of treatment. However, this was not discovered until we spoke with the collateral source during the third neuropsychological evaluation.

SUMMARY

The symptomatology of early-onset dementias can overlap with primary psychiatric disorders. Diagnosing early-onset dementias with atypical presentations can be challenging. Anxiety and mood disorders can be risk factors for developing dementia and therefore a detailed evaluation and necessary testing need to be considered when symptoms do not improve or when the suspicion for an underlying dementing process is high.

The following are key points and recommendations regarding early-onset dementia that may be useful to clinicians:

- The phenotypic expressions of dementias are diverse and complex and they may not always conform to the textbook model.
- Dementias can first present with psychiatric manifestations or with worsening of preexisting psychiatric symptoms and patterns.
- Even common dementias can have atypical presentations. The expression or presentations of dementias can change over time and therefore patients might need to be reevaluated as needed.
- Given that chronic anxiety and depression are risk factors for the later development of dementia, one should always consider an underlying dementing process as a potential etiology in individuals with a chronic or long-standing history of depression or anxiety that is associated with cognitive deficits, worsening of psychiatric symptoms, or both.
- Always attempt to interview a collateral source. Consider using neuropsychological testing to help define cognitive functioning and psychiatric symptomatology and especially consider repeat testing. A detailed history is extremely important. In-depth querying about not only previous psychiatric treatment history, but understanding their personality style may be critical. Is your patient a chronic worrier, perfectionist, or described as always feeling stressed? These may be useful clues in determining risk factors. The diagnoses of various dementias is often dependent on ruling out other factors and rarely does one have the "smoking gun" finding that "rules in" a dementia. Being able to detect risk factors that otherwise might not have been detected can help with differential diagnosis and determine dementia etiology.

REFERENCES

1. Langenecker SC, Lee HJ, Bieliauskas LA. Neuropsychology of depression and related mood disorders. In: Grant I, Adams K, editors. Neuropsychological assessment of neuropsychiatric and neuromedical disorders. United Kingdom: Oxford University Press; 2009. p. 523–59.
2. Biessels GJ, Staekenborg S, Brunner E, et al. Risk of dementia in diabetes mellitus: a systematic review. Lancet Neurol 2006;5:64–74.
3. Solomon A, Kivipelto M, Wolozin B, et al. Midlife serum cholesterol and increased risk of Alzheimer's and vascular dementia three decades later. Dement Geriatr Cogn Disord 2009;28:75–80.
4. Qui C, Winblad B, Fratiglioni L. The age-dependent relation of blood pressure to cognitive function and dementia. Lancet Neurol 2005;4:487–99.

5. Nalivaevaa NN, Fisk L, Kochkina EG, et al. Effect of hypoxia/ischemia and hypoxic reconditioning/reperfusion on expression of some amyloid-degrading enzymes. Ann N Y Acad Sci 2004;1035:21–33.
6. Sierksma AS, Van den Hove DL, Steinbusch WM, et al. Major depression, cognitive dysfunction and Alzheimer's disease: is there a link? Eur J Pharmacol 2010;626:72–82.
7. Dong H, Yuede CM, Yoo HS, et al. Corticosterone and related receptor expression are associated with increased β-amyloid plaques in isolated Tg2576 mice. Neuroscience 2008;155:154–63.
8. Jeong YH, Park CH, Yoo J, et al. Chronic stress accelerates learning and memory impairments and increases amyloid deposition in APP V7171-CT100 transgenic mice, and Alzheimer's disease model. FASEB J 2006;20:729–31.
9. Rothman SM, Mattson MP. Adverse stress, hippocampal networks, and Alzheimer's disease. Neuromolecular Med 2010;12:56–70.
10. Csermansky JG, Dong H, Fagan AM, et al. Plasma cortisol and progression of dementia in subjects with Alzheimer-type dementia. Am J Psychiatry 2006;163:2164–9.
11. Sousa N, Lukoyanov NV, Madeira MD, et al. Reorganization of the morphology of hippocampal neurites and synapses after stress-induced damage correlates with behavioral improvement. Neuroscience 2000;97:253–66.
12. Coffey CE, Wilkinson WE, Weiner RD, et al. Quantitative cerebral atrophy in depression: a controlled magnetic resonance imaging study. Arch Gen Psychiatry 1993;50:7–16.
13. MacQueen G, Frodl T. The hippocampus in major depression: evidence for the convergence of the bench and bedside in psychiatric research. Mol Psychiatry 2010. [Epub ahead of print].
14. Ownby RL, Crocco E, Acevedo A, et al. Depression and risk for Alzheimer's disease: systematic review, meta-analysis, and metaregression analysis. Arch Gen Psychiatry 2006;63:530–8.
15. Green RC, Cupples LA, Kurz A, et al. Depression as a risk factor for Alzheimer disease: the MIRAGE study. Arch Neurol 2003;60:753–9.
16. Geerlings MI, den Heijer T, Koudstaal PJ, et al. History of depression, depressive symptoms, and medial temporal lobe atrophy and the risk of Alzheimer's disease. Neurology 2008;70:1258–64.
17. McKinnon MC, Yucel K, Nazarov A. A meta-analysis examining clinical predictors of hippocampal volume in patients with major depressive disorder. J Psychiatry Neurosci 2009;34:41–54.
18. Myint AM, Kim YK, Verkerk R, et al. Kynurenine pathway in major depression; evidence of impaired neuroprotection. J Affect Disord 2007;98:143–51.
19. Vythilingam M, Vermetten E, Anderson GM, et al. Hippocampal volume, memory, and cortisol status in major depressive disorder: effects of treatment. Biol Psychiatry 2004;56:101–12.
20. Hickie I, Naismith S, Ward PB, et al. Reduced hippocampal volumes and memory loss in patients with early- and late-onset depression. Br J Psychiatry 2005;186:197–202.
21. Aihara M, Ida I, Yuuki N, et al. HPA axis dysfunction in unmedicated major depressive disorder and its normalization by pharmacotherapy correlates with alteration of neural activity in prefrontal cortex and limbic/paralimbic regions. Psychiatry Res 2007;155:245–56.
22. Korczyn AD, Halperin I. Depression and dementia. J Neurol Sci 2009;283:139–42.
23. Kunugi H, Ida I, Owashi T, et al. Assessment of the dexamethasone/CRH test as a state-dependent marker for hypothalamic-pituitary-adrenal (HPA) axis

abnormalities in major depressive episode: a multicenter study. Neuropsychopharmacology 2006;31:212–20.

24. Van Londen L, Goekoop JG, Zwinderman AH, et al. Neuropsychological performance and plasma cortisol, arginine vasopressin and oxycontin in patients with major depression. Psychol Med 1998;28:275–84.

25. Karege F, Vaudan G, Schwald M, et al. Neurotrophin levels in postmortem brains of suicide victims and the effects of antemortem diagnosis and psychotropic drugs. Brain Res Mol Brain Res 2005;136:29–37.

26. Xu H, Chen Z, He J, et al. Synergetic effects of quetiapine and venlafaxine in preventing the chronic restraint stress-induced decrease in cell proliferation and BDNF expression in rat hippocampus. Hippocampus 2006;16:551–9.

27. Laske C, Stransky E, Fritsche A, et al. Inverse association of cortisol serum levels with T-tau, P-tau 181 and P-tau 231 peptide levels and T-tau/Abeta 1–42 ratios in CSF in patients with mild Alzheimer's disease dementia. Eur Arch Psychiatry Clin Neurosci 2009;259:80–5.

28. Weiner MF, Vobach S, Olsson K, et al. Cortisol secretion and Alzheimer's disease. Biol Psychiatry 1997;42:1030–8.

29. Stern Y. What is cognitive reserve? Theory and research application of the reserve concept. J Int Neuropsychol Soc 2002;8:448–60.

30. Tsolaki M, Papaliagkas V, Kounti F, et al. Severely stressful events and dementia: a study of an elderly Greek demented population. Psychiatry Res 2010;176:51–4.

31. Villarreal G, Hamilton DA, Petropoulos H, et al. Reduced hippocampal volume and total white matter volume in posttraumatic stress disorder. Biol Psychiatry 2002;52:119–25.

32. Bremner JD, Randall P, Scott TM, et al. MRI-based measurement of hippocampal volume in patients with combat-related posttraumatic stress disorder. Am J Psychiatry 1995;152:973–81.

33. Qureshi SU, Kimbrell T, Pyne JM, et al. Greater prevalence and incidence of dementia in older veterans with posttraumatic stress disorder. J Am Geriatr Soc 2010;58:1627–33.

34. Martland HS. Punch drunk. JAMA 1928;91:1103–7.

35. McKee AC, Cantu RC, Nowinski CJ, et al. Chronic traumatic encephalopathy in athletes: progressive tauopathy after repetitive head injury. J Neuropathol Exp Neurol 2009;68:709–35.

36. Jordan BD. Brain injury in boxing. Clin Sports Med 2009;28:561–78.

37. Mendez MF. The neuropsychiatric aspects of boxing. Int J Psychiatry 1995;25: 249–62.

38. Mann DM, Brown AM, Prinja D, et al. A morphological analysis of senile plaques in the brains of non-demented persons of different ages using silver, immunocytochemical and lectin histochemical staining techniques. Neuropathol Appl Neurobiol 1990;16:17–25.

39. Welsh-Bohmer KA. Defining "prodromal" Alzheimer's disease, frontotemporal dementia, and Lewy body dementia: are we there yet? Neuropsychol Rev 2008;18:70–2.

40. Folstein MF, Folstein SE. McHugh PR. Mini-mental state: a practical method for grading the cognitive state of patients for the clinician. J Psychiatr Res 1975; 12:189–98.

41. Nasreddine ZS, Phillips NA, Bedirian V, et al. The Montreal cognitive assessment, MoCA: a brief screening tool for mild cognitive impairment. J Am Geriatr Soc 2005;53:695–9.

42. Tariq SH, Tumosa N, Chibnall JT, et al. Comparison of the Saint Louis University mental status examination and the mini-mental state examination for detecting dementia and mild neurocognitive disorder—a pilot study. Am J Geriatr Psychiatry 2006;14:900–10.
43. Crum RM, Anthony JC, Bassett SS, et al. Population-based norms for the mini-mental state examination by age and education level. JAMA 1993;269:2386–91.
44. Ostrosky-Solis F, Lopez-Arango G, Ardila A. Sensitivity and specificity of the mini-mental state examination in a Spanish-speaking population. Appl Neuropsychol 2000;7:25–31.
45. Roselli M, Tappen R, Williams C, et al. The relation of education and gender on the attention items of the mini-mental state examination in Spanish-speaking Hispanic elders. Arch Clin Neuropsychol 2006;21:677–86.
46. Hoops S, Nazem S, Siderowf AD, et al. Validity of the MoCA and MMSE in the detection of MCI and dementia in Parkinson disease. Neurology 2009;73: 1738–45.
47. Salmon DP, Bondi MW. Neuropsychology of Alzheimer's disease. In: Terry RD, Katzman R, Bick KL, et al, editors. Alzheimer's disease. Philadelphia: Lippincott Williams & Wilkins; 1999. p. 39–56.
48. Podell K, Keller JM. Neuropsychological assessment. In: Coffey CE, Cummings JL, editors. The American Psychiatric Publishing Textbook of Geriatric Neuropsychiatry. 3rd edition. Arlington: American Psychiatric Publishing, Inc; 2011. p. 155–84.
49. Troster A. Neuropsychological characteristics of dementia with Lewy bodies and Parkinson's disease with dementia: differentiation, early detection, and implications for "mild cognitive impairment" and biomarkers. Neuropsychol Rev 2008; 18:103–19.
50. Claasen DO, Josephs KA, Ahskog JE, et al. REM sleep behavior disorder preceding other aspects of synucleinopathies by up to half a century. Neurology 2010;75:494–9.
51. Kirshner HS. Frontotemporal dementia and primary progressive aphasia: an update. Curr Neurol Neurosci Rep 2010;10:504–11.
52. Wittenberg D, Possin KL, Rascovskyc K, et al. The early neuropsychological and behavioral characteristics of frontotemporal dementia. Neuropsychol Rev 2008; 18:91–102.
53. Heilbronner RL, Bush SS, Ravdin LD, et al. Neuropsychological consequences of boxing and recommendations to improve safety: a National Academy of Neuropsychology Education paper. Arch Clin Neuropsychol 2009;24:11–9.
54. Sachdev PS, Smith JS, Angus-Lepan H, et al. Pseudodementia twelve years on. J Neurol Neurosurg Psychiatr 1990;53:254–9.
55. Porter RJ, Gallagher P, Thompson JM, et al. Neurocognitive impairment in drug-free patients with major depressive disorder. Br J Psychiatry 2003;182:214–20.
56. Airaksinen E, Larsson M, Forsell Y. Neuropsychological functions in anxiety disorders in population-based samples: evidence of episodic memory dysfunction. J Psychiatr Res 2005;39:207–14.
57. Goldberg E. The new executive brain: frontal lobes in a complex world. New York: Oxford University Press; 2009.

The Assessment of Decisional Capacity

Teresa Lim, MD, MSc[a], Deborah B. Marin, MD[b,c],*

KEYWORDS

- Decisional capacity • Assessment • Capacity instruments
- Sliding scale

CASE VIGNETTE

A 68-year-old man with medical history significant for hypertension and diabetes mellitus type 2 presented to the emergency department with sudden onset of left-sided weakness of 1-hour duration. The patient was accompanied by his wife, who informed the physician that she was the agent of his health care proxy. The patient was alert, and oriented to person and place. Physical examination was significant for motor and sensory deficits on the left face and left upper and lower extremities. Workup for an acute stroke was initiated including laboratory testing and a noncontrast head computed tomogram (CT). The head CT showed no edema or hemorrhage. Time from symptom onset was within the 3-hour window for fibrinolytic therapy and therefore the stroke team presented to the patient and his wife the treatment options. The patient refused to give consent for fibrinolytic treatment despite the stroke team's strong recommendation that the treatment benefit outweighed the risks.

INTRODUCTION

Intravenous recombinant tissue plasminogen activator (rtPA) for treatment of acute ischemic stroke[1] has been shown to significantly reduce disability at 3 months after stroke,[2] but many trials have demonstrated that this treatment is associated with an increased risk of intracranial hemorrhage.[3,4] Given the potential adverse outcome associated with intravenous rtPA, clinicians must be certain that patients who are

---

The authors have nothing to disclose.

[a] Department of Psychiatry, Mount Sinai School of Medicine, 1 Gustave L Levy Place, Box 1230, New York, NY 10029, USA

[b] Department of Geriatrics and Palliative Medicine, Mount Sinai School of Medicine, New York, NY 10029, USA

[c] Department of Psychiatry, Mount Sinai School of Medicine, 1425 Madison Avenue, 5th Floor Room 5-38, New York, NY 10029, USA

* Corresponding author. Department of Psychiatry, Mount Sinai School of Medicine, 1425 Madison Avenue, 5th Floor Room 5-38, New York, NY 10029.

E-mail address: deborah.marin@mssm.edu

being offered this treatment give informed consent.[5–8] This case vignette illustrates the dilemma confronting clinicians in determining whether patients have the capacity to make an informed decision, especially when their decision is counter to what the physicians believe is their best choice. The vignette also illustrates the urgency and importance of accurate, rapid, and reliable determination of a patient's capacity status in a situation where delivery of treatment is time sensitive.

The main objective of informed consent is to protect a patient's autonomy. There are 3 criteria that must be met for informed consent to be considered valid[9]:

1. A physician must convey the details of the treatment or procedure, including the risks, benefits, and alternatives of the proposed treatment or procedure in an understandable manner
2. The patient has to voluntarily agree to the treatment or procedure
3. The patient has to have intact decisional capacity.

Decisional capacity status is determined by a physician's clinical assessment.[10] Impaired decisional capacity can be caused by a wide variety of diseases including, but not limited to, psychiatric illnesses, delirium, and dementia.[11–14] The prevalence of impaired capacity in acute medically ill, hospitalized patients has been found to be as high as 31%[15] and the prevalence of delirium at the time of hospital admission ranges from 10% to 31% with the rate of development of new-onset delirium in hospitalized patients ranging between 3% and 29%.[16] It is estimated that the geriatric population will increase to 72 million by 2030, making up 19% of the total population in the United States.[17,18] Because the elderly are particularly vulnerable to developing delirium[19] and dementia, 2 conditions that are associated with cognitive compromise,[20] physicians will be treating an increasing number of patients who are at risk of having impaired capacity. As such, the accurate assessment of capacity is essential for appropriate clinical care.

ACCURACY AND RELIABILITY OF PHYSICIAN ASSESSMENT OF DECISIONAL CAPACITY

Physicians are often involved in the assessment of capacity of their patients, and it has been shown that at least in some systems, clinicians are limited in their ability to perform these assessments.[21] Several studies suggest that clinicians have a tendency to overestimate the capacity of patients in different clinical settings.[15,22–26] Fitten and Waite[23] found that 28% of medically ill hospitalized patients (age 65 years and older) were not identified by their physicians to have compromised decisional capacity. These patients did not have known neurologic or psychiatric histories and appeared grossly cognitively intact, as suggested by their Mini Mental Status Exam (MMSE) score (27.6 $\pm$ 1.9).[23] This finding was supported by Etchells and colleagues,[24] who reported that both MMSE scores and the medical residents' clinical impressions of capacity status were on the whole inaccurate. Similarly, a study of 44 nursing home residents found that 35% of residents who were identified by a structured capacity instrument to lack capacity were not identified to have impaired decisional capacity by their clinicians.[22] In addition, a longitudinal study showed that there were inconsistencies in physicians' judgments of capacity status in patients with Alzheimer disease.[26] Clinicians with extensive experience in capacity assessments had an agreement rate of 98% for healthy control subjects (kappa = 1.0) but only had a 56% (kappa = 0.14; P = .44) judgment agreement for patients with mild or moderate Alzheimer dementia. The lack of a structured instrument to aid in the assessment of decisional capacity may contribute to the low interrater reliability of capacity assessments. Physicians were found to use their idiosyncratic criteria in their determination of capacity in patients, leading to poor interrater agreement, as evidenced in a study by Marson and colleagues.[27]

FOUR COMPONENTS OF CAPACITY

The inconsistencies in the criteria used by physicians in the assessment of capacity can be minimized by the use of a structured instrument.[28,29] Many of the currently available instruments use 1 or more of the 4 components of capacity that are derived from aspects of legal competence: expression of a choice, understanding the information that is presented regarding the proposed treatment, appreciation of the situation as it pertains to the patient, and rational manipulation of information.[30] Work by Roth, Appelbaum, and Grisso[31-33] was pivotal in establishing the major elements of capacity that reflected patients' functional abilities.

Ability to Communicate a Choice

The ability to communicate a choice is the least stringent of the 4 components of capacity and thus offers the greatest protection for patient autonomy. A patient has to be able to reach a decision and to express his or her choice to fulfill this standard. This fact implies that a patient who is unable to make up his or her mind or who is so indecisive to the point where a treatment decision cannot be reached does not have the ability to make a decision. Patients who are either comatose or in a vegetative state are considered to not have met this criterion.[34]

Ability to Understand Relevant Information

This ability requires that a patient not only be able to indicate his or her choice but to also understand the information that is presented regarding his or her treatment. Roth, Appelbaum, and Grisso suggested that understanding can be demonstrated by the patient's ability to paraphrase what has been told to him or her regarding the diagnosis, the recommended treatment, benefits, risks, and alternatives to the treatment. Being able to paraphrase, however, does not necessarily demonstrate one's ability to personally relate the information to his or her situation. Thus a patient's ability to understand and to appreciate his or her medical situation is determined independently of each other.

Ability to Appreciate the Nature of the Situation and the Possible Consequences

The patient's ability to relate the information to his or her circumstance is a key concept of this particular standard, and this includes having insight into and acceptance of the illness. Refusing treatment, however, does not necessarily indicate that a patient is incompetent. For example, a patient can refuse to have his or her gangrenous leg amputated,[35] yet this patient can be considered to have capacity if there is awareness that he or she suffered from gangrene, and could potentially die if one does not receive surgery, and if he or she understands the implications of their decision.

Ability to Manipulate Information Rationally

This component of capacity focuses on the thought process applied by the patient to arrive at his or her decision. The ability to rationally manipulate information is intricately related to one's understanding and appreciation of the information. Patients who exhibit adequate understanding and appreciation can still be considered incompetent because they did not follow a logical thought process to arrive at their decision. This element of capacity does not take into account the outcome of the decision. As a result, patients who make a choice that may not be considered "reasonable" can have capacity if they are able to demonstrate that they employed a logical thought process to arrive at their decision.

SLIDING-SCALE CONCEPT OF DECISIONAL CAPACITY

Accurate and reliable determination of a patient's capacity status is of great importance to avoid 2 errors, both of which could have dire consequences: (a) incorrectly identifying a capable patient as lacking capacity, and (b) incorrectly identifying an incapable patient as having capacity. The likelihood of either of these 2 errors occurring is dependent on the stringency of the standards employed in the determination of capacity. Raising the standards will result in a greater proportion of patients identified as impaired, while lowering the standards will lead patients with significant cognitive impairments to make inappropriate decisions.

One approach to avoid such errors is to recognize that determination of capacity is specific to a situation and decision. It has been proposed that the stringency of criteria used to assess capacity should vary according to the situation: that is, the more serious the consequences of the decision, the more stringent the criteria for intact capacity.[10,36,37] Drane[36] proposed a model that includes 3 different standards, each corresponding to varying severity of the consequences of the treatment decision. The first standard is the least stringent of the three. It is applicable to clinical scenarios in which the proposed treatment is effective, carries minimal risk, and there are few or no alternatives. In this situation, the only stipulation that is required to be considered capable of giving consent is that the patient is "aware of what is going on." Drane defined awareness as "the sense of orientation or being conscious of the general situation." Thus a patient in this clinical situation whose cognitive ability may be impaired secondary to his or her illness can be still be considered to have the capacity to give informed consent. The second and more stringent standard would be applied in a clinical setting that has the following characteristics: (a) the proposed treatment carries a greater than minimal risk; (b) the proposed treatment has less definitive benefit; and (c) there are alternatives to the proposed treatment. In this situation, the patient must not only be able to express a choice but must also exhibit an understanding of the proposed treatment, the risk, benefits, and alternatives to the treatment. The third and most stringent standard is to be applied in clinical situations whereby an effective and life-saving treatment is available and refusal of treatment could result in severe morbidity and mortality. According to this criterion, patients must satisfy the most rigorous standard of capacity—they must exhibit an appreciation of the nature and consequences of their decisions as it pertains to their situation and demonstrate an ability to rationally manipulate the information. This standard does not require that a patient make a "reasonable" decision but, given the severe consequences of refusing treatment, it must be evident to the treating physician that the patient fully understands and appreciates the consequences of refusing treatment. In addition, the patient must be able to demonstrate that he or she arrived at the decision through a logical thought process.

CAPACITY INSTRUMENTS

The 4 components of capacity are not only used in the sliding scale described above but are often used in instruments designed to aid in the evaluation of decisional capacity. There has been a growing interest in the development of reliable and valid tools to aid in capacity assessment. These instruments were tested in various patient populations and clinical settings. Studies have been done to determine and to compare the format, validity, and reliability of these tools,[38–42] and some of these instruments are discussed briefly here and summarized in **Table 1**.

MacArthur Competence Assessment Tool for Treatment

The MacArthur Competence Assessment Tool for Treatment (MacCAT-T) is one of the more widely used and studied instruments.[40,43] It is a semistructured interview that was developed to assess all 4 aspects of capacity, and has been used in psychiatric patients (schizophrenia, major depressive disorder, anorexia nervosa), patients with dementia, and hospitalized medically ill patients.[44–47] Several studies indicated that this instrument has high interrater reliability (intraclass correlation coefficient [ICC] = 0.82–0.99 and 0.75–0.87[42,44]), and construct validity has been demonstrated in a variety of populations. This instrument is relatively quick to administer, requiring approximately 15 to 20 minutes. It requires the clinician to use the patient's clinical information, thus individualizing the MacCAT-T to each patient.

Capacity to Consent to Treatment Instrument

The Capacity to Consent to Treatment Instrument (CCTI) is a semistructured assessment that involves 2 hypothetical vignettes.[48] It assesses the 4 aspects of capacity, with the addition of another element of capacity: reasonableness of the decision. The authors used this tool to compare the capacity status of patients with mild to

Table 1 Capacity instruments				
Instrument	**Elements Measured**	**Length of Administration**	**Patient Population**	**Reliability**
MacCAT-T	Expression of a choice, Understanding, Appreciation, Reasoning	15–20 min	Medical inpatients; schizophrenia; dementia; depression; psychosis; anorexia nervosa; normal controls	High interrater reliability
CCTI	Expression of a choice, Understanding, Appreciation, Reasoning	20–25 min	Alzheimer disease (mild and moderate); Parkinson's disease; normal controls	High interrater reliability
HCAT	Understanding	10 min	Medical inpatients; Alzheimer disease; nursing home residents; psychotic patients in outpatient setting; normal controls	High interrater reliability
ACE	Expression of a choice, Understanding, Appreciation	15 min	Medical inpatients	High interrater reliability

Abbreviations: ACE, Aid to Capacity Evaluation; CCTI, Capacity to Consent to Treatment Instrument; HCAT, Hopkins Competency Assessment Test II; MacCAT-T, MacArthur Competence Assessment Tool for Treatment.

moderate Alzheimer disease with that of normal elderly control subjects, thus evidencing construct validity. Marson and colleagues[28] demonstrated that the use of this tool led to improved interrater agreement between a physician's judgment and expert assessment (increase in interrater agreement from 56% to 73%, with a kappa value of 0.14 and 0.48, respectively).

Hopkins Competency Assessment Test II

The Hopkins Competency Assessment Test (HCAT) is a semistructured interview that involves presenting patients with an essay (worded at the sixth, eighth, or thirteenth grade level) describing the process of informed consent and durable power of attorney.[49] Patients are then presented with 6 questions about the material that was discussed. Unlike the MacCAT-T and CCTI, this instrument only assesses understanding. It was tested in different patient populations including hospitalized medically ill patients, psychiatric patients in the outpatient setting, Alzheimer patients, and nursing home residents.[22,49,50] HCAT has been shown to have high interobserver reliability (Pearson product-moment correlation coefficient = 95%),[49] and it is easy and quick to administer (10 minutes). This instrument is not situation specific and only assesses understanding, thus limiting its use.

Aid to Capacity Evaluation

The Aid to Capacity Evaluation (ACE) is a semistructured interview that focuses on the understanding and appreciation aspects of capacity with specific attention to[29]: (a) the ability to understand the diagnosis, proposed treatment, alternatives to treatment, and option of refusing treatment; (b) the ability to recognize the consequences of accepting treatment or refusing treatment; and (c) that the patient's final decision is not significantly affected by delusions, hallucinations, and major depression. This instrument was tested in medical inpatients and was found to have an interrater agreement of 93% (kappa = 0.79).[29] ACE results also had high agreement with those of expert assessment. Similar to the MacCAT-T, this tool can be individualized to each patient, with a mean administration time of 15 minutes.

ADVANTAGE OF USING CAPACITY INSTRUMENTS

The process of deciding which instrument to use can initially appear challenging because of the variations between the instruments, in that they measure different domains of capacity, have different rating scales, and have been tested in different patient populations. In addition, there are limitations to establishing reliability and validity of these instruments. Most capacity assessment instruments demonstrated good interrater reliability, but very few instruments have been evaluated for test-retest reliability.[40,51–53] Establishing validity of these instruments has also been limited due to the lack of a "gold standard" against which these tools can be validated. Nonetheless, studies have demonstrated that the use of a structured instrument to aid in the assessment of capacity improves the reliability of a physician's assessment of capacity. The practice of a physician's clinical assessment of capacity that is shaped by the clinical interview, brief mental status examination, and medical record review,[23] has been shown to be idiosyncratic and unreliable; thus the use of an instrument helps to ensure that a physician has covered the important aspects of capacity determination and aids in guiding and structuring a physician's reasoning. There is evidence suggesting that the use of such instruments increases the reliability, decreases the inconsistencies of a clinician's evaluation of capacity, and improves interrater agreement amongst physicians.[28,29,54] For example, the use of the CCTI in the assessment of capacity status in patients with mild to moderate Alzheimer disease led to an increase in interrater agreement from 56% to 73%, with a kappa value of 0.14 and 0.48, respectively.[28] Etchells and colleagues[29] conducted a study in which medical students and residents were trained to use the ACE instrument to aid in the assessment of capacity. This study demonstrated that the capacity status of medically ill, hospitalized patients, as determined by the medical students and residents who were using the ACE instrument, had high agreement with that of physicians who had extensive experience in capacity determination (expert assessment).

Although capacity instruments have been shown to improve the reliability of physicians' assessments of capacity, these capacity instruments do not replace clinical assessment but aid the physician in the evaluation of capacity status. The use of an instrument helps to structure the evaluation and ensures that all key points are covered in the assessment. If the use of a capacity instrument is not feasible, structuring the evaluation to include questions that assess the 4 components of capacity can increase the accuracy of a physician's assessment. An article by Appelbaum[55] outlined the components of capacity and questions to address in the assessment of capacity. Alternative wording to some of the questions outlined by Appelbaum are included in **Table 2**.

UTILITY OF THE FOLSTEIN MINI MENTAL STATUS EXAM

Although the Folstein MMSE is not one of the instruments discussed above, it is currently often used in the assessment of capacity. The MMSE was developed to measure general cognitive abilities, and is often used as part of the capacity assessment because it can be easily and rapidly administered. Despite its advantages and widespread use, some studies have shown that this instrument may not be an appropriate measure of capacity.[24,56,57] This proposal was illustrated by Fitten and Waite,[23] who evaluated the cognitive function of elderly, medically ill hospitalized patients using the MMSE. The study showed that despite having normal scores on MMSE, these patients were identified to have significantly greater deficits in their understanding of the treatment, risks, benefits, and alternatives to the proposed treatment when compared with healthy controls. Cassell and colleagues[57] also found that medically ill, hospitalized patients performed significantly poorer on cognitive tasks than healthy controls despite having MMSE scores within the normal range. The results of these studies suggest that the MMSE might not be a sensitive instrument in detecting specific cognitive dysfunction related to impaired capacity. It can, however, aid in the identification of patients whose capacity status might be questionable.

OTHER CONSIDERATIONS WHEN ASSESSING CAPACITY

Decisional capacity is situation and decision specific. Patients who have impaired capacity to make decisions regarding their medical treatment do not necessarily lack capacity to make decisions regarding other aspects of their lives. In addition, capacity status may not be permanent and could change over time. For example, a patient with delirium might lack capacity during his or her acute episode of illness but might regain capacity when the underlying medical condition is treated. Understanding is often one of the components of capacity that is assessed, but the patient's understanding of the proposed treatment, risks, benefits, and alternatives is dependent on the information that is presented to him or her by the treatment team. Dunn and Jeste[58] showed that information presented in a brief and organized manner improved patients' understanding. Patients' cultural backgrounds[59] and stage in

Table 2	
Questions to assess the 4 components of capacity	
Component of Capacity	**Possible Questions**
Expressing a choice	Were you able to give some thought to what we had talked about (ie, proposed treatment, risks, benefits and alternatives)? Have you come to a decision? What is your decision?
Understanding of the information regarding treatment	Are you aware of your diagnosis? What have you been told about your diagnosis? Could you please tell me what treatment was recommended and what is your understanding as to how this treatment can improve the condition? What are the benefits of getting this treatment? What are the risks involved in getting this treatment? Are there alternatives to the treatment that were recommended and if so what are the alternatives?
Appreciation of the situation as it pertains to the patient	What are your thoughts about what is wrong with your health? Do you think that you require treatment for your current condition? How do you think the recommended treatment can help you? If you decide to not receive treatment, how will this decision affect you?
Rational manipulation of the information	What are your thoughts regarding your decision? How is it that you arrived at your decision? What helped you to come to your decision? Are there any beliefs that affected your decision to accept/reject your decision (to assess for delusions and hallucination)?

life[60,61] could also affect how they make health-related decisions. Such issues should be taken into account when assessing a patient's capacity status.

CONCLUSION TO THE CLINICAL VIGNETTE

The clinical vignette described at the beginning of this article illustrates the importance of rapid, reliable, and accurate determination of capacity status. Using the sliding-scale concept, the patient is able to give consent for hematological workup and head CT even if his cognitive ability may be impaired, because these procedures involve relatively low risks and have the benefit of aiding the treatment team in determining the cause of the patient's symptoms. The proposed treatment of intravenous rtPA, however, carries the risk of intracranial hemorrhage and thus the patient will have to meet more stringent standards of capacity to be considered to have the capacity to give informed consent. The patient may initially appear to have intact cognition, given that he is alert, oriented to person and place, and does not have severe speech deficits, but he might be found to have impaired capacity on a more comprehensive evaluation.[62] Information regarding the patient's medical condition, the purpose, risks, benefits, and alternatives to the proposed treatment, including the option of receiving no treatment, must be presented in a comprehensive but understandable manner. After this information is presented to the patient, the treating team should then determine his capacity status, either with the aid of a capacity instrument or through a series of detailed and exploratory questions[55] to assess the 4 aspects of capacity.

The patient may have initially appeared to have full capacity because he was alert, and oriented to person and place. When asked to repeat back what a stroke is, the patient correctly paraphrased that a stroke meant decreased blood flow to a certain region of his brain. He was also able to repeat that the doctors had proposed a treatment that involved administering an agent intravenously that could break up the blood clot in the artery. However, the patient did not agree with the physician in that he did not believe he had suffered a stroke.

According to the 4 components of capacity, the patient was able to clearly express the choice of not wanting to be treated. The patient, however, could not relate this information as it pertained to his situation. He did not appreciate the severity of his illness as demonstrated by the lack of insight into his medical condition. In addition, the patient was unable to manipulate the information in a rational manner because of his distorted view of his medical condition. According to this assessment, the medical team decided that this patient had impaired capacity. Decisions regarding the patient's medical care and treatment were thus directed toward the patient's wife, who was identified as the agent of his health care proxy.

SUMMARY

Physicians are often faced with the issue of whether a patient has the capacity to give informed consent for treatment. Given that many disease states and clinical settings could result in impaired capacity, it is essential that physicians are able to accurately and reliably assess capacity. The practice of assessing capacity based on the physician's clinical judgment has been found to result in the overestimation of intact capacity and poor interrater reliability. The use of capacity instruments to aid in the assessment has been shown to improve the accuracy of these evaluations. When the use of an instrument is not possible, one should structure the clinical interview to include questions that assess the 4 components of capacity. These steps can help to minimize the idiosyncrasies of clinical assessment of capacity and allow the treatment team to arrive at an accurate determination of the patient's capacity status.

REFERENCES

1. The National Institute of Neurological Disorders rt-PA Stroke Study Group. Tissue plasminogen activator for acute ischemic stroke. N Engl J Med 1995;333:1581–7.
2. Hacke W, Donnan G, Fieschi C, et al. Association of outcome with early stroke treatment: pooled analysis of ATLANTIS, ECASS, and NINDS rt-PA stroke trials. Lancet 2004;363:768–74.
3. Lansberg M, Thijs V, Bammer R, et al. Risk factors of symptomatic intracerebral hemorrhage after tPA therapy for acute stroke. Stroke 2007;38:2275–8.
4. Tsivgoulis G, Frey J, Flaster M, et al. Pre-tissue plasminogen activator blood pressure levels and risk of symptomatic intracerebral hemorrhage. Stroke 2009; 40:3631–4.

5. Adams HP Jr, Adams RJ, Brott T, et al. Guidelines for the early management of patients with ischemic stroke: a scientific statement from the Stroke Council of the American Stroke Association. Stroke 2003;34:1056–83.
6. Fleck LM, Hayes OW. Ethics and consent to treat issues in acute stroke therapy. Emerg Med Clin North Am 2002;20:703–15, vii, viii.
7. Ciccone A, Bonito V, Italian Neurological Society's Study Group for Bioethics and Palliative Care in Neurology, et al. Thrombolysis for acute ischemic stroke: the problem of consent. Neurol Sci 2001;22:339–44.
8. Rosenbaum J, Bravata D, Concato J, et al. Informed consent for thrombolytic therapy for patients with acute ischemic stroke treated in routine clinical practice. Stroke 2004;35:e353–5.
9. Nelson-Marten P, Rich R. Informed consent in clinical practice and research. Semin Oncol Nurs 1999;15(2):81–8.
10. Buchanan A. Mental capacity, legal competence and consent to treatment. J R Soc Med 2004;97(9):415–20.
11. Demarquay G, Derex L, Nighoghossian N, et al. Ethical issues of informed consent in acute stroke. Cerebrovasc Dis 2005;19:65–8.
12. Van Staden C, Kruger C. Incapacity to give informed consent owing to mental disorder. J Med Ethics 2003;29:41–3.
13. Lavelle-Jones C, Byrne D, Rice P, et al. Factors affecting quality of informed consent. BMJ 1993;306:885–90.
14. Bial A, Schilsky R, Sachs G. Evaluation of cognition in cancer patients: special focus on the elderly. Crit Rev Oncol Hematol 2006;60:242–55.
15. Raymont V, Bingley W, Buchanan A, et al. Prevalence of mental incapacity in medical inpatients and associated risk factors: cross-sectional study. Lancet 2004;364:1421–7.
16. Siddiqui N, House A, Holmes J. Occurrence and outcome of delirium in medical in patients: a systematic literature review. Age Ageing 2006;35:350–62.
17. Plassman B, Langa K, Fisher K, et al. Prevalence of dementia in the United States: The ageing, demographics, and memory study. Neuroepidemiology 2007;29:125–32.
18. Administration on aging. Available at: http://www.aoa.gov/AoARoot/Aging_Statistics/future_growth/future_growth.aspx. Accessed June 23, 2010.
19. Young J, Inouye S. Delirium in older people. BMJ 2007;334:842–6.
20. Inouye S. The dilemma of delirium: clinical and research controversies regarding delirium in hospitalized elderly medical patients. Am J Med 1994;97:278–88.
21. Jackson E, Warner J. How much do doctors know about consent and capacity? J R Soc Med 2002;95:601–3.
22. Barton C Jr, Mallik H, Orr W, et al. Clinicians' judgment of capacity of nursing home patients to give informed consent. Psychiatr Serv 1996;47(9):956–60.
23. Fitten L, Waite M. Impact of medical hospitalization in treatment decision-making capacity in the elderly. Arch Intern Med 1990;150:1717–21.
24. Etchells E, Katz M, Schuchman M, et al. Accuracy of clinical impressions and mini-mental state exam scores for assessing capacity to consent to major medical treatment. Comparison with criterion-stand psychiatric assessment. Psychosomatics 1997;38:239–45.
25. Folstein M, Folstein S, McHugh PR. Mini-Mental State: a practical method of grading the cognitive state of patients for the clinicians. J Psychiatr Res 1975;12:189–98.
26. Marson D, McInturff B, Hawkins L, et al. Consistency of physician judgments of capacity to consent in mild Alzheimer's disease. J Am Geriatr Soc 1997;45(4):453–7.

27. Marson D, Hawkins L, McInturff B, et al. Cognitive models that predict physician judgments of capacity to consent in mild Alzheimer's disease. J Am Geriatr Soc 1996;45:458–64.
28. Marson D, Earnst K, Jamil F. Consistency of physicians' legal standard and personal judgments of competency in patients with Alzheimer's disease. J Am Geriatr Soc 2000;48(8):911–8.
29. Etchells E, Darzins P, Silberfeld M, et al. Assessment of patient capacity to consent to treatment. J Gen Intern Med 1999;14:27–34.
30. Berg J, Appelbaum P, Grisso T. Constructing competence: Formulating standards of legal competence to make medical decisions. Rutgers Law Rev 1996; 48:345–96.
31. Roth L, Meisel A, Lidz C. Tests of competency to consent to treatment. Am J Geriatr Psychiatry 1977;134:279–84.
32. Appelbaum P, Roth L. Competency to consent to research. A psychiatric overview. Arch Gen Psychiatry 1982;39:951–8.
33. Appelbaum P, Grisso T. Assessing patients' capacities to consent to treatment. N Engl J Med 1988;319:1635–8.
34. Morgan v Olds, 417 NW2d 232, 235 (Iowa Ct App 1987).
35. Lane v Candura, 376 NE2d 1232 (Mass App Ct 1978).
36. Drane J. Competency to give and informed consent: A model for making clinical assessment. JAMA 1984;252:925–7.
37. Tancredi L. Competency for informed consent. Int J Law Psychiatry 1982;5:51–63.
38. Dunn L, Nowrangi M, Palmer B, et al. Assessing decisional capacity for clinical research or treatment: a review of instruments. Am J Psychiatry 2006;163: 1323–34.
39. Moye J, Gurrera R, Karel M. Empirical advances in the assessment of the capacity to consent to medical treatment: clinical implications and research needs. Clin Psychol Rev 2006;26:1054–77.
40. Sturman E. The capacity to consent to treatment and research: a review of standardized assessment tools. Clin Psychol Rev 2005;25:954–74.
41. Sullivan K. Neuropyschological assessment of mental capacity. Neuropsychol Rev 2004;14(3):131–42.
42. Vellinga A, Smit J, van Leeuwen E, et al. Instruments to assess decision-making capacity: an overview. Int Psychogeriatr 2004;16(4):397–419.
43. Grisso T, Appelbaum P, Hill-Fotouhi C. The MacCAT-T: a clinical tool to assess patient's capacities to make treatment decisions. Psychiatr Serv 1997;48:1415–9.
44. Palmer B, Nayak G, Dunn L, et al. Treatment-related decision-making capacity in middle-aged and older patients with psychosis: a preliminary study using the MacCAT-T and HCAT. Am J Geriatr Psychiatry 2002;10:207–11.
45. Vollman J, Bauer A, Danker-Hope H, et al. Competence of mentally ill patients: a comparative empirical study. Psychol Med 2003;33:1463–71.
46. Lapid M, Rummans T, Poole K, et al. Decisional capacity of severely depressed patients requiring electroconvulsive therapy. J ECT 2003;19:67–72.
47. Moye J, Karel M, Azar A, et al. Capacity to consent to treatment: empirical comparison of three instruments in older adults with and without dementia. Gerontologist 2004;44:166–75.
48. Marson D, Ingram K, Cody H, et al. Assessing the competency of patients with Alzheimer's disease under different legal standards. Arch Neurol 1995;52:949–54.
49. Janofsky J, McCarthy R, Folstein M. The Hopkins Competency Assessment Test: a brief method for evaluating patients' capacity to give informed consent. Hosp Community Psychiatry 1992;42:132–6.

50. Palmer B, Dunn L, Appelbaum P, et al. Correlates of treatment-related decision-making capacity among middle-aged and older patients with schizophrenia. Arch Gen Psychiatry 2004;61:230–6.
51. Bean G, Nishisato S, Rector N, et al. The psychometric properties of the Competency Interview Schedule. Can J Psychiatry 1994;39:368–76.
52. Appelbaum P, Grisso T. The MacArthur treatment competence study: I. Mental illness and competence to consent to treatment. Law Hum Behav 1995;19: 105–26.
53. Saks E, Dunn L, Marshall B, et al. The California Scale of Appreciation: a new instrument to measure the appreciation component of capacity to consent to research. Am J Geriatr Psychiatry 2002;10:166–74.
54. Cairns R, Maddock C, Buchanan A, et al. Reliability of mental capacity assessments in psychiatric in-patients. Br J Psychiatry 2005;187:372–8.
55. Appelbaum P. Assessment of patients' competence to consent to treatment. N Engl J Med 2007;357:1834–40.
56. Kim S, Caine E. Utility and limits of the mini mental state examination in evaluating consent capacity in Alzheimer's disease. Psychiatr Serv 2002;53(10):1322–4.
57. Cassell E, Leon A, Kaufman S. Preliminary evidence of impaired thinking in sick patients. Ann Intern Med 2001;134(12):1120–3.
58. Dunn L, Jeste D. Enhancing informed consent for research and treatment. Neuropsychopharmacology 2001;24:595–607.
59. Cattarinich X, Gibson N, Cave A. Assessing mental capacity in Canadian Aboriginal seniors. Soc Sci Med 2001;53:1469–79.
60. Rodin M, Mohile S. Assessing decisional capacity in the elderly. Semin Oncol 2008;35(6):625–32.
61. Elkin E, Kim S, Capser E, et al. Desire for information and involvement in treatment decisions: elderly cancer patients' preferences and their physicians' perceptions. J Clin Oncol 2007;33(25):5275–80.
62. Akinsanya J, Diggory P, Heitz E, et al. Assessing capacity and obtaining consent for thrombolysis for acute stroke. Clin Med 2009;9(30):239–41.

Movement Disorders Induced by Antipsychotic Drugs: Implications of the CATIE Schizophrenia Trial

Stanley N. Caroff, MD[a,b,*], Irene Hurford, MD[a,b],
Janice Lybrand, MD[a], E. Cabrina Campbell, MD[a,b]

KEYWORDS

- Antipsychotic drugs • Schizophrenia • Tardive dyskinesia
- Catatonia • Neuroleptic malignant syndrome • Akathisia
- Parkinsonism • Dystonia

From its inception, the pharmacology of antipsychotic drugs was inextricably linked to the movement-inhibiting or "neuroleptic" properties of these agents.[1] Chlorpromazine and other early antipsychotics were originally thought to be useful primarily for calming psychomotor excitement rather than specific antipsychotic effects.[2] Parkinsonism and other extrapyramidal side effects (EPS) were observed frequently but were considered to be indicators that therapeutic doses of antipsychotics had been achieved.

This material is based on work supported in part by the Department of Veterans Affairs, Veterans Health Administration, Office of Research Development, with resources and the use of facilities at the Philadelphia Veterans Affairs Medical Center. The content of this work does not represent the views of the Department of Veterans Affairs or the United States Government. Data cited from the Clinical Antipsychotic Trials of Intervention Effectiveness (CATIE) project were based on work supported by the National Institute of Mental Health (NO1 MH90001).

Disclosure: S.N.C. served as a consultant for Eli Lilly & Company and received research grants from Ortho-McNeil Neurologics and Bristol-Myers Squibb. The other authors have nothing to disclose.

[a] Department of Psychiatry, Veterans Affairs Medical Center-116A, University & Woodland Avenues, Philadelphia, PA 19104, USA
[b] University of Pennsylvania School of Medicine, 3400 Spruce Street, Philadelphia, PA 19104, USA
* Corresponding author. Department of Psychiatry, Veterans Affairs Medical Center-116A, University & Woodland Avenues, Philadelphia, PA 19104.
E-mail address: stanley.caroff@va.gov

However, it soon became clear that EPS can be mistaken for or worsen psychotic symptoms, are sometimes irreversible or lethal, necessitate additional burdensome side effects from antiparkinsonian agents, can be disfiguring and stigmatizing, and have been shown to influence compliance, relapse, and rehospitalization.[2–4] As a result, EPS dominated concerns about tolerability of antipsychotic drugs and fueled efforts for new drug research and development.

In 1988, Kane and colleagues[5] reported that clozapine had broader efficacy in schizophrenia with negligible EPS, stimulating the search for other second-generation antipsychotics (SGAs) with less toxicity. Industry-sponsored clinical trials suggested that newer SGAs were superior to first-generation antipsychotics (FGAs) in reducing psychotic symptoms and causing fewer EPS.[6–13] Cumulative and convincing evidence confirming reduced liability for EPS with SGAs contributed to their market dominance and fostered the concept of "atypicality" in their mechanism of action.[14–21]

Subsequent studies raised questions about the advantages of SGAs seen in earlier trials. Although haloperidol was a very reasonable choice as a comparator in industry-sponsored trials because of its widespread use in clinical practice, new evidence suggested that the advantages of SGAs in reducing EPS were diminished when lower doses or lower-potency FGAs are used, or if prophylactic antiparkinsonian drugs are administered.[19,22–27]

In view of these conflicting findings, the Clinical Antipsychotic Trials of Intervention Effectiveness (CATIE) Schizophrenia Trial offered an opportunity to address the liability for movement disorders between first- and second-generation antipsychotics.[28–30] The strengths of the CATIE study include its large sample size, diverse representation of clinical settings, independence from industry sponsorship, and a well-controlled, double-blind, head-to-head treatment comparison. The rationale, design, methods, and statistical analysis of the CATIE trial have been described previously.[28] In brief, CATIE was designed to address the overall effectiveness between 4 SGAs (olanzapine, risperidone, quetiapine, and ziprasidone) and a mid-potency FGA (perphenazine), including the influence of specific EPS on tolerability and effectiveness.

Although EPS have been extensively reviewed, here the authors provide an update on diagnosis and management with insights derived from the CATIE trial. In addition, the often neglected movement disorders of drug-induced catatonia and neuroleptic malignant syndrome (NMS) are discussed.

DYSTONIA

Dystonia is an acute, alarming involuntary movement disorder that can be painful and distressing, and erodes patient trust and compliance.[31] Dystonia is characterized by briefly sustained or intermittent spasms or contractions of antagonistic muscle groups, resulting in twisting and repetitive movements or postures. Drug-induced dystonia can affect any muscle group, but most commonly involves the head, neck, jaw, eyes, and mouth, resulting in spasmodic torticollis, retro- or anterocollis, trismus and dental trauma, forced jaw-opening or dislocation, grimacing, blepharospasm, tongue biting, protrusion or twisting, and distortion of the lips.[32–34] Dystonia is not action dependent or sensory stimulus dependent. More subtle signs, including muscle cramps or tightness of the jaw and tongue with difficulty speaking or chewing, may precede dystonia or occur alone. At the other extreme, dystonia may present as an oculogyric crisis or with other forced eye movements, or with dysarthria, dysphagia, and potentially lethal respiratory stridor if pharyngeal or laryngeal musculature is affected. Less frequently observed, dystonia may affect axial, truncal, or limb movements, occasionally leading to camptocormia, pleurothotonus (Pisa syndrome), or opisthotonus.

The differential diagnosis of dystonia is extensive, comprising primary genetic disorders and secondary forms including neurodegenerative disorders, structural abnormalities of the brain, and metabolic and toxic etiology.[34–37] Drug-induced dystonia is distinguished by recent antipsychotic treatment, negative family history, focal and nonprogressive course, and absence of associated neurologic signs. The co-occurrence of dystonia or other EPS with behavioral disturbances narrows the differential to disorders associated with both features, for example, Huntington disease, Wilson disease, and neuroacanthocytosis. Although most often associated with the initiation of antipsychotics, dystonia may also be seen if dosages are increased, if a second antipsychotic is added, or for the few days each time after long-acting injectable antipsychotics are administered,[34] if another drug (eg, paroxetine) is added that inhibits antipsychotic metabolism, or following the discontinuation of antiparkinsonian agents. Dystonia also occurs in a tardive form, which may respond to anticholinergic treatment, but first appears or worsens rather than resolves when antipsychotic drugs are discontinued. The relationship between the acute and tardive forms is unknown. Apart from antipsychotic drugs, dopamine antagonists used as antiemetics or sedatives (prochlorperazine, metoclopramide), anticonvulsants, antimalarials, stimulants, and serotonergic agents have been implicated. Dystonias are encountered with levodopa during the course of treatment of Parkinson disease. Toxins (manganese, carbon monoxide, carbon disulfide) have also been implicated. Finally, dystonia was erroneously ascribed to psychogenic factors for much of the twentieth century, and patients with drug-induced dystonia still may be dismissed as hysterical if clinicians are unaware that it is often intermittent and fluctuates with stress and relaxation. However, some patients may feign symptoms to avoid taking antipsychotic drugs or to obtain anticholinergic drugs for euphoric effects.[33]

Dystonia is the earliest EPS to be seen after antipsychotic drug administration. Usually observed within a few hours of a single dose, especially following parenteral administration, dystonias may appear after a delay of several hours to a few days.[32] In 95% of cases, dystonia appears within the first 5 days of treatment after a drug is started or increased in dosage.[32,33] Dystonic reactions last a few seconds or several hours and are often recurrent even after a single drug dose. After drug discontinuation, dystonia resolves within 24 to 48 hours.[34]

Dystonia is less frequent than parkinsonism or akathisia, occurring in 2% to 5% of patients generally.[32–34] However, in young men receiving high-potency antipsychotics parenterally, the frequency approaches 90% in some series.[32]

Patient risk factors for dystonia include age, male sex, race, previous dystonic reactions, family history of dystonia, cocaine use, mood disorders, hypocalcemia, hypoparathyroidism, hyperthyroidism, and dehydration.[33,34,38] Children and young adults are highly vulnerable, whereas drug-induced dystonia is rare in persons older than 45 years.[33]

Drug dosage and potency have been associated with risk of dystonia.[33,34,39] Moderate to high doses of antipsychotics are associated with dystonia, whereas low or very high doses are less often involved.[38] Antipsychotics with weak dopamine antagonism and prominent anticholinergic effects diminish the risk of dystonia, while the newer SGAs appear to have reduced liability as well.[14,15] In a sample of published industry-sponsored trials, haloperidol had up to 4 times greater risk of causing dystonia than SGAs,[6,8,40] with clozapine unlikely to cause it at all.

There were only 6 cases of acute dystonia in the CATIE trial (6/1460 or 0.4%) that were not present at baseline, 4 of which resulted in treatment discontinuation. Of these 6 patients, none were receiving olanzapine, 1 was receiving perphenazine, 1 was receiving quetiapine, 1 was receiving risperidone, and 3 were receiving ziprasidone.[30]

The CATIE data suggest that in older patients with chronic schizophrenia, use of a mid-potency FGA at modest doses presents no greater risk for dystonia than SGAs.

Moreover, Satterthwaite and colleagues[31] performed a meta-analysis of studies comparing intramuscular haloperidol versus 3 injectable SGAs, and found that although the SGAs were significantly less likely to induce dystonia, this advantage was abolished when an anticholinergic agent was administered with haloperidol. However, the use of prophylactic anticholinergic medications to prevent dystonia had been controversial before the introduction of the SGAs due to atropinic side effects. But in young or other high-risk patients receiving parenteral, high-potency antipsychotics, or in paranoid or other patients ambivalent about treatment, the benefits of preventing a dystonic reaction far outweigh potential risks.[41]

Dystonia is responsive within 10 to 20 minutes to anticholinergic or antihistaminic agents administered intramuscularly and repeated if necessary. Intravenous administration is necessary only in an emergency, for example, for laryngeal stridor. Benzodiazepines have been used in some cases. If response is not achieved, a search for underlying disorders, for example, hypocalcemia, should be conducted or tardive dystonia considered.[42] After dystonia is suppressed, oral anticholinergics are continued for 24 to 48 hours if the antipsychotic is discontinued, or for at least several days if antipsychotic treatment is continued with gradual tapering to prevent recurrence. However, at-risk patients who tolerate anticholinergic drugs may need continued prophylaxis.

The pathophysiology of drug-induced dystonia is unknown.[32,35,43] It remains unclear whether excessive dopaminergic activity from a compensatory increase in turnover following drug-induced receptor blockade causes dystonia as antipsychotic drug levels diminish, or whether dystonia results from dopamine antagonism per se.[32] Recent clarification of the genetics of primary dystonia may shed light on mechanisms of drug-induced forms in light of some reports suggesting familial predisposition.[34,37]

PARKINSONISM

Drug-induced parkinsonism is a subacute syndrome that mimics Parkinson disease. Though less alarming than dystonia, it is more common, more difficult to treat, and can be the cause of significant disability during maintenance treatment especially in the elderly. Bradykinesia is accompanied by masked facies, reduced arm swing, slowed initiation of activities, soft speech, and flexed posture.[32] Bilateral and symmetric rigidity of neck, trunk, and extremities appears with cog-wheeling. Resting or action tremors are also observed symmetrically, and can be generalized or take the form of a focal perioral tremor (rabbit syndrome). Patients may also experience sialorrhea, and postural or gait disturbances.

It is important to differentiate drug-induced parkinsonism from negative or withdrawal symptoms of schizophrenia and psychomotor retardation associated with depression. It can be difficult to distinguish drug-induced from idiopathic Parkinson disease. Parkinson disease is usually asymmetric in symptom presentation, has a slow progressive course, may have associated dysautonomia, should precede treatment and not resolve after antipsychotic drugs are discontinued, and may show nigrostriatal degeneration on dopamine transporter scans and sympathetic dysregulation on ^{123}I-metaiodobenzylguanidine cardiac scintigraphy.[44] Of note, olfactory deficits have recently been reported in drug-induced parkinsonism.[45] The differential diagnosis also includes essential tremor and other causes of parkinsonism, including vascular parkinsonism that also tends to be asymmetric, and parkinsonism caused by other drugs including antiemetics, tetrabenazine, and reserpine.

Although dopamine receptor blockade occurs within a few hours after administration of antipsychotic drugs, the onset of parkinsonism may be delayed from days to weeks, with 50% to 75% of cases occurring within 1 month and 90% within 3 months.[32] Parkinsonism may also occur after doses are increased, a second antipsychotic is added, anticholinergic drugs are discontinued, or another drug is added that reduces central dopamine activity or increases plasma levels of the antipsychotic. In most cases, symptoms are reversible in days or weeks, but occasionally, especially in the elderly, or if long-acting injectable antipsychotics are used, symptoms may last for months. In about 15% of cases parkinsonism may persist, raising the possibility of underlying Parkinson disease.[44]

The incidence of drug-induced parkinsonism is variable depending on risk of the population studied, sensitivity of diagnosis, and potency of the drugs used, but has been estimated to occur in at least 10% to 15% of patients treated in routine practice with FGAs.[32] It is the second most common cause of parkinsonism after Parkinson disease. The risk of drug-induced parkinsonism has been associated with increasing age, female gender, dementia, human immunodeficiency virus infection, and preexisting extrapyramidal disease or family history of Parkinson disease.[32,44,46]

Although parkinsonism has correlated with increased dosages, potency, and reduced anticholinergic properties of antipsychotics,[47] dose-response relationships have not always been clear in view of differences in individual susceptibility. In industry-sponsored trials, haloperidol has been associated with 2 to 4 times the risk of parkinsonism compared with SGAs (22% to 38% vs 4% to 14%).[6,8,14,15,40,48,49] However, judging by severe motor worsening experienced by patients with Parkinson disease after receiving antipsychotics, even SGAs may cause significant parkinsonism in susceptible individuals except for clozapine and quetiapine.[14,15] Patients with Lewy body dementia may experience a potentially lethal "neuroleptic sensitivity syndrome" when exposed to FGAs or SGAs.

In contrast to previous studies using haloperidol as the representative FGA, there were no significant differences in the CATIE trial between perphenazine and SGAs in the proportion of patients exhibiting parkinsonism defined as a mean score of 1 or more on the Simpson-Angus Extrapyramidal Signs Scale (SAS) (**Table 1**).[28,50] However, significantly more patients discontinued perphenazine (8%) than SGAs (2% to 4%) as a result of all EPS combined, and perphenazine (10%) had a significantly higher rate of concomitant anticholinergic drug use relative to SGAs (3% to 9%). Quetiapine itself was associated with a higher rate of anticholinergic side effects (31% vs 20%–25%), and conversely, had the lowest rate of concomitant anticholinergic drugs.

In a more sensitive analysis of the CATIE data, examination of the proportion of patients showing no evidence of parkinsonism at baseline who met at least 1 of 3 criteria for parkinsonism (scored at least one moderate symptom or two mild symptoms on the SAS scale, treatment discontinuation for parkinsonism, treatment with antiparkinsonian medication) revealed again no significant differences between treatment groups (**Table 2**).[29,30] Rates of parkinsonism were 37% to 44% among the 4 SGAs and 37% for the FGA perphenazine.

Prophylaxis of parkinsonism with anticholinergic drugs is less compelling than for dystonia and introduces a significant risk of atropinic toxicity. Given the delayed onset, close monitoring for parkinsonian symptoms with prompt consideration of lowering dosages or switching to lower risk antipsychotics takes precedence, albeit with attendant risk of relapse. If a given antipsychotic is effective and cannot be changed and if parkinsonism persists, treatment may include anticholinergic drugs or amantadine. However, there is limited controlled evidence for the use of these agents.[42] Specific dopaminergic therapy is ineffective, due to ongoing drug-induced blockade of

Table 1
Initial analysis of CATIE outcome measures related to EPS

Outcome	Olanzapine	Quetiapine	Risperidone	Perphenazine	Ziprasidone	P Value
Discontinuations due to extrapyramidal symptoms[a]						
	8/336 (2)	10/337 (3)	11/341 (3)	22/261 (8)	7/185 (4)	0.002
Extrapyramidal side effects[a,b]						
Parkinsonism	16/240 (7)	10/247 (4)	20/238 (8)	15/243 (6)	6/129 (5)	0.50
Akathisia	12/234 (5)	12/248 (5)	12/240 (6)	16/241 (7)	13/132 (10)	0.19
Tardive dyskinesia	32/236 (14)	30/236 (13)	38/238 (16)	41/237 (17)	18/126 (14)	0.23
Anticholinergic side effects[a,c]						
	79/336 (24)	105/337 (31)	84/341 (25)	57/261 (22)	37/185 (20)	<0.01
Anticholinergic medications added[a]						
	25/336 (7)	11/337 (3)	32/341 (9)	26/261 (10)	14/185 (8)	0.01

[a] Number/total number of patients (%).
[b] Parkinsonism percentages = the number of patients with an Simpson-Angus Extrapyramidal Signs Scale (SAS) mean score ≥1, with a mean score <1 at baseline, and at least one post-baseline assessment; akathisia percentages = the number of patients with a Barnes Akathisia Rating Scale (BAS) global score ≥3, with a global score <3 at baseline, and at least one post-baseline assessment; tardive dyskinesia (TD) percentages = the number of patients with an Abnormal Involuntary Movement Scale (AIMS) global score ≥2, with a global score <2 at baseline, and at least one post-baseline assessment. Patients with TD at baseline were excluded from all EPS assessments.
[c] Urinary hesitancy, dry mouth, constipation.
Data from Lieberman JA, Stroup TS, McEvoy JP, et al. Effectiveness of antipsychotic drugs in patients with chronic schizophrenia. N Engl J Med 2005;353(12):1209–23; and Caroff SN, Miller DD, Rosenheck RA. Extrapyramidal side effects. In: Stroup TS, Lieberman JA, editors. The Clinical Antipsychotic Trials of Intervention Effectiveness (CATIE) Schizophrenia Trial: how does it inform practice, policy, and research? Cambridge: Cambridge University Press; 2010. p. 156–72.

dopamine receptors, and raises the risk of worsening psychotic symptoms. Once patients have been maintained on adjunctive antiparkinsonian therapy for 3 to 6 months, cautious tapering may be attempted.[32] However, several studies have shown that 62% to 96% of patients may experience worsening parkinsonism following antiparkinsonian drug discontinuation.[51]

The mechanisms underlying drug-induced parkinsonism parallel Parkinson disease. Antipsychotics induce a functional dopamine deficiency in the corpus striatum by blocking dopamine receptors. Their liability for inducing parkinsonism therefore is the product of dopamine receptor binding affinity balanced by affinity for blocking muscarinic cholinergic receptors.[47] Several causative genes and susceptibility factors for Parkinson disease have been identified recently implicating various proteinopathies, but these have not been studied in drug-induced variants.[52]

AKATHISIA

Akathisia is another common EPS.[32,46,53–55] Akathisia is distinct in being defined by subjective as well as objective features, more often affecting the lower extremities, remaining a problem even with SGAs, and being less responsive to treatment. Patients subjectively complain of inner tension, restlessness, anxiety, urge to move and inability to sit still, and drawing sensations in the legs. Observable motor features are complex, semi-purposeful, and repetitive, including foot shuffling or tapping, shifting of weight, rocking, pacing incessantly, and even running. Although the severity of

Table 2 Second analysis of observed EPS events for patients without the events at baseline					
Extrapyramidal Event	Olanzapine	Quetiapine	Risperidone	Perphenazine	Ziprasidone
Any parkinsonian event	70/201 (35)[a]	55/187 (29)	71/191 (37)	48/160 (30)	31/98 (32)
Any akathisia event	52/238 (22)	42/250 (17)	61/244 (25)	51/207 (25)	26/130 (20)
Tardive dyskinesia (S-K)	2/182 (1)	8/179 (5)	4/179 (2)	6/183 (3)	3/89 (3)
Tardive dyskinesia (mS-K)	20/216 (9)	19/222 (9)	21/220 (10)	26/221 (12)	10/120 (8)

Any parkinsonian event includes meeting SAS score criteria, discontinuing treatment, or adding a medication for parkinsonism.
Any akathisia event includes meeting BAS score criteria, discontinuing treatment, or adding a medication for akathisia.
Abbreviations: S-K, Schooler-Kane criteria; mS-K, modified Schooler Kane criteria requiring only one post-baseline assessment.[89]
[a] Number/total number of patients without the extrapyramidal symptom at baseline (%).
Data from Miller DD, Caroff SN, Davis SM, et al. Extrapyramidal side effects of antipsychotics in a randomised trial. Br J Psychiatry 2008;193(4):279–88; and Caroff SN, Miller DD, Rosenheck RA. Extrapyramidal side effects. In: Stroup TS, Lieberman JA, editors. The Clinical Antipsychotic Trials of Intervention Effectiveness (CATIE) Schizophrenia Trial: how does it inform practice, policy, and research? Cambridge: Cambridge University Press; 2010. p. 156–72.

these sensations varies with stress and arousal, they can become intolerable and have been associated with violence and suicide.[53,55]

Acute drug-induced akathisia must be distinguished from tardive akathisia, neuro-degenerative conditions, and drug intoxication and withdrawal states. Restlessness can be observed with other medications including serotonin uptake inhibitors, calcium channel blockers, antiemetics, antivertigo agents, or sedatives. Akathisia resembles restless legs syndrome (Ekbom syndrome), which occurs during relaxation, rest, or sleep mostly in the evening or night. Misdiagnosis of restless legs syndrome can lead to inappropriate prescription of dopamine agonists that could worsen psychosis, leading to increased antipsychotic use and further compounding akathisia.[54] Finally, distinguishing akathisia from agitation and anxiety is challenging but crucial in determining whether to continue antipsychotic treatment.

Akathisia may begin within several days after treatment but usually increases with duration of treatment, occurring in up to 50% of cases within 1 month and 90% of cases within 3 months.[32] Akathisia should resolve after drug discontinuation, but could temporarily worsen or persist in withdrawal or tardive forms.

Estimates of the incidence of akathisia vary between 21% and 75% across studies of FGAs, with an estimated prevalence on average of at least 20% to 35% of patients in routine practice, depending on the susceptibility of the sample population, sensitivity of diagnosis, and the potency of drug treatment.[53]

Patient risk factors for akathisia have not been well established, but increasing age, female sex, negative symptoms, cognitive dysfunction, iron deficiency, prior akathisia, concomitant parkinsonism, and mood disorders may entail greater risk.[54,55] In most but not all clinical trials, SGAs have resulted in a significantly lower incidence of akathisia compared with FGAs.[53] In a representative sample of trials, akathisia developed at an incidence rate of about 2 to 7 times higher with haloperidol (15%–40%) compared with SGAs (0%–12%).[6,8,14,15,40,48,49]

In the CATIE study, there were no significant differences among treatment groups in the incidence of akathisia as defined by scores of 3 or more on the global assessment of the Barnes Akathisia Rating Scale (BAS) (see **Table 1**).[28,56] On subsequent analysis, examination of the proportion of patients showing no evidence of akathisia at baseline who met at least 1 of 3 criteria for akathisia (scored at least mild symptoms on the BAS global item, akathisia given as the reason for starting any medication, or discontinued antipsychotic medication because of akathisia) revealed no significant differences between treatment groups (see **Table 2**).[29,30] Rates of akathisia ranged from 26% to 34% for the SGAs and 35% for perphenazine.

There are no data on prophylaxis and given akathisia's subacute onset, close observation for early signs is the best preventive measure. Once developed, akathisia should prompt reassessment of antipsychotic therapy, with reduction in dosage, discontinuation, or switching to a less potent dopamine antagonist, all of which incur the risk of psychotic exacerbation or relapse. Evidence of treatments derives mostly from small, short-term clinical trials without active comparative groups.[55,57] β-Adrenergic blockers that are lipophilic and target β_2-receptors have been effective in some studies though limited by hypotension, bradycardia, and medical contraindications. Anticholinergics have been used, but are felt to be most effective in the presence of concomitant parkinsonism. Benzodiazepines have been useful due to their anxiolytic and sedative properties. Amantadine may be effective in some cases. Recently, 5-HT_{2A} receptor antagonists have attracted interest, with mirtazepine showing equal efficacy in treating akathisia compared with propranolol, with better tolerability.[55]

The pathophysiology of akathisia remains unknown, but dopamine antagonism underlying antipsychotic-induced akathisia and treatment of restless legs syndrome with dopamine agonists underscore the importance of dopamine-dependent mechanisms. Responses to anticholinergics, and β-adrenergic and serotonergic blockers, suggest a role for other neurotransmitters as well. Apart from exploratory reports of dopamine receptor polymorphisms in drug-induced akathisia, there have been preliminary studies of genetic predisposition to restless legs syndrome, which is highly familial and may shed light on underlying mechanisms.[58,59]

CATATONIA

Catatonia is the least recognized movement disorder associated with antipsychotic drugs. The neglect is not surprising, given the lack of consensus on the definitions of behaviors considered catatonic and the boundaries of the syndrome itself.[60] Jaspers[61] defined catatonia as constituting "psychomotor" behaviors that fall between those with clear motor origins on the one hand, for example, tremor, and behaviors stemming from known psychological states, for example, hyperactivity in mania. Catatonia is conceptualized as a syndrome comprised of disorders of movement, speech, and volition.

Catatonic symptoms that have been associated with antipsychotics include akinesia, stupor, and mutism (akinetic mutism), and less often catalepsy and waxy flexibility.[62,63] The more complex and qualitative catatonic behaviors typical of schizophrenia (stereotypies, echophenomena, verbigeration, automatic obedience) are rarely seen in drug-induced cases. In an unknown percentage of patients, antipsychotics could transform preexisting catatonia into a more malignant form, consistent with NMS.[64,65]

The differential diagnosis of catatonia includes a broad range of neurodegenerative, developmental, metabolic, toxic, infectious, and structural conditions affecting brain function.[66] Catatonia overlaps and may be obscured by drug-induced parkinsonism. Catatonia also occurs in schizophrenia and mood disorders, leading to the conundrum of the "catatonic dilemma,"[67] in which it may be difficult to distinguish catatonia due to the psychiatric disorder requiring antipsychotic drugs from the treatment itself. This condition is best resolved by discontinuing antipsychotics, leading to resolution of the iatrogenic cases.

Acute catatonia develops within hours to days after drug exposure and is expected to resolve in a similar period of time after drug discontinuation. In some cases, for example, after resolution of NMS, mixed catatonic/parkinsonian features may persist for weeks or even months if not treated with electroconvulsive therapy (ECT).[68] The onset of catatonia has been reported to occur with antipsychotics after discontinuation of benzodiazepines or antiparkinsonian agents. The incidence of drug-induced catatonia is unknown. Stubner and colleagues[69] reported only 5 cases of "catatonic neuroleptic syndrome" among 86,439 patients receiving antipsychotics in a retrospective drug surveillance program.

Patient-related risk factors for drug-induced catatonia include past episodes and preexisting catatonic symptoms observed in schizophrenia or mood disorders. Catatonia is mostly observed in association with high-potency drugs.[63] The relative liability between FGAs and SGAs has not been studied. However, SGAs are not without risk, considering published case reports documenting both occurrence or worsening of catatonia with the newer drugs.[14] However, SGAs have also been proposed as treatments for catatonia.[70] In animal models, SGAs show an advantage over FGAs in reducing the risk of catalepsy,[14] raising the possibility that these newer agents would be less likely to cause catatonia, and may be particularly useful in patients with preexisting risk of catatonia. In fact, use of SGAs in trials that included patients with catatonic schizophrenia did not result in adverse effects in this subgroup and was beneficial in 2 of the studies.[14]

There are no data on whether prophylaxis with benzodiazepines or other agents would prevent catatonia in vulnerable patients. A more conservative approach would be to avoid using antipsychotics and specifically treat preexisting catatonia with benzodiazepines or ECT in patients presenting with the syndrome. For patients at risk based on history, clinicians should consider using other agents for the underlying psychiatric disorder, for example, lithium for mania. However, patients who require antipsychotic treatment merit careful observation and monitoring for incipient symptoms. Treatment of drug-induced catatonia has not been rigorously studied, but must include prompt discontinuation of the offending agent as patients with immobility and nonresponsiveness are at high risk for medical complications, or may progress to NMS. Specific treatment includes benzodiazepines, but recent evidence has reinforced the utility of amantadine or memantine.[63,71] Use of direct dopaminergic agonists have not been studied. Patients who fail to respond to these measures may benefit from ECT, which offers the advantage of resolving both catatonia and the underlying psychosis or mood disorder.

The pathophysiology of drug-induced catatonia is unknown, but may involve drug effects on parallel dopamine pathways in basal ganglia-thalamocortical circuits subserving motor, arousal, volitional, and imitative behaviors.[72] The efficacy in anecdotal reports of benzodiazepines, amantadine, and memantine suggest potential interactions with γ-aminobutyric acid (GABA)-ergic and glutamate pathways. Several investigators have studied the genetic underpinnings of different types of catatonia that may correspond to drug sensitivity,[73,74] while Kanes[75] has reported intriguing findings of genetic influences on sensitivity to drug-induced catatonia in strains of mice, mapped to chromosomes 4, 9, and 15.

NEUROLEPTIC MALIGNANT SYNDROME

NMS represents an extremely rare but potentially lethal form of EPS, combining features of advanced parkinsonism and catatonia.[4,76–78] NMS was initially misdiagnosed as an idiopathic form of catatonia stemming from psychosis, often leading to tragic consequences of continued or even more aggressive antipsychotic treatment, with recognition as a drug-induced side effect delayed until the late 1950s, and then not accepted worldwide until the 1980s.[4] Classic signs are elevated temperatures from moderate to life-threatening hyperthermia, generalized rigidity with tremors, altered consciousness with catatonia, and autonomic instability. Rigidity is described as "lead-pipe," tremors are often generalized, and other motor findings have included dyskinesias, myoclonus, dysarthria, and dysphagia. In extreme form, NMS presents as a hypermetabolic crisis with muscle enzyme elevations (creatine phosphokinase, median elevations 800 IU/L),[79] myoglobinuria, leukocytosis, metabolic acidosis, hypoxia, elevated serum catecholamines, and low serum iron levels.[77]

The differential diagnosis of NMS includes other disorders with elevated temperatures and encephalopathy, such as malignant catatonia due to psychosis,[65] central nervous system infections,[80] benign extrapyramidal side effects, agitated delirium, heatstroke,[81] serotonin syndrome, and withdrawal from dopamine agonists, sedatives, or alcohol. In the perioperative setting, NMS may be confused with malignant hyperthermia of anesthesia.[82] NMS may result from treatment with dopamine antagonists used in medical settings. Although no laboratory test is diagnostic for NMS, thorough assessment and neuroimaging studies are often necessary to exclude other serious medical conditions.

NMS may develop explosively within hours but usually evolves over days; about two-thirds of cases occur during the first 1 to 2 weeks after drug initiation.[77] Once dopamine-blocking drugs are withheld, two-thirds of NMS cases resolve within 1 to 2 weeks, with an average duration of 7 to 10 days. Patients may experience prolonged symptoms if injectable long-acting drugs are implicated. Occasional patients develop a residual catatonic/parkinsonian state after acute metabolic symptoms subside that can last for weeks to months unless ECT is administered.[68] NMS is potentially fatal when associated with renal failure, sudden cardiorespiratory arrest, disseminated intravascular coagulation, pulmonary emboli, or aspiration pneumonia.

The incidence of NMS is about 0.02% among patients treated with antipsychotic drugs.[77] Potential risk factors have been investigated in small case control studies, and include dehydration, exhaustion, agitation, catatonia, previous episodes, and high doses of high-potency drugs given parenterally at a rapid rate. The effect of concurrent administration of multiple antipsychotics, lithium, and selective serotonin or serotonin-norepinephrine reuptake inhibitors in enhancing the risk of NMS has been suggested but is unproven.[83] Most of these factors are common in psychiatric practice and are therefore of limited value in predicting the rare occurrence of NMS, and do not outweigh the value of antipsychotic drugs when indicated.

NMS has been associated with all currently marketed antipsychotic drugs, but correlates with the use of high-potency agents. Haloperidol has accounted for about half of all reported cases. The SGAs have also been implicated in isolated case reports, but a few large-scale surveys suggest reduced risk compared with FGAs.[77] There are reports of atypical or milder forms of NMS associated with SGAs, but in fact NMS has always varied in severity even with FGAs.

Treatment consists of early diagnosis, discontinuing dopamine antagonists, and supportive medical care. Benzodiazepines, dopamine agonists, dantrolene, and ECT have been advocated, but randomized controlled trials comparing these agents with supportive care have not been done and may not be feasible because NMS is rare, often self-limited after drug discontinuation, and heterogeneous in presentation, course, and outcome.[76] The authors have proposed that these agents may be considered empirically in individual cases, based on symptoms, severity, and duration of the episode.[76]

Several lines of evidence strongly implicate drug-induced dopamine receptor blockade as the primary triggering mechanism in the pathogenesis of NMS.[72] Such evidence includes the dopaminergic antagonist properties of all triggering agents, correlation of risk with increased drug potency, reports of beneficial effects of dopamine agonists, reduced cerebrospinal fluid levels of homovanillic acid in affected patients, correlations of NMS symptoms with dopamine pathways in basal ganglia-thalamocortical neurocircuits, and most convincingly, that NMS is clinically indistinguishable from the "parkinsonian-hyperthermia syndrome" resulting from discontinuation or loss of efficacy of dopaminergic agents in patients with Parkinson disease. However, other neurotransmitter systems, autonomic, and peripheral neuromuscular hypotheses have also been proposed.[84] Genetic studies have been reported in a small number of cases, examining associations between NMS and genetic polymorphisms for ryanodine and dopamine receptors, and the cytochrome oxidase system, but without consistent results.

TARDIVE DYSKINESIA

In contrast to acute EPS, tardive dyskinesia (TD) is insidious in onset, arises only after prolonged treatment, and is often masked by ongoing treatment. In addition, TD is irreversible in most cases but usually mild, whereas acute EPS are transient but unmistakable and incapacitating. Even so, TD can become socially disfiguring and severe enough to compromise eating, speaking, breathing, or ambulation.

TD presents as a polymorphous involuntary movement disorder.[32,85,86] In its most common form, TD is characterized by involuntary, nonrhythmic, repetitive, purposeless hyperkinetic movements. Most often, TD affects orofacial and lingual musculature (buccolinguomasticatory syndrome) with chewing or bruxism of the jaw, protrusion, curling or twisting of the tongue, lip smacking, puckering, sucking and pursing, retraction, grimacing or bridling of the mouth, bulging of the cheeks, or eye blinking and blepharospasm. Choreoathetoid movements of the fingers, hands, and upper or lower extremities are common. Axial symptoms affecting the neck, shoulders, spine, or pelvis may be observed. Dyskinesias can affect breathing, swallowing, or speech.

TD may present with other than choreoathetoid symptoms that can be difficult to distinguish from acute EPS. These symptoms may coexist with those of classic TD, but represent separate subtypes with increased risk of progression, persistence, and severe disability. For example, tardive dystonia, estimated to occur in up to 1% to 4% of treated patients,[42] may be more generalized and disabling than TD, and may respond to anticholinergic agents. Akathisia and other movement disorders also occur as tardive variants.[87] Dyskinesias increase with emotional arousal, activation, or distraction, and diminish with relaxation, sleep, or volitional effort. As a result, symptoms of TD fluctuate over time, such that repeated measurements are necessary for reliable assessment of severity and persistence.

Although different diagnostic schemes for TD have been proposed, criteria proposed by Schooler and Kane[88] have been widely accepted. These investigators require at least 3 months of exposure to antipsychotics, ratings of at least moderate severity in one or more body areas, or ratings of at least mild severity in 2 or more body areas, and the absence of other conditions that might cause dyskinesias. Ratings are obtained using the Abnormal Involuntary Movement Scale (AIMS).[89]

A careful neurologic evaluation is indicated for all patients with new-onset dyskinesias. Clues to neurologic causes include family history, sudden onset or progressive course, associated medical or neurologic abnormalities, and asymmetry. The differential diagnosis of TD includes acute EPS, transient withdrawal dyskinesias, spontaneous dyskinesias associated with schizophrenia and aging, Wilson disease, Huntington disease, Sydenham chorea, chorea gravidarum, Fahr syndrome, systemic lupus, senile chorea, Meige syndrome, edentulous chorea, infarction or lesions of the basal ganglia, postanoxic and encephalitic states, Tourette syndrome, torsion dystonia, spasmodic torticollis, hyperthyroidism, hypoparathyroidism, and conversion disorder. Several drugs and toxins are associated with dyskinesias including caffeine, phenytoin, estrogens, levodopa, antidepressants, antihistamines, stimulants, and manganese poisoning.

The onset of TD occurs insidiously over 3 months or more of treatment and may begin with tic-like movements or increased eye-blink frequency. TD is often suppressed or masked by ongoing antipsychotic treatment, becoming apparent only when treatment is reduced, switched, or discontinued.

The natural course of TD is unclear. Early studies showed that withdrawal of antipsychotics may lead to an initial worsening of TD in 33% to 53% of patients (unmasking or withdrawal dyskinesia), but with long-term follow-up 36% to 55% of patients eventually improve, which led to recommendations for drug reduction or withdrawal.[90] However, complete and permanent reversibility beyond the withdrawal period is rare; Glazer and colleagues[91,92] found that only 2% of patients showed complete reversal of TD after drug discontinuation. In a meta-analysis of treatments for TD, Soares and McGrath[93] reported that 37.3% of patients assigned to placebo across studies showed some improvement in TD, but concluded that insufficient evidence existed to support drug cessation or reduction as effective treatments for TD, especially when contrasted with robust evidence for the risk of psychotic relapse.[94]

Data on the change in prevalence of TD during continued treatment have been inconclusive, with some studies showing an increase, others a decrease, and still others no change at all.[95] However, prevalence rates obscure the dynamics of TD in individual patients. Roughly 50% of patients have persistent TD symptoms, 10% to 30% have a reduction in symptoms, and 10% to 30% show increased symptoms during treatment.[96] Long-term studies estimated that from 2% to 23% of patients show loss of observable TD symptoms during treatment with FGAs.[95] Similarly, studies of SGAs have shown reduction of TD ratings, with some showing greater reduction, less reduction, or no difference as compared with first-generation agents.[95] Improved outcome of TD correlates in some studies with younger age, lower doses, reduced duration of drug treatment and dyskinesia, and increased length of follow-up.

In the CATIE trial, there was a significant decline in ratings of TD severity among 200 patients with TD at baseline, but there were no significant differences between SGAs in the decline in AIMS scores.[95] Fifty-five percent of these patients met criteria for TD at 2 consecutive visits post-baseline, 76% met criteria at some or all post-baseline visits, 24% did not meet criteria at any subsequent visit, 32% showed 50% or greater decrease, and 7% showed 50% or greater increase in AIMS scores. Thus, similar to past evidence on the course of TD during treatment with FGAs or SGAs, most patients showed either persistence or fluctuation in observable symptoms.

The frequency of TD occurrence has been extensively studied but with varying results affected by spontaneous dyskinesias, sensitivity and definitions of diagnosis, susceptibility of the patient sample, fluctuation in TD symptoms, the dynamics of emergence and remission, and the influence of drug treatment on suppression and unmasking of TD. Estimates of the cross-sectional prevalence of TD with FGA antipsychotics range from 3% to 62% with a mean of 24%.[85,97] Several studies have shown a cumulative incidence of TD of about 5% annually.[85] In studies of first-episode patients with limited prior drug exposure, the incidence of TD was 6% to 12% in the first year even when low doses of antipsychotics were used.[98,99] The annual incidence of TD in patients older than 45 years was 25% to 30% after 1 year of treatment.[100]

Previous studies of TD risk have suggested an association with increasing age, female gender, psychiatric diagnosis, longer duration of antipsychotic treatment, higher cumulative drug doses, concomitant drug treatments, higher ratings of negative symptoms and thought disorder, greater cognitive impairments, presence of acute EPS, and diabetes. The patients with TD at baseline in the CATIE trial were found to be significantly older and had been treated with an antipsychotic significantly longer, were more likely to be currently treated with an FGA and to be currently treated with an anticholinergic agent, had greater neurocognitive impairment, higher levels of psychopathology, and higher ratings of parkinsonism and akathisia compared with non-TD patients.[101] Gender, race, and ethnicity were not differentially distributed between patients with TD versus those without TD. Patients with diabetes or hypertension did not have higher rates of TD. However, alcohol and drug abuse or dependence were significantly associated with TD.

Differences in liability for TD between FGAs and SGAs have been studied extensively. In contrast to the incidence of TD with FGAs, numerous industry-sponsored trials of SGAs found a significant 6- to 12-fold reduction in risk for TD.[12,27,102–104] Correll and colleagues,[12,27] in a meta-analysis, found a 4.6% reduction in the risk of TD for SGAs compared with studies using haloperidol, but later found only a 1.6% difference in attributable risk when studies using mid-potency FGAs were included.[27] It remains unlikely that clozapine causes TD.[105]

In contrast to industry studies using haloperidol, there were no significant differences among groups in the CATIE trial receiving perphenazine or 4 SGAs in the incidence of TD defined by scores of 2 or more on the AIMS global severity score (see **Table 1**).[28] In a second analysis, patients were considered to have persistent TD if they met full Schooler-Kane (S-K) criteria.[29,88] Analyses were also conducted using modified S-K criteria such that meeting the AIMS criteria on only one assessment was required, that is, "probable" TD. Few patients who had no evidence of TD at baseline met full S-K TD criteria during treatment (1.1%–4.5% receiving SGAs and 3.3% receiving perphenazine; see **Table 2**). The proportion of patients who met modified S-K TD criteria ranged from 8.3% to 9.6% with SGAs and 11.8% for perphenazine. There were no statistically significant differences between treatment groups on any TD indicator.

Because there is no uniformly effective treatment for TD, it is important to minimize the risk of TD by early detection (**Fig. 1**). Some preventive principles are to confirm the indication for antipsychotics, use conservative doses opting for lower potency agents, inform patients and caregivers of risk, assess on a regular basis for incipient signs, consider differential diagnosis, and reconsider drug treatment if symptoms emerge.

The first step in treatment is the decision on antipsychotic treatment. Although drug withdrawal had been recommended in the past as increasing the odds of resolution of TD, about 33% to 53% of patients will experience worsening of dyskinesias initially, 36% to 55% may show improvement over time,[90] but few will show complete resolution of symptoms,[92] and the risk of psychotic relapse is 53% within 9 months.[94]

A second option in a patient with good control of psychotic symptoms is to decide not to change the antipsychotic, try to gradually reduce the dose, inform patients and caregivers of risks, document the decision, and monitor carefully. In most cases, TD is not progressive even with continued antipsychotic treatment, although symptoms may worsen in a few cases (7% in the CATIE trial).[95] Another alternative is to switch antipsychotics; more potent antipsychotics, such as haloperidol, can be used to suppress disabling symptoms of TD in about 67% of patients.[96] SGAs have also

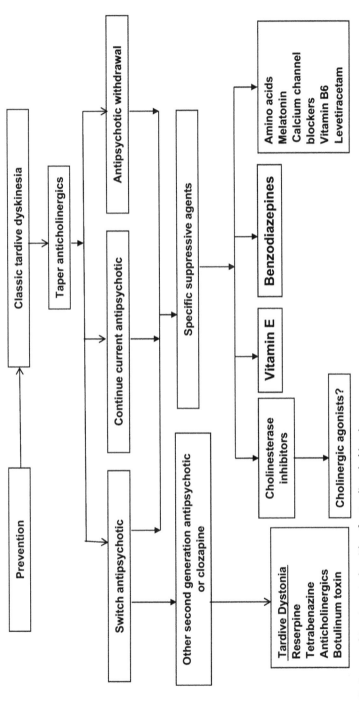

Fig. 1. Proposed treatment algorithm for tardive dyskinesia.

been associated with reduction of TD symptoms[14,15]; results of the CATIE trial indicated that whereas most patients treated with SGAs show a persistent (34%) or fluctuating course (42%), 24% did not meet criteria on any visit at follow-up, and 32% showed greater than 50% reduction in AIMS scores.[95] Clozapine has been recommended for suppressing tardive dystonia. While there have been speculations that SGAs may increase the possibility of remission on an active or passive basis, existing data are inconclusive regarding whether recovery rather than suppression occurs during treatment with SGAs or FGAs.

After discontinuing or optimizing antipsychotic therapy, there are a large number of agents that have been tested in the treatment of TD (see **Fig. 1**).[96,106] These treatments include dopamine-depleting agents, dopamine agonists, noradrenergic agonists and antagonists, GABAergic drugs (benzodiazepines, valproate, baclofen, levetiracetam), lithium, calcium channel blockers, serotonergic drugs, vitamins (vitamin E), branched-chain amino acids, neuropeptides, cholinergic precursors and cholinesterase inhibitors, ECT, and botulinum toxin or surgical intervention (for tardive dystonia). Anticholinergic agents can worsen TD (expect for tardive dystonia), with improvement noted in 60% of cases after discontinuation.[96]

Several hypotheses have been proposed to explain the pathophysiology of TD including dopamine receptor hypersensitivity, GABA insufficiency, and structural damage resulting from increased catecholamine metabolism and oxidative free radical production.[107] Another hypothesis proposes that TD results from damage to striatal cholinergic interneurons caused by the loss of dopamine mediated inhibition.[108] If correct, this implies that cholinesterase inhibitors or cholinergic agonists may be effective in suppressing TD by directly enhancing postsynaptic cholinergic activity, thereby compensating for the loss of presynaptic cholinergic neurons. Several preliminary trials have explored the use of cholinesterase inhibitors, with mixed results.[109–111] However, this hypothesis is supported by animal and human evidence correlating cholinergic mechanisms with the delay in onset, irreversibility, age-related risk, worsening with anticholinergic drugs, and reduced risk with the newer SGA drugs, suggesting that further investigation of cholinergic mechanisms may be worthwhile.

As a genetic basis for TD has been assumed, an increasing number of candidate genes have been selected for study. Using the CATIE trial sample, a total of 128 candidate genes selected from the literature were studied in 710 subjects (207 or 29.2% with TD).[112] No single marker or haplotype association reached statistical significance after adjustment for multiple comparisons, therefore providing no support for either novel or prior associations from the literature. In a genome-wide association study of the CATIE sample, Aberg and colleagues[113] genotyped 738 schizophrenia patients for 492K SNPs in association with scale scores for EPS, and found 2 SNPs and 1 SNP reaching genome-wide significance for parkinsonism and TD, respectively. Although these findings require replication, they demonstrate the potential of candidate gene and genome-wide association studies to discover genetic pathways that mediate TD.

SUMMARY

Whether the newer SGA drugs have reduced liability for EPS because of weaker dopamine receptor binding affinity or a more complex "atypical" mechanism affecting multiple neurotransmitters, their dominance in clinical practice has effectively and significantly reduced the frequency of these side effects. However, the association between antipsychotic drugs and EPS remains important for several reasons: (1) questions about the cost effectiveness of the SGAs, that is, whether their reduced liability for EPS outweighs their higher costs, are legitimate; (2) tens of thousands of patients previously exposed to more potent agents have TD, which remains untreatable and irreversible; (3) there is some risk of acute EPS and TD with SGAs; (4) haloperidol and other FGAs are still used in psychiatry, in medical settings for delirium and agitation, and in developing nations; (5) better understanding of the pathophysiology of these disorders may provide insights into the mechanism of action of antipsychotics and the bases of psychotic disorders.

Regarding specific EPS, dystonia is less frequent than before but may be encountered with high-potency drugs. Parkinsonism is debilitating but is more likely to be seen when antipsychotics are used in elderly patients. Akathisia remains a problem even with newer SGA drugs. TD is most often mild but irreversible, with limited options for treatment. Catatonia is rare and is associated with high-potency drugs. NMS is extremely rare, but early diagnosis is crucial for a positive outcome. EPS are less likely to occur with SGAs than with haloperidol, but clozapine and quetiapine, perhaps because of fast dissociation of dopamine receptor binding, are least likely to induce EPS.

Finally, the CATIE schizophrenia trial has provided an additional perspective on the relative risks and clinical value of the SGAs and FGAs. The study showed that perphenazine, a mid-potency FGA used at modest doses, was not significantly different from 4 SGAs in the risk of developing EPS. It is fair to conclude that the significant advantages of SGAs over haloperidol regarding risk of EPS shown in previous trials are diminished when modest doses of a low or mid-potency FGA are used as the comparator. This conclusion is now supported by several published studies.[19,22,23,26,27] These findings imply that haloperidol is not synonymous with "FGA," and by extension, the dichotomy between FGAs and SGAs and the concept of "atypicality" based on EPS liability may be oversimplified. Instead, antipsychotic drugs could be conceptualized as a single drug class with a spectrum of risk for EPS depending on receptor-binding affinities, especially for dopamine and acetylcholine receptors, and individual patient susceptibility.

REFERENCES

1. Preskorn SH. The evolution of antipsychotic drug therapy: reserpine, chlorpromazine, and haloperidol. J Psychiatr Pract 2007;13(4):253–7.
2. Rifkin A. Extrapyramidal side effects: a historical perspective. J Clin Psychiatry 1987;48(Suppl):3–6.
3. Van Putten T. Why do schizophrenic patients refuse to take their drugs? Arch Gen Psychiatry 1975;31:67–72.
4. Caroff S. The neuroleptic malignant syndrome. J Clin Psychiatry 1980;41:79–83.
5. Kane J, Honigfeld G, Singer J, et al. Clozapine for the treatment-resistant schizophrenic. A double-blind comparison with chlorpromazine. Arch Gen Psychiatry 1988;45(9):789–96.
6. Arvanitis LA, Miller BG. Multiple fixed doses of "Seroquel" (quetiapine) in patients with acute exacerbation of schizophrenia: a comparison with haloperidol and placebo. The Seroquel Trial 13 Study Group. Biol Psychiatry 1997; 42(4):233–46.
7. Potkin SG, Saha AR, Kujawa MJ, et al. Aripiprazole, an antipsychotic with a novel mechanism of action, and risperidone vs placebo in patients with schizophrenia and schizoaffective disorder. Arch Gen Psychiatry 2003;60(7):681–90.
8. Tollefson GD, Beasley CM Jr, Tran PV, et al. Olanzapine versus haloperidol in the treatment of schizophrenia and schizoaffective and schizophreniform

disorders: results of an international collaborative trial. Am J Psychiatry 1997; 154(4):457–65.

9. Marder SR, Meibach RC. Risperidone in the treatment of schizophrenia. Am J Psychiatry 1994;151(6):825–35.

10. Daniel DG, Zimbroff DL, Potkin SG, et al. Ziprasidone 80 mg/day and 160 mg/day in the acute exacerbation of schizophrenia and schizoaffective disorder: a 6-week placebo-controlled trial. Ziprasidone Study Group. Neuropsychopharmacology 1999;20(5):491–505.

11. Dossenbach M, Arango-Davila C, Silva Ibarra H, et al. Response and relapse in patients with schizophrenia treated with olanzapine, risperidone, quetiapine, or haloperidol: 12-month follow-up of the Intercontinental Schizophrenia Outpatient Health Outcomes (IC-SOHO) study. J Clin Psychiatry 2005;66(8):1021–30.

12. Correll CU, Leucht S, Kane JM. Lower risk for tardive dyskinesia associated with second-generation antipsychotics: a systematic review of 1-year studies. Am J Psychiatry 2004;161(3):414–25.

13. Tenback DE, van Harten PN, Slooff CJ, et al. Effects of antipsychotic treatment on tardive dyskinesia: a 6-month evaluation of patients from the European Schizophrenia Outpatient Health Outcomes (SOHO) Study. J Clin Psychiatry 2005;66(9):1130–3.

14. Caroff SN, Mann SC, Campbell EC, et al. Movement disorders associated with atypical antipsychotic drugs. J Clin Psychiatry 2002;63(Suppl 4):12–9.

15. Tarsy D, Baldessarini RJ, Tarazi FI. Effects of newer antipsychotics on extrapyramidal function. CNS Drugs 2002;16(1):23–45.

16. Kane JM, Woerner M, Lieberman J. Tardive dyskinesia: prevalence, incidence, and risk factors. J Clin Psychopharmacol 1988;8(4 Suppl):52S–6S.

17. Glazer WM. Expected incidence of tardive dyskinesia associated with atypical antipsychotics. J Clin Psychiatry 2000;61(Suppl 4):21–6.

18. Glazer WM. Extrapyramidal side effects, tardive dyskinesia, and the concept of atypicality. J Clin Psychiatry 2000;61(Suppl 3):16–21.

19. Leucht S, Pitschel-Walz G, Abraham D, et al. Efficacy and extrapyramidal side-effects of the new antipsychotics olanzapine, quetiapine, risperidone, and sertindole compared to conventional antipsychotics and placebo. A meta-analysis of randomized controlled trials. Schizophr Res 1999;35(1):51–68.

20. Meltzer HY. The mechanism of action of novel antipsychotic drugs. Schizophr Bull 1991;17(2):263–87.

21. Davis JM, Chen N, Glick ID. A meta-analysis of the efficacy of second-generation antipsychotics. Arch Gen Psychiatry 2003;60(6):553–64.

22. Geddes J, Freemantle N, Harrison P, et al. Atypical antipsychotics in the treatment of schizophrenia: systematic overview and meta-regression analysis. BMJ 2000;321(7273):1371–6.

23. Leucht S, Wahlbeck K, Hamann J, et al. New generation antipsychotics versus low-potency conventional antipsychotics: a systematic review and meta-analysis. Lancet 2003;361(9369):1581–9.

24. Rosenheck R, Perlick D, Bingham S, et al. Effectiveness and cost of olanzapine and haloperidol in the treatment of schizophrenia: a randomized controlled trial. JAMA 2003;290(20):2693–702.

25. Hugenholtz GW, Heerdink ER, Stolker JJ, et al. Haloperidol dose when used as active comparator in randomized controlled trials with atypical antipsychotics in schizophrenia: comparison with officially recommended doses. J Clin Psychiatry 2006;67(6):897–903.

26. Jones PB, Barnes TR, Davies L, et al. Randomized controlled trial of the effect on Quality of Life of second- vs first-generation antipsychotic drugs in schizophrenia: Cost Utility of the Latest Antipsychotic Drugs in Schizophrenia Study (CUtLASS 1). Arch Gen Psychiatry 2006;63(10):1079–87.

27. Correll CU, Schenk EM. Tardive dyskinesia and new antipsychotics. Curr Opin Psychiatry 2008;21(2):151–6.

28. Lieberman JA, Stroup TS, McEvoy JP, et al. Effectiveness of antipsychotic drugs in patients with chronic schizophrenia. N Engl J Med 2005;353(12):1209–23.

29. Miller DD, Caroff SN, Davis SM, et al. Extrapyramidal side-effects of antipsychotics in a randomised trial. Br J Psychiatry 2008;193(4):279–88.

30. Caroff SN, Miller DD, Rosenheck RA. Extrapyramidal side effects. In: Stroup TS, Lieberman JA, editors. The Clinical Antipsychotic Trials of Intervention Effectiveness (CATIE) Schizophrenia Trial: how does it inform practice, policy, and research? Cambridge (United Kingdom): Cambridge University Press; 2010. p. 156–72.

31. Satterthwaite TD, Wolf DH, Rosenheck RA, et al. A meta-analysis of the risk of acute extrapyramidal symptoms with intramuscular antipsychotics for the treatment of agitation. J Clin Psychiatry 2008;69(12):1869–79.

32. Tarsy D. Neuroleptic-induced extrapyramidal reactions: classification, description, and diagnosis. Clin Neuropharmacol 1983;6(Suppl 1):S9–26.

33. van Harten PN, Hoek HW, Kahn RS. Acute dystonia induced by drug treatment. BMJ 1999;319(7210):623–6.

34. Rupniak NM, Jenner P, Marsden CD. Acute dystonia induced by neuroleptic drugs. Psychopharmacology (Berl) 1986;88(4):403–19.

35. Tarsy D, Simon DK. Dystonia. N Engl J Med 2006;355(8):818–29.

36. Marsden CD, Quinn NP. The dystonias. BMJ 1990;300(6718):139–44.

37. Nemeth AH. The genetics of primary dystonias and related disorders. Brain 2002;125(Pt 4):695–721.

38. Keepers GA, Casey DE. Prediction of neuroleptic-induced dystonia. J Clin Psychopharmacol 1987;7(5):342–5.

39. Keepers GA, Clappison VJ, Casey DE. Initial anticholinergic prophylaxis for neuroleptic-induced extrapyramidal syndromes. Arch Gen Psychiatry 1983; 40(10):1113–7.

40. Simpson GM, Lindenmayer JP. Extrapyramidal symptoms in patients treated with risperidone. J Clin Psychopharmacol 1997;17(3):194–201.

41. Arana GW, Goff DC, Baldessarini RJ, et al. Efficacy of anticholinergic prophylaxis for neuroleptic-induced acute dystonia. Am J Psychiatry 1988;145(8): 993–6.

42. Dayalu P, Chou KL. Antipsychotic-induced extrapyramidal symptoms and their management. Expert Opin Pharmacother 2008;9(9):1451–62.

43. Berardelli A, Rothwell JC, Hallett M, et al. The pathophysiology of primary dystonia. Brain 1998;121(Pt 7):1195–212.

44. Thanvi B, Treadwell S. Drug induced parkinsonism: a common cause of parkinsonism in older people. Postgrad Med J 2009;85(1004):322–6.

45. Bovi T, Antonini A, Ottaviani S, et al. The status of olfactory function and the striatal dopaminergic system in drug-induced parkinsonism. J Neurol 2010. [Epub ahead of print].

46. Gelenberg AJ. General principles of treatment of extrapyramidal syndromes. Clin Neuropharmacol 1983;6(Suppl 1):S52–6.

47. Snyder S, Greenberg D, Yamamura HI. Antischizophrenic drugs and brain cholinergic receptors. Affinity for muscarinic sites predicts extrapyramidal effects. Arch Gen Psychiatry 1974;31(1):58–61.

48. Hirsch SR, Kissling W, Bauml J, et al. A 28-week comparison of ziprasidone and haloperidol in outpatients with stable schizophrenia. J Clin Psychiatry 2002; 63(6):516–23.

49. Barnes TR, McPhillips MA. Critical analysis and comparison of the side-effect and safety profiles of the new antipsychotics. Br J Psychiatry Suppl 1999;38: 34–43.

50. Simpson GM, Angus JWS. A rating scale for extrapyramidal side effects. Acta Psychiatr Scand 1970;212:11–9.

51. Gelenberg AJ. Treating extrapyramidal reactions: some current issues. J Clin Psychiatry 1987;48(Suppl):24–7.

52. Bras JM, Singleton A. Genetic susceptibility in Parkinson's disease. Biochim Biophys Acta 2009;1792(7):597–603.

53. Kane JM, Fleischhacker WW, Hansen L, et al. Akathisia: an updated review focusing on second-generation antipsychotics. J Clin Psychiatry 2009;70(5): 627–43.

54. Bratti IM, Kane JM, Marder SR. Chronic restlessness with antipsychotics. Am J Psychiatry 2007;164(11):1648–54.

55. Poyurovsky M. Acute antipsychotic-induced akathisia revisited. Br J Psychiatry 2010;196(2):89–91.

56. Barnes TR. A rating scale for drug-induced akathisia. Br J Psychiatry 1989;154: 672–6.

57. Miller CH, Fleischhacker WW. Managing antipsychotic-induced acute and chronic akathisia. Drug Saf 2000;22(1):73–81.

58. Eichhammer P, Albus M, Borrmann-Hassenbach M, et al. Association of dopamine D3-receptor gene variants with neuroleptic induced akathisia in schizophrenic patients: a generalization of Steen's study on DRD3 and tardive dyskinesia. Am J Med Genet 2000;96(2):187–91.

59. Pichler I, Hicks AA, Pramstaller PP. Restless legs syndrome: an update on genetics and future perspectives. Clin Genet 2008;73(4):297–305.

60. Ungvari GS, Caroff SN, Gerevich J. The catatonia conundrum: evidence of psychomotor phenomena as a symptom dimension in psychotic disorders. Schizophr Bull 2010;36(2):231–8.

61. Jaspers K. General psychopathology. Manchester (England): Manchester University Press; 1963.

62. Lopez-Canino A, Francis A. Drug-induced catatonia. In: Caroff SN, Mann SC, Francis A, et al, editors. Catatonia: from psychopathology to neurobiology. Washington, DC: American Psychiatric Press, Inc; 2004. p. 129–39.

63. Gelenberg AJ, Mandel MR. Catatonic reactions to high-potency neuroleptic drugs. Arch Gen Psychiatry 1977;34(8):947–50.

64. White DA, Robins AH. An analysis of 17 catatonic patients diagnosed with neuroleptic malignant syndrome. CNS Spectr 2000;5(7):58–65.

65. Mann SC, Caroff SN, Bleier HR, et al. Lethal catatonia. Am J Psychiatry 1986; 143(11):1374–81.

66. Gelenberg AJ. The catatonic syndrome. Lancet 1976;1(7973):1339–41.

67. Brenner I, Rheuban WJ. The catatonic dilemma. Am J Psychiatry 1978;135(10): 1242–3.

68. Caroff SN, Mann SC, Keck PE Jr, et al. Residual catatonic state following neuroleptic malignant syndrome. J Clin Psychopharmacol 2000;20(2):257–9.

69. Stubner S, Rustenbeck E, Grohmann R, et al. Severe and uncommon involuntary movement disorders due to psychotropic drugs. Pharmacopsychiatry 2004;37(Suppl 1):S54–64.

70. Van Den Eede F, Van Hecke J, Van Dalfsen A, et al. The use of atypical antipsychotics in the treatment of catatonia. Eur Psychiatry 2005;20(5–6):422–9.

71. Carroll BT, Goforth HW, Thomas C, et al. Review of adjunctive glutamate antagonist therapy in the treatment of catatonic syndromes. J Neuropsychiatry Clin Neurosci 2007;19(4):406–12.

72. Mann SC, Caroff SN, Fricchione G, et al. Central dopamine hypoactivity and the pathogenesis of neuroleptic malignant syndrome. Psychiatr Ann 2000;30: 363–74.

73. Stober G. Genetics. In: Caroff SN, Mann SC, Francis A, et al, editors. Catatonia: from psychopathology to neurobiology. Washington, DC: American Psychiatric Press, Inc; 2004. p. 173–87.

74. Kaiser R, Konneker M, Henneken M, et al. Dopamine D4 receptor 48-bp repeat polymorphism: no association with response to antipsychotic treatment, but association with catatonic schizophrenia. Mol Psychiatry 2000;5(4):418–24.

75. Kanes SJ. Animal models. In: Caroff SN, Mann SC, Francis A, et al, editors. Catatonia: from psychopathology to neurobiology. Washington, DC: American Psychiatric Press, Inc; 2004. p. 189–200.

76. Strawn JR, Keck PE Jr, Caroff SN. Neuroleptic malignant syndrome. Am J Psychiatry 2007;164(6):870–6.

77. Caroff SN. Neuroleptic malignant syndrome. In: Mann SC, Caroff SN, Keck PE Jr, et al, editors. Neuroleptic malignant syndrome and related conditions. 2nd edition. Washington, DC: American Psychiatric Press, Inc; 2003. p. 1–44.

78. Caroff SN, Mann SC, Campbell EC, et al. Severe drug reactions. In: Ferrando SJ, Levenson JL, Owen JA, editors. Clinical manual of psychopharmacology in the medically ill. Washington, DC: American Psychiatric Press, Inc; 2010. p. 39–77.

79. Meltzer HY, Cola PA, Parsa M. Marked elevations of serum creatine kinase activity associated with antipsychotic drug treatment. Neuropsychopharmacology 1996;15(4):395–405.

80. Caroff SN, Mann SC, McCarthy M, et al. Acute infectious encephalitis complicated by neuroleptic malignant syndrome. J Clin Psychopharmacol 1998; 18(4):349–51.

81. Mann SC, Boger WP. Psychotropic drugs, summer heat and humidity, and hyperpyrexia: a danger restated. Am J Psychiatry 1978;135(9):1097–100.

82. Caroff SN, Rosenberg H, Mann SC, et al. Neuroleptic malignant syndrome in the perioperative setting. Am J Anesthesiol 2001;28:387–93.

83. Stevens DL. Association between selective serotonin-reuptake inhibitors, second-generation antipsychotics, and neuroleptic malignant syndrome. Ann Pharmacother 2008;42(9):1290–7.

84. Gurrera RJ. Sympathoadrenal hyperactivity and the etiology of neuroleptic malignant syndrome. Am J Psychiatry 1999;156(2):169–80.

85. Kane JM. Tardive dyskinesia: epidemiological and clinical presentation. In: Bloom FE, Kupfer DJ, editors. Psychopharmacology: the fourth generation of progress. New York: Raven Press; 1995. p. 1485–95.

86. Casey DE. Neuroleptic drug-induced extrapyramidal syndromes and tardive dyskinesia. Schizophr Res 1991;4(2):109–20.

87. Burke RE, Kang UJ, Jankovic J, et al. Tardive akathisia: an analysis of clinical features and response to open therapeutic trials. Mov Disord 1989;4(2):157–75.

88. Schooler NR, Kane JM. Research diagnoses for tardive dyskinesia. Arch Gen Psychiatry 1982;39(4):486–7.

89. Guy W. Abnormal involuntary movement scale (AIMS). ECDEU assessment manual for psychopharmacology revised. Rockville (MD): Alcohol, Drug Abuse and Mental Health Administration, National Institute of Mental Health; 1976. p. 534–7.

90. Casey DE, Gerlach J. Tardive dyskinesia: what is the long-term outcome? In: Casey DE, Gardos G, editors. Tardive dyskinesia and neuroleptics: from dogma to reason. Washington, DC: American Psychiatric Press, Inc; 1986. p. 76–97.

91. Glazer WM, Moore DC, Schooler NR, et al. Tardive dyskinesia. A discontinuation study. Arch Gen Psychiatry 1984;41(6):623–7.

92. Glazer WM, Morgenstern H, Schooler N, et al. Predictors of improvement in tardive dyskinesia following discontinuation of neuroleptic medication. Br J Psychiatry 1990;157:585–92.

93. Soares KV, McGrath JJ. The treatment of tardive dyskinesia—a systematic review and meta-analysis. Schizophr Res 1999;39(1):1–16 [discussion: 17–8].

94. Gilbert PL, Harris MJ, McAdams LA, et al. Neuroleptic withdrawal in schizophrenic patients. A review of the literature. Arch Gen Psychiatry 1995;52(3):173–88.

95. Caroff SN, Davis VG, Miller DD, et al. Treatment outcomes of patients with tardive dyskinesia and chronic schizophrenia. J Clin Psychiatry 2010. [Epub ahead of print].

96. Egan MF, Apud J, Wyatt RJ. Treatment of tardive dyskinesia. Schizophr Bull 1997;23(4):583–609.

97. Woerner MG, Kane JM, Lieberman JA, et al. The prevalence of tardive dyskinesia. J Clin Psychopharmacol 1991;11(1):34–42.

98. Chakos MH, Alvir JM, Woerner MG, et al. Incidence and correlates of tardive dyskinesia in first episode of schizophrenia. Arch Gen Psychiatry 1996;53(4):313–9.

99. Oosthuizen PP, Emsley RA, Maritz JS, et al. Incidence of tardive dyskinesia in first-episode psychosis patients treated with low-dose haloperidol. J Clin Psychiatry 2003;64(9):1075–80.

100. Jeste DV. Tardive dyskinesia in older patients. J Clin Psychiatry 2000;61(Suppl 4): 27–32.

101. Miller DD, McEvoy JP, Davis SM, et al. Clinical correlates of tardive dyskinesia in schizophrenia: baseline data from the CATIE schizophrenia trial. Schizophr Res 2005;80(1):33–43.

102. Beasley CM, Dellva MA, Tamura RN, et al. Randomised double-blind comparison of the incidence of tardive dyskinesia in patients with schizophrenia during long-term treatment with olanzapine or haloperidol. Br J Psychiatry 1999;174: 23–30.

103. Jeste DV, Lacro JP, Bailey A, et al. Lower incidence of tardive dyskinesia with risperidone compared with haloperidol in older patients. J Am Geriatr Soc 1999;47(6):716–9.

104. Kane JM. Tardive dyskinesia circa 2006. Am J Psychiatry 2006;163(8):1316–8.

105. Kane JM, Woerner MG, Pollack S, et al. Does clozapine cause tardive dyskinesia? J Clin Psychiatry 1993;54(9):327–30.

106. Jeste DV, Lohr JB, Clark K, et al. Pharmacological treatments of tardive dyskinesia in the 1980s. J Clin Psychopharmacol 1988;8(4 Suppl):38S–48S.

107. Casey DE. Tardive dyskinesia: pathophysiology and animal models. J Clin Psychiatry 2000;61(Suppl 4):5–9.

108. Miller R, Chouinard G. Loss of striatal cholinergic neurons as a basis for tardive and L-dopa-induced dyskinesias, neuroleptic-induced supersensitivity psychosis and refractory schizophrenia. Biol Psychiatry 1993;34(10):713–38.

109. Caroff SN, Campbell EC, Havey J, et al. Treatment of tardive dyskinesia with donepezil: a pilot study. J Clin Psychiatry 2001;62(10):772–5.
110. Caroff SN, Walker P, Campbell C, et al. Treatment of tardive dyskinesia with galantamine: a randomized controlled crossover trial. J Clin Psychiatry 2007;68(3):410–5.
111. Caroff SN, Martine R, Kleiner-Fisman G, et al. Treatment of levodopa-induced dyskinesias with donepezil. Parkinsonism Relat Disord 2006;12(4):261–3.
112. Tsai HT, Caroff SN, Miller DD, et al. A candidate gene study of tardive dyskinesia in the CATIE schizophrenia trial. Am J Med Genet B Neuropsychiatr Genet 2009;5(153B):336–40.
113. Aberg K, Adkins DE, Bukszar J, et al. Genomewide association study of movement-related adverse antipsychotic effects. Biol Psychiatry 2010;67(3):279–82.

Differentiating Frontal Lobe Epilepsy from Psychogenic Nonepileptic Seizures

W. Curt LaFrance Jr, MD, MPH[a,b,*], Selim R. Benbadis, MD[c,d]

KEYWORDS

- Seizures • Psychogenic nonepileptic seizures
- Frontal lobe epilepsy • Diagnosis • Video EEG

The erroneous diagnosis of epilepsy is common. At a typical epilepsy center, 20% to 40% of patients previously diagnosed with epilepsy, and whose seizures are not responding to drugs, are found to be misdiagnosed.[1–3] Most patients who are misdiagnosed as having epilepsy are eventually shown to have psychogenic nonepileptic seizures (PNES), or (more rarely) syncope[4] or parasomnias.[5] Occasionally, other paroxysmal conditions can be misdiagnosed as epilepsy, but they are uncommonly seen in a seizure monitoring unit (SMU). Once the diagnosis of seizures is made, it is easily perpetuated without being questioned, which explains the usual diagnostic delay[6,7] and its cost.[8–10]

PNES are time-limited, paroxysmal changes in movements, sensations, behaviors, or consciousness, that can resemble epileptic seizures, but they are not associated with epileptiform activity. Of the 1% of the US population diagnosed with seizures, presumed to be epilepsy, 5% to 20% have PNES.[11] On average, 7 years elapse between a patient's onset of PNES and the correct diagnosis.[6] The misdiagnosis of PNES is costly to patients, the health care system, and to society. Repeated workups and treatments for what is mistakenly believed to be epilepsy are estimated to incur

Disclosures: Dr LaFrance has received grants from the NINDS, and the Epilepsy Foundation, American Epilepsy Society and receives editor's royalties for Schachter SC, LaFrance Jr WC, editors. Gates and Rowan's Nonepileptic Seizures. 3rd edition. Cambridge (NY): Cambridge University Press; 2010.
Dr Benbadis serves as a consultant or a speaker for Cyberonics, GSK, Lundbeck, Pfizer, Sleepmed, UCB pharma, and XLTEK.
[a] Division of Neuropsychiatry and Behavioral Neurology, Rhode Island Hospital, 593 Eddy Street, Potter 3, Providence, RI 02903, USA
[b] Departments of Psychiatry and Neurology, Brown Medical School, Providence, RI, USA
[c] Tampa General Hospital, 4 Columbia Drive, Suite 730, Tampa, FL 33606, USA
[d] University of South Florida, Tampa, FL, USA
* Corresponding author. Division of Neuropsychiatry and Behavioral Neurology, Rhode Island Hospital, 593 Eddy Street, Potter 3, Providence, RI 02903.
E-mail address: william_lafrance_Jr@brown.edu

Neurol Clin 29 (2011) 149–162
doi:10.1016/j.ncl.2010.10.005
0733-8619/11/$ – see front matter © 2011 Elsevier Inc. All rights reserved.

neurologic.theclinics.com

$100 to $900 million per year in medical services.[9] Patients with PNES are prescribed antiepileptic drugs (AEDs) that do not treat, and may exacerbate PNES,[12] have multiple tests performed, and may not receive the necessary mental health care that could benefit them. Delayed diagnosis could lead to adverse effects from unneeded AEDs, iatrogenic complications from invasive procedures in continuous PNES (nonepileptic psychogenic status),[13] medical costs from unnecessary hospitalization treatment and workup, delayed referral to appropriate psychiatric treatment, and employment difficulties and disability.[14]

The first step in PNES treatment is proper diagnosis. Video electroencephalography (EEG) remains the gold standard for PNES diagnosis. Certain seizure types, such as those seen in frontal lobe epilepsy (FLE), may mimic PNES semiology, and, conversely, ictal characteristics of PNES may resemble epileptic seizures (ES). New diagnostic techniques may help distinguish stereotypic semiology seen in FLE that are not seen in PNES. Bedside observations may also be of benefit in augmenting the video EEG interpretation to establish the PNES diagnosis. The use of other diagnostic measures to augment video EEG diagnosis is examined in this article. The safety of discontinuing AEDs in lone NES is discussed.

Nonepileptic seizures (NES) can be physiologic or psychogenic in origin and can be difficult to distinguish from ES, with both seizure types showing alterations in behavior, consciousness, sensation, and perception.[15] Recent research has yielded clinically useful differentiating features at bedside and on video EEG. Appropriate diagnosis then informs potential treatments.

DIAGNOSIS: DISTINGUISHING NES FROM ES

The diagnosis and treatment of patients with PNES has long confounded neurologists, psychiatrists, and emergency physicians. As an adjunct to anamnesis and video EEG, ictal semiology, neurophysiologic tests, patient characteristics, and neuropsychological testing contribute to making the diagnosis of PNES.

Differentiating NES from ES is the first step in appropriate treatment.[16] PNES can appear similar to ES, and, to distinguish the 2 types of seizures, the gold standard is video EEG.[17] Because there is no tissue confirmation against which to measure the accuracy of video EEG, the next best measure is interrater reliability (IRR). Video EEG has been shown to have substantial IRR for epilepsy and moderate IRR for PNES, as discussed later.[18] The IRR would almost certainly be higher when incorporating supplemental information including history, physical, and more ictal segments. Other techniques can be used as adjuncts to make the diagnosis of NES,[19] but admission to an SMU is the key. Video EEG not only provides a definitive diagnosis in almost 90% of patients but also rectifies an incorrect diagnosis of epilepsy, and results in treatment change in 79% of patients.[20] Monitoring a patient with seizures in the SMU may also help to identify the 10% of patients with PNES who also have epilepsy.[21] Higher numbers of mixed ES/PNES were given in the literature in the past, but these seem to have been overestimates based on less-stringent criteria for differentiating epilepsy from PNES.

Some physical observations of the ictal semiology used in differentiating PNES from epilepsy are noted later (**Table 1**).[22]

Eye and Facial Findings

Using data from video EEG monitoring, researchers found that 50 of 52 patients with PNES (96%) closed their eyes during the seizure, compared with 152 of 156 of patients with ES (97%), who had their eyes open at the beginning of their seizure.[23] This

Table 1
Behaviors to distinguish between psychogenic nonepileptic and epileptic seizures

Observation	PNES	ES
Situational onset	Common	Rare
Gradual onset	Common	Rare
Precipitated by stimuli (noise, light)	Occasional	Rare
Purposeful movements	Occasional	Very rare
Opisthotonus (arc de cercle)	Occasional	Very rare
Tongue biting (tip)	Occasional	Rare
Tongue biting (side)	Very Rare	Common
Prolonged ictal atonia	Occasional	Very rare
Vocalization during tonic-clonic phase	Occasional	Very rare
Reactivity during unconsciousness	Occasional	Very rare
Rapid postictal reorientation	Common	Unusual
Undulating motor activity	Common	Very rare
Asynchronous limb movements	Common	Rare
Rhythmical pelvic movements	Occasional	Rare
Side-to-side head shaking	Common	Rare
Ictal crying	Occasional	Very rare
Ictal stuttering	Occasional	Rare
Postictal whispering	Occasional	Not present
Closed mouth in tonic phase	Occasional	Very rare
Closed eyelids during seizure onset	Very common	Rare
Convulsion >2 min	Common	Very rare
Resisted lid opening	Common	Very rare
Pupillary light reflex	Usually retained	Commonly absent
Cyanosis	Rare	Common
Ictal grasping	Rare	Occurs in FLE and TLE
Postictal nose rubbing	Not present	Can occur in TLE
Stertorous breathing postictally	Not present	Common
Self-injury	May be present (especially excoriations)	May be present (especially lacerations)
Incontinence	May be present	May be present

Abbreviations: FLE, frontal lobe epilepsy; TLE, temporal lobe epilepsy.

Reproduced from Benbadis SR, LaFrance WC Jr. Clinical features and the role of video-EEG monitoring. In: Schachter SC, LaFrance WC Jr, editors. Gates and Rowan's Nonepileptic Seizures. 3rd edition. Cambridge: Cambridge University Press; 2010. p. 38–50. Chapter 4; with permission.
Data from Refs. [22–32,36–40]

information may help clinicians differentiate between PNES and ES, particularly when the 2 types of seizures occur in the same patient. Also, other observers, such as family members, could report to physicians whether the patient's eyes were open or closed during the ictal event. However, this observation has been challenged by other investigators, who prospectively assessed whether observer or self-report eye closure could predict NES, before video EEG monitoring.[24] In the monitoring unit, 112 met study criteria and had either PNES (n = 43, 38.4%) or epilepsy (n = 84, 75%). The investigators recorded eye closure as a percentage of episode duration, rather than the previously studied dichotomous, absent or present. Self-report of eye closure more accurately predicted actual videorecorded eye closure than observer report. The study confirmed that video-recorded eye closure was 92% specific for PNES identification, but not as sensitive (only 64%) as previously reported.

Patients with PNES may also exhibit geotropic eye movements, in which the eyes deviate downward to the side that the head is turned.[25] Eyelids are typically closed for a longer duration (20 seconds) compared with temporal lobe epilepsy (TLE) or FLE (~2 seconds).[26] Weeping is also a characteristic with PNES.[27,28]

Ictal stuttering and postictal whispering voice are seen in PNES.[29,30] Postictal nose rubbing and cough have been observed in TLE but not in PNES.[31] Similarly, noisy or stertorous breathing can be seen after ictus in epileptic convulsions but was not observed following PNES convulsions.[32] Although it helps to differentiate convulsive epilepsy from convulsive PNES, this finding does not apply to partial seizures.

Pelvic thrusting is reportedly as common in FLE as in PNES.[33–35] Other ictal features associated with PNES are out-of-phase or side-to-side oscillatory movements or chaotic and disorganized thrashing.[15] In contrast, seizures of FLE typically arise from sleep, are brief, and often involve vocalization and quick tonic posturing.[36,37] Occasionally, whole body trembling may be observed with PNES. These behaviors may wax and wane (including stop and go), and vary in direction and rhythm, which is atypical for ES (ES tend to follow a stereotyped evolution).

Physical injury during an ictus was once believed to occur only in patients with epilepsy, but research shows that more than 50% of patients with PNES are injured during seizures.[38] The character of the injury is helpful in differentiating ES from PNES. Excoriations on long bone surfaces, such as the arm, leg, or cheek, are seen in PNES,[39] as opposed to lacerations from epilepsy. Tongue biting, self-injury, and incontinence are commonly associated with ES but are also reported by up to two-thirds of patients with PNES, rendering these signs less specific than was once believed,[40] especially when they are reported rather than documented. Objectively documented injuries or incontinence are of higher diagnostic value (specificity).

Observing what the patients bring into the SMU also has some value. One group found that, of those admitted for monitoring, patients with PNES brought a toy stuffed animal with them.[41] In their study, 381 patients with PNES were compared with 453 patients with epilepsy. Of 23 patients (2.5%) who had toy animals during admission, 20 were diagnosed with PNES, and 3 were diagnosed with epilepsy (P<.001). The 3 patients with epilepsy had a history of a psychiatric disorder. Sensitivity was 5.2% and specificity was 99.3%, with a positive predictive power of 87%, and a negative predictive power of 55%. The investigators proposed that such behaviors may represent nonverbal expressions of attachment desires, dependency needs, or other psychological traits.

DIAGNOSTIC MEASURES
EEG

NES diagnosis is most accurately established by coregistering EEG neurophysiologic testing with video. Video EEG, in which the patient's seizure is observed visually with simultaneous EEG, allows data about behavior to be coupled with EEG rhythms. With the history and examination, the absence of expected epileptiform patterns before, during, and after the ictus points to a NES diagnosis. Occasionally, EEG-negative epilepsy on scalp EEG occurs, in which a simple partial seizure, a frontal lobe epileptic seizure, or a deep temporal lobe epileptic seizure does not generate an ictal epileptiform pattern.[42] The EEG can also be uninterpretable because of movement or electromyographic artifact. Without video EEG, neurologists' ability to differentiate ES from NES by history alone has a specificity of 50%.[43]

One study described a method for diagnosing frontal lobe epileptic seizures by comparing the video EEGs in a synchronized, side-by-side view.[44] Split-screen synchronized display was found to be a simple and valid technique for studying and presenting particular semiological aspects of ES. Using this methodology to diagnose NES may also be of value. Research suggests that magnetoencephalography (MEG) may be useful for identification and localization of FLE,[45] and MEG studies are attempting to develop optimal procedures for localizing interictal epileptiform discharges of patients with localization-related FLE. For the scalp EEG–negative cases in which the differential diagnosis of FLE versus PNES is present, future research could examine the potential to screen for spikes in FLE that are not seen in PNES.

Neurohumoral Measures

The use of serum prolactin (PRL) drawn within 30 minutes of the ictus onset is helpful for differentiating generalized tonic-clonic (GTC) epileptic seizures and complex partial epileptic seizures (CPS) from PNES, as summarized in a report from the Therapeutics and Technology Assessment Subcommittee of the American Academy of Neurology.[46] Trimble[47] first showed that GTC epileptic seizures, but not PNES, raised serum PRL. Pooling the available data of the 10 studies meeting inclusion criteria, the subcommittee investigators found a sensitivity of 60% for GTC and 46% for CPS, and a specificity of 96% for both. They found a positive predictive value of 93% to 99%. Cragar and colleagues[19] similarly found lack of PRL increase has an average 89% sensitivity to PNES. Clinically, this translates into a strong confirmation of a diagnosis of ES when an increased PRL is found in patients with GTC- or CPS-like events suspected of being PNES. The investigators concluded that an increase in serum PRL level is probably a useful adjunct to differentiate GTC or CPS from PNES. However, PRL is of limited usefulness for differentiating FLE of any semiology from PNES.

Neuroimaging

Structural neuroimaging abnormalities neither confirm nor exclude ES or PNES. PNES can occur in the presence of structural lesions,[48] and about 10% of patients with PNES alone have structural abnormalities on magnetic resonance imaging scans.[49] Functional imaging is not useful for the diagnosis of PNES versus FLE. A negative ictal single-photon emission computed tomography (SPECT) scan does not imply a diagnosis of PNES nor does an abnormal scan mean epilepsy is present. A small series of ictal and interictal SPECT scans of patients with PNES revealed a few scans with lateralized perfusion abnormalities, but the findings did not change when the ictal and interictal images were compared.[50] In contrast, patients with epilepsy have dynamic changes when ictal and interictal changes are compared on functional neuroimaging.

CHARACTERISTICS OF PATIENTS WITH PNES AND EPILEPSY
Neuropsychological Measures

Many studies exist describing the cognitive, emotional, personality, and psychomotor differences between the ES and PNES groups. Cragar and colleagues[19] reviewed the literature on adjunctive tests for diagnosing PNES and reported sensitivity and specificity of the different measures. A summary of their findings noted that patients with ES and PNES perform roughly the same on neuropsychological (NP) measures but worse than healthy controls. PNES tended to perform better than patients with ES on certain NP tests, as described later.

A summary of studies examining intelligence, psychomotor function, motivational measures, and personality features in PNES[51] suggests that, for cognitive measures, patients with ES and PNES show no significant differences on tests of intelligence, learning, and memory but score lower than healthy control subjects.[52] On psychomotor measures, patients with PNES show reduced motor speed and grip strength, compared with healthy controls.[53] Motivational measures reveal that patients with PNES score lower than patients with ES on some motivational measures, perhaps reflecting a lack of psychological resources necessary to persist with a challenging NP battery. Some studies show comparable failure rates in PNES and ES groups on symptom validity batteries. Frank malingering is believed to occur rarely in PNES,[54–56] but malingering is probably underdiagnosed in general, because it is an accusation rather than a diagnosis. The Minnesota Multiphasic Personality Inventory (MMPI) has been used for more than 20 years in assessing patients with PNES. Personality testing performed with instruments such as MMPI-2 studies show increases in hypochondria, hysteria, and depression scores in PNES.[19,57]

Intelligence Measures and Cognitive Testing

Comparing patients with PNES with those with ES, Binder and colleagues[52] found no significant differences on tests of intelligence or learning and memory, including the Wechsler Adult Intelligence Scale - Revised, Wisconsin Card Sort Test, or Rey Auditory Verbal Learning Test. Control subjects were significantly superior to the PNES and the ES group. Bortz and colleagues[58] studied the California Verbal Learning Test results in patients with PNES and ES and the investigators suggested that "failure to explicitly recognize words following repeated exposure" may be reflective of a negative response bias and psychological denial in patients with PNES.

Psychomotor Measures

Kalogjera-Sackellares and Sackellares[53] evaluated patients with PNES compared with matched normal controls and found reduced motor speed and grip strength in the patients with PNES. Some have interpreted this as a manifestation of motivation, which is discussed later. Dodrill and Holmes[59] reported that patients with PNES performed better than those with ES on measures from the Halstead-Reitan Battery, with differences between Tactual Performance Test, Seashore Tonal Memory, and Trailmaking Part B. Although finger tapping and grooved pegboard differed between controls compared with PNES and ES groups, Binder and colleagues[52] did not find differences between the ES and PNES groups on these measures.

Motivational Measures

Motivational tests include the Portland Digit Recognition Test (PDRT), the Test of Memory Malingering (TOMM), and others, and are used to detect inadequate performance on NP testing. The presence of unconscious psychological stress is hypothesized as an explanation for variable effort in patients with PNES.[60] Binder and colleagues[52,54] found that patients with PNES performed poorly compared with patients with ES on the PDRT. The investigators noted that frank malingering occurs rarely in PNES, and that the poorer performance in PNES may reflect a lack of psychological resources necessary to persist with a challenging NP battery. More recent symptom validity tests of patients with PNES and patients with ES show discrepant findings. Drane and colleagues[55] concluded that many patients with PNES do not put forth maximal effort on neuropsychological tests, based on the Word Memory

Test failure rate in their sample (51.2% in NES, vs 8.1% in ES). More extensive batteries, including the Digit Memory Test, Letter Memory Test, TOMM, and PDRT, failed to show differences between the ES and PNES groups, with 22% of patients with epilepsy and 24% of patients with PNES performing suboptimally on 1 or more effort measures.[56]

Personality Testing: MMPI/MMPI-2 and Clinical Psychological Profiles

The MMPI has been used for more than 20 years in assessing patients with PNES. Most MMPI studies in PNES report the conversion V profile, with increases in scales 1 (Hs [hypochondriasis]) and 3 (Hy [hysteria]), and depressions in Scale 2 (D [depression]).[19] Cragar and colleagues[19] also reported an average sensitivity of 70% and specificity of 73% to PNES diagnosis using MMPI-2 decision rules. Using the MMPI-2 and clinical variables yielded 80% sensitivity and specificity for PNES diagnosis between 57 patients with ES and 51 with PNES.[57] Along with others, the study shows the MMPI-2 to be a useful adjunct to video EEG diagnosis.

The dramatic personality of patients with PNES was illustrated in a blinded pilot study of artwork drawn by patients with ES and NES.[61] The investigators calculated that an 80% positive predictive value for PNES existed if subjects used 10 or more colors to draw their seizures. Galimberti and colleagues[62] administered the cognitive behavioral assessment (CBA) psychometric battery to patients with lone NES, mixed ES/PNES, and ES controls. The CBA, which assesses personality characteristics and emotional adjustment, comprises scales rating introversion-extroversion, neuroticism, psychoticism, state-trait anxiety, psychophysiologic distress, and depressive and other anxiety symptoms, and found that the mean scores on the psychophysiologic distress scale for the PNES and the ES/PNES groups were higher than the mean scores of the ES control group.

Family and Patient Traits

Studies comparing family functioning in patients with ES and PNES reveal that individuals with PNES consider their families to be more dysfunctional, particularly in regard to communication, and that family members of patients with PNES reported difficulties defining roles.[63] Individuals with PNES score higher on symptom checklists (a measure of somatic complaints) compared with other patients with seizures.[64] Pain disorders are also common in patients with PNES. Among patients in epilepsy clinics, a diagnosis of fibromyalgia or chronic pain has an 85% positive predictive value for PNES.[65] PNES could be described as a disorder of communication, in which internal distress is conveyed somatically rather than verbally.

Patients with PNES have several psychiatric diagnosis comorbidities, including depression, anxiety, posttraumatic stress disorder, or a personality disorder. Bowman and colleagues[66] found that up to half of patients with PNES had 1 of these diagnoses on clinical interview using the DSM-III-R. We found similar results using DSM-IV criteria in patients with PNES.[67] The simultaneous presence of depression, a history of abuse, and a personality disorder may portend a worse prognosis for patients with PNES.[68] Comparisons between outcomes and prognosis in patients with ES and in patients with PNES could be of benefit to discern the effect of comorbidities on seizures.

To summarize, compared with healthy controls, patients with ES and with PNES perform worse on several NP measures, but there are few differences between ES and PNES groups on tests that would reliably differentiate ES from PNES. The impairments are believed to be caused by at least 3 factors: (1) patients with both ES and PNES were on AEDs, which may affect cognition; (2) structural lesions in the patients with ES and in some of the patients with PNES and ES, and (3) emotional factors contributing to cognitive impairment in the PNES group.[60] The psychological makeup of patients with PNES seems to be that they have personalities with anxiety, cognitive, and somatic distress. Along with these comorbidities, they have difficulty expressing and communicating distress verbally; they express themselves somatically. Family dysfunction is also present in PNES.

Overall, neuropsychological measures are not useful to make a diagnosis of PNES (vs epilepsy), because they are neither sensitive nor specific. However, psychological testing may be a useful adjunct once the diagnosis of PNES has been made, to characterize the psychopathology and mechanisms underlying the symptoms and clarify the psychiatric diagnosis (eg, somatoform disorder, dissociation).

LIMITATIONS AND PITFALLS OF VIDEO EEG

In most cases, the diagnosis of PNES with video EEG is clear and can be made with a high degree of confidence. There are limitations to video EEG, and it is important to be familiar with them to avoid serious diagnostic errors.

Ictal EEG has limitations because it may be negative in simple partial ES[69,70] and in some complex partial ES, especially those of frontal lobe onset.[67] Ictal EEG may also be uninterpretable or difficult to read if movements generate excessive artifact. Knowing what type of clinical seizures may be unaccompanied by ictal EEG changes is critical. The most common types of ES that are unaccompanied by ictal EEG changes are those without impairment of awareness (ie, simple partial ES). This type includes all simple partial ES with subjective phenomena (ie, auras), which can involve the 5 senses as well as psychic or experiential sensations.

The other types of simple partial ES that are commonly unaccompanied by ictal EEG changes are brief tonic phenomena such as those typical of frontal lobe ES. These phenomena are typically brief (5–30 seconds) and tonic, and may be hypermotor, but not usually as dramatically flailing or thrashing as PNES. In hypermotor seizures in which semiology is suspected of being psychogenic, given that both FLE and PNES are scalp EEG–negative, it can be impossible to prove based on EEG that such episodes are psychogenic. Brief episodes of *deja vu*, or fear, or tonic stiffening with no EEG changes, can be epileptic. Conversely, in favor of PNES is when the events never progress to clear ES, and if there is suggestibility (triggering them with placebo maneuvers). This situation is similar to psychogenic movement disorders (PMD), in which the diagnosis rests solely on phenomenology (ie, there is no equivalent of the EEG in PMD), and response to placebo or suggestion is considered a diagnostic criterion for a definite psychogenic mechanism.[68] A solid rule is that psychogenic events do not occur out of physiologic sleep, so that events that arise out of EEG-verified sleep are related to neurologic disorders (ES or parasomnias). ES with altered awareness and no EEG changes are rare, and if the clinical events are strongly suggestive of seizures, it is best to err on the side of treating them as epileptic, at least initially. More recently, video split-screen techniques have been shown to be helpful in diagnosing ES.[44]

Lack of ictal EEG changes only indicates that the episodes are nonepileptic, and nonepileptic does not always mean psychogenic. Other diagnoses must be considered before making a diagnosis of PNES. The most common diagnoses to consider are physiologic nonepileptic events, such as syncope, for episodes that occur during waking, and parasomnias for episodes that occur in sleep. When syncope (convulsive or not) is recorded on video EEG, the EEG proceeds through a stereotyped pattern of changes (delta slowing and suppression caused by lack of cerebral blood flow).[71,72]

Occasionally, in the absence of ictal EEG changes, the differentiation between seizure and parasomnia can be difficult. Hypnic jerks or sleep starts are benign myoclonic jerks that everyone has experienced on occasion. Although they resemble the jerks of myoclonic seizures, their occurrence only on falling asleep defines them as benign nonepileptic phenomena. Parasomnias are easily identified on video EEG by their occurrence in waking to stage 1 transition and having no EEG correlate associated with the jerks.[73] Restless legs syndrome and periodic limb movements of sleep also may interfere with sleep; however, no ictal EEG changes are seen with these disorders.

A common myth is that a recorded episode with a negative EEG is all that is required to make a diagnosis of PNES, and this is grossly inaccurate. A negative EEG can only be interpreted in the context of the semiology of the event in question. Thus, both the video and EEG must be available. (The diagnosis could be more accurate with video alone than with EEG alone, when differences in ictal semiology are classified by the informed observer.)

Unlike the definitive diagnosis of brain tumors, the closest test to a biopsy for distinguishing epilepsy from PNES would be intracranial monitoring. The risk and morbidity associated with craniotomy and grid or depth electrode placement outweighs the use in patients with a suspicion of PNES. In the absence of the definitive confirmation of the diagnosis, there is no way to prove that the PNES diagnosis is correct even when there is a high degree of certainty. Ramsay and colleagues[74] described the limitations of scalp EEG and reported the use of depth electrodes on scalp-negative EEGs. Subsequent EEG monitoring revealed that patients with epilepsy had an epileptic focus in either the mesial (n = 8) or inferior frontal (n = 2) areas.

As noted earlier, we conducted a study of the interrater reliability of the diagnosis by video EEG,[18] sampling a group of epileptologists, and found that, for the diagnosis of epilepsy, there was substantial agreement (κ = 0.69, 95% confidence interval [CI] 0.51–0.86). For the diagnosis of PNES, there was moderate agreement (κ = 0.57, 95% CI 0.39–0.76). For physiologic nonepileptic events, the agreement was low (κ = 0.09, 95% CI 0.02–0.27). The overall κ statistic across all 3 diagnostic categories was moderate at 0.56 (95% CI 0.41–0.73).[18] The investigators noted that the diagnosis in this study was, intentionally but artificially, based solely on video EEG recordings, which does not reflect clinical reality, whereas the actual diagnosis of PNES is made by a combination of patient history (neurologic and psychiatric), examination, and video EEG monitoring. The study underscored that there is a certain component of subjective, artful judgment. When used properly, video EEG allows the diagnosis of paroxysmal seizure–like events, and in particular the diagnosis of PNES, with a high degree of confidence.

False Positives in EEG

Having a report of a prior abnormal EEG is a common problem. Many patients with PNES seen at epilepsy centers have had previous EEGs interpreted as epileptiform. A common error is that the episodic symptoms are not really suggestive of seizures (ie, nonspecific symptoms such as light-headedness, dizziness, and numbness), and the diagnosis of seizures is entirely based on the (over-read) EEG. In this situation, it is essential to obtain and review the tracing previously read as epileptiform, because no amount of normal subsequent EEGs will cancel the previous "abnormal" one. When reviewed, most will turn out to show normal variants that were overinterpreted as epileptiform.[75–77] However, obtaining prior EEGs can be difficult. First, records are not always available or accessible, and second, not all digital EEG systems are compatible. In this regard, software that allows one to read any digital EEG format is valuable. The most common errors in EEG interpretation, and the main source of over-reading, are benign temporal sharp transients, or wicket spikes.[77] In general, the threshold for considering a sharp transient epileptiform must be high. Criteria include asymmetric contour (upslope steeper than downslope), different frequency and ampli-tude than ongoing background, diphasic or triphasic morphology, after-going slow wave, and disruption background. In addition, contrary to a common misconception, phase reversal is not one of the criteria. Phase reversals only reflect the maximum location of a discharge.[75–77] In children, an additional issue is the frequent coexisting benign focal epileptiform discharges (BFEDC), which are frequently seen in asymp-tomatic children.

THE USEFULNESS OF AEDS FOR REFRACTORY SEIZURES

Treatment of PNES is beyond the scope of this article [78]; however, given that patients with FLE can be refractory to AEDs, and that AEDs do not treat PNES[79] and can exac-erbate PNES,[12] it does address the recent research on AEDs. One pharmacologic question that has been addressed recently has been the effect of withdrawing AEDs from patients with lone PNES. Given that most patients with PNES are prescribed AEDs, Oto and colleagues[80] studied whether withdrawal of AEDs can be performed safely in patients with PNES in a prospective evaluation of safety and outcome. Seventy-eight patients with PNES who satisfied a standardized set of criteria for excluding the diagnosis of coexisting or underlying epilepsy had their AEDs withdrawn (64 as outpatients, 14 as inpatients). PNES frequency declined in the group as a whole during the period of the study (follow-up 6–12 months) in all individuals except for 8 patients in whom there was a transient increase. Fourteen patients reported new physical symptoms after withdrawal; however, no serious adverse events were reported. The investigators concluded that, with appropriate diagnostic investigation and surveillance during follow-up, withdrawal of AED can be achieved safely in patients with PNES.

SUMMARY

Differentiating PNES from FLE can be challenging, and the diagnosis of PNES can be difficult to distinguish by history alone. Physical signs, patient characteristics, and neuropsychological testing are helpful adjuncts to the video EEG to confirm the diag-nosis. The first phase of treatment begins with the neurologist, as the findings of the video EEG monitoring are shared in a positive nonpejorative manner. Neurologists, psychiatrists, and psychologists must then continue to work together to diagnose comorbidities and effectively treat this difficult population. Interdisciplinary research and discussion, along with collaborative sponsorship between neurologic and psychi-atric institutes, will help move the field forward to address these difficult-to-treat pop-ulations with seizures.

REFERENCES

1. Benbadis SR, O'Neill E, Tatum WO, et al. Outcome of prolonged video-EEG moni-toring at a typical referral epilepsy center. Epilepsia 2004;45(9):1150–3.
2. Smith D, Defalla BA, Chadwick DW. The misdiagnosis of epilepsy and the management of refractory epilepsy in a specialist clinic. QJM 1999;92(1):15–23.
3. Scheepers B, Clough P, Pickles C. The misdiagnosis of epilepsy: findings of a population study. Seizure 1998;7(5):403–6.

4. Zaidi A, Clough P, Cooper P, et al. Misdiagnosis of epilepsy: many seizure-like attacks have a cardiovascular cause. J Am Coll Cardiol 2000;36(1):181–4.
5. Tinuper P, Provini F, Bisulli F, et al. Movement disorders in sleep: guidelines for differentiating epileptic from non-epileptic motor phenomena arising from sleep. Sleep Med Rev 2007;11(4):255–67.
6. Reuber M, Fernandez G, Bauer J, et al. Diagnostic delay in psychogenic nonepileptic seizures. Neurology 2002;58(3):493–5.
7. Carton S, Thompson PJ, Duncan JS. Non-epileptic seizures: patients' understanding and reaction to the diagnosis and impact on outcome. Seizure 2003; 12(5):287–94.
8. Nowack WJ. Epilepsy: a costly misdiagnosis. Clin Electroencephalogr 1997; 28(4):225–8.
9. Martin RC, Gilliam FG, Kilgore M, et al. Improved health care resource utilization following video-EEG-confirmed diagnosis of nonepileptic psychogenic seizures. Seizure 1998;7(5):385–90.
10. LaFrance WC Jr, Alper K, Babcock D, et al. Nonepileptic seizures treatment workshop summary. Epilepsy Behav 2006;8(3):451–61.
11. Gates JR, Luciano D, Devinsky O. The classification and treatment of nonepileptic events. In: Devinsky O, Theodore WH, editors. Epilepsy and behavior. New York: Wiley-Liss; 1991. p. 251–63. Chapter 18.
12. Niedermeyer E, Blumer D, Holscher E, et al. Classical hysterical seizures facilitated by anticonvulsant toxicity. Psychiatr Clin (Basel) 1970;3(2):71–84.
13. Dworetzky BA, Bubrick EJ, Szaflarski JP, et al. Nonepileptic psychogenic status: markedly prolonged psychogenic nonepileptic seizures. Epilepsy Behav 2010; 19(1):65–8.
14. LaFrance WC Jr, Benbadis SR. Avoiding the costs of unrecognized psychological nonepileptic seizures. Neurology 2006;66(11):1620–1.
15. Gates JR, Ramani V, Whalen S, et al. Ictal characteristics of pseudoseizures. Arch Neurol 1985;42(12):1183–7.
16. LaFrance WC Jr, Devinsky O. Treatment of nonepileptic seizures. Epilepsy Behav 2002;3(5 Suppl 1):S19–23.
17. Alsaadi TM, Thieman C, Shatzel A, et al. Video-EEG telemetry can be a crucial tool for neurologists experienced in epilepsy when diagnosing seizure disorders. Seizure 2004;13(1):32–4.
18. Benbadis SR, LaFrance WC Jr, Papandonatos GD, et al. Interrater reliability of EEG-video monitoring. Neurology 2009;73(11):843–6.
19. Cragar DE, Berry DT, Fakhoury TA, et al. A review of diagnostic techniques in the differential diagnosis of epileptic and nonepileptic seizures. Neuropsychol Rev 2002;12(1):31–64.
20. Smolowitz JL, Hopkins SC, Perrine T, et al. Diagnostic utility of an epilepsy monitoring unit. Am J Med Qual 2007;22(2):117–22.
21. Benbadis SR, Agrawal V, Tatum WO IV. How many patients with psychogenic nonepileptic seizures also have epilepsy? Neurology 2001;57(5):915–7.
22. Benbadis SR, LaFrance WC Jr. Clinical features and the role of video-EEG monitoring. In: Schachter SC, LaFrance WC Jr, editors. Gates and Rowan's Nonepileptic Seizures. 3rd edition. Cambridge: Cambridge University Press; 2010. p. 38–50. Chapter 4.
23. Chung SS, Gerber P, Kirlin KA. Ictal eye closure is a reliable indicator for psychogenic nonepileptic seizures. Neurology 2006;66(11):1730–1.
24. Syed TU, Arozullah AM, Suciu GP, et al. Do observer and self-reports of ictal eye closure predict psychogenic nonepileptic seizures? Epilepsia 2008;49(5):898–904.

25. Henry JA, Woodruff GHA. A diagnostic sign in states of apparent unconsciousness. Lancet 1978;2(8096):920–1.
26. Donati F, Kollar M, Pihan H, et al. Eyelids position - during epileptic versus psychogenic seizures [abstract: OPL145]. J Neurol Sci 2005;238(Suppl 1):S82–3.
27. Flügel D, Bauer J, Kaseborn U, et al. Closed eyes during a seizure indicate psychogenic etiology: a study with suggestive seizure provocation. J Epilepsy 1996;9(3):165–9.
28. Bergen D, Ristanovic R. Weeping as a common element of pseudoseizures. Arch Neurol 1993;50(10):1059–60.
29. Vossler DG, Haltiner AM, Schepp SK, et al. Ictal stuttering: a sign suggestive of psychogenic nonepileptic seizures. Neurology 2004;63(3):516–9.
30. Chabolla DR, Shih JJ. Postictal behaviors associated with psychogenic nonepileptic seizures. Epilepsy Behav 2006;9(2):307–11.
31. Wennberg R. Postictal coughing and noserubbing coexist in temporal lobe epilepsy. Neurology 2001;56(1):133–4.
32. Sen A, Scott C, Sisodiya SM. Stertorous breathing is a reliably identified sign that helps in the differentiation of epileptic from psychogenic non-epileptic convulsions: an audit. Epilepsy Res 2007;77(1):62–4.
33. Gröppel G, Kapitany T, Baumgartner C. Cluster analysis of clinical seizure semiology of psychogenic nonepileptic seizures. Epilepsia 2000;41(5):610–4.
34. Geyer JD, Payne TA, Drury I. The value of pelvic thrusting in the diagnosis of seizures and pseudoseizures. Neurology 2000;54(1):227–9.
35. Saygi S, Katz A, Marks DA, et al. Frontal lobe partial seizures and psychogenic seizures: comparison of clinical and ictal characteristics. Neurology 1992;42(7):1274–7.
36. Kanner AM, Morris HH, Luders H, et al. Supplementary motor seizures mimicking pseudoseizures: some clinical differences. Neurology 1990;40(9):1404–7.
37. Jobst BC, Williamson PD. Frontal lobe seizures. Psychiatr Clin North Am 2005;28(3):635–51.
38. Reuber M, Pukrop R, Bauer J, et al. Outcome in psychogenic nonepileptic seizures: 1 to 10-year follow-up in 164 patients. Ann Neurol 2003;53(3):305–11.
39. Trimble MR. Non-epileptic seizures. In: Halligan PW, Bass CM, Marshall JC, editors. Contemporary approaches to the study of hysteria: clinical and theoretical perspectives. Oxford: Oxford University Press; 2001. p. 143–54. Chapter 10.
40. de Timary P, Fouchet P, Sylin M, et al. Non-epileptic seizures: delayed diagnosis in patients presenting with electroencephalographic (EEG) or clinical signs of epileptic seizures. Seizure 2002;11:193–7.
41. Burneo JG, Martin R, Powell T, et al. Teddy bears: an observational finding in patients with non-epileptic events. Neurology 2003;61(5):714–5.
42. Devinsky O, Kelley K, Porter RJ, et al. Clinical and electroencephalographic features of simple partial seizures. Neurology 1988;38(9):1347–52.
43. Deacon C, Wiebe S, Blume WT, et al. Seizure identification by clinical description in temporal lobe epilepsy: how accurate are we? Neurology 2003;61(12):1686–9.
44. Tinuper P, Grassi C, Bisulli F, et al. Split-screen synchronized display. A useful video-EEG technique for studying paroxysmal phenomena. Epileptic Disord 2004;6(1):27–30.
45. Ossenblok P, de Munck JC, Colon A, et al. Magnetoencephalography is more successful for screening and localizing frontal lobe epilepsy than electroencephalography. Epilepsia 2007;48(11):2139–49.

46. Chen DK, So YT, Fisher RS. Use of serum prolactin in diagnosing epileptic seizures: report of the Therapeutics and Technology Assessment Subcommittee of the American Academy of Neurology. Neurology 2005;65(5):668–75.
47. Trimble MR. Serum prolactin in epilepsy and hysteria. Br Med J 1978;2(6153): 1682.
48. Lowe MR, De Toledo JC, Rabinstein AA, et al. Correspondence: MRI evidence of mesial temporal sclerosis in patients with psychogenic nonepileptic seizures. Neurology 2001;56(6):821–3.
49. Reuber M, Fernandez G, Helmstaedter C, et al. Evidence of brain abnormality in patients with psychogenic nonepileptic seizures. Epilepsy Behav 2002;3(3): 249–54.
50. Ettinger AB, Coyle PK, Jandorf L, et al. Postictal SPECT in epileptic versus nonepileptic seizures. J Epilepsy 1998;11:67–73.
51. LaFrance WC Jr. Psychogenic nonepileptic seizures. Curr Opin Neurol 2008; 21(2):195–201.
52. Binder LM, Kindermann SS, Heaton RK, et al. Neuropsychologic impairment in patients with nonepileptic seizures. Arch Clin Neuropsychol 1998;13(6): 513–22.
53. Kalogjera-Sackellares D, Sackellares JC. Impaired motor function in patients with psychogenic pseudoseizures. Epilepsia 2001;42(12):1600–6.
54. Binder LM, Salinsky MC, Smith SP. Psychological correlates of psychogenic seizures. J Clin Exp Neuropsychol 1994;16(4):524–30.
55. Drane DL, Williamson DJ, Stroup ES, et al. Cognitive impairment is not equal in patients with epileptic and psychogenic nonepileptic seizures. Epilepsia 2006; 47(11):1879–86.
56. Cragar DE, Berry DT, Fakhoury TA, et al. Performance of patients with epilepsy or psychogenic non-epileptic seizures on four measures of effort. Clin Neuropsychol 2006;20(3):552–66.
57. Schramke CJ, Valeri A, Valeriano JP, et al. Using the Minnesota Multiphasic Inventory 2, EEGs, and clinical data to predict nonepileptic events. Epilepsy Behav 2007;11(3):343–6.
58. Bortz JJ, Prigatano GP, Blum D, et al. Differential response characteristics in nonepileptic and epileptic seizure patients on a test of verbal learning and memory. Neurology 1995;45(11):2029–34.
59. Dodrill CB, Holmes MD. Part summary: psychological and neuropsychological evaluation of the patient with non-epileptic seizures. In: Gates JR, Rowan AJ, editors. Non-epileptic seizures. 2nd edition. Boston: Butterworth-Heinemann; 2000. p. 169–81. Chapter 13.
60. Swanson SJ, Springer JA, Benbadis SR, et al. Cognitive and psychological functioning in patients with non-epileptic seizures. In: Gates JR, Rowan AJ, editors. Non-epileptic Seizures. 2nd edition. Boston: Butterworth-Heinemann; 2000. p. 123–37. Chapter 9.
61. Anschel DJ, Dolce S, Schwartzman A, et al. A blinded pilot study of artwork in a comprehensive epilepsy center population. Epilepsy Behav 2005;6(2): 196–202.
62. Galimberti CA, Ratti MT, Murelli R, et al. Patients with psychogenic nonepileptic seizures, alone or epilepsy-associated, share a psychological profile distinct from that of epilepsy patients. J Neurol 2003;250(3):338–46.
63. Krawetz P, Fleisher W, Pillay N, et al. Family functioning in subjects with pseudoseizures and epilepsy. J Nerv Ment Dis 2001;189(1):38–43.

64. van Merode T, Twellaar M, Kotsopoulos IA, et al. Psychological characteristics of patients with newly developed psychogenic seizures. J Neurol Neurosurg Psychiatry 2004;75(8):1175–7.
65. Benbadis SR. A spell in the epilepsy clinic and a history of "chronic pain" or "fibromyalgia" independently predict a diagnosis of psychogenic seizures. Epilepsy Behav 2005;6(2):264–5.
66. Bowman ES, Markand ON. Psychodynamics and psychiatric diagnoses of pseudoseizure subjects. Am J Psychiatry 1996;153(1):57–63.
67. LaFrance WC Jr, Syc S. Depression and symptoms affect quality of life in psychogenic nonepileptic seizures. Neurology 2009;73(5):366–71.
68. Kanner AM, Parra J, Frey M, et al. Psychiatric and neurologic predictors of psychogenic pseudoseizure outcome. Neurology 1999;53(5):933–8.
69. Devinsky O, Sato S, Kufta CV, et al. Electroencephalographic studies of simple partial seizures with subdural electrode recordings. Neurology 1989;39(4):527–33.
70. Sperling MR, O'Connor MJ. Auras and subclinical seizures: characteristics and prognostic significance. Ann Neurol 1990;28(3):320–8.
71. Benbadis SR, Chichkova R. Psychogenic pseudosyncope: an underestimated and provable diagnosis. Epilepsy Behav 2006;9(1):106–10.
72. Sheldon RS, Koshman ML, Murphy WF. Electroencephalographic findings during presyncope and syncope induced by tilt table testing. Can J Cardiol 1998;14(6):811–6.
73. Montagna P, Liguori R, Zucconi M, et al. Physiological hypnic myoclonus. Electroencephalogr Clin Neurophysiol 1988;70(2):172–6.
74. Ramsay RE, Cohen A, Brown MC. Coexisting epilepsy and non-epileptic seizures. In: Rowan AJ, Gates JR, editors. Non-epileptic Seizures. 1st edition. Stoneham (MA): Butterworth-Heinemann; 1993. p. 47–54. Chapter 6.
75. Benbadis SR, Tatum WO. Overintepretation of EEGs and misdiagnosis of epilepsy. J Clin Neurophysiol 2003;20(1):42–4.
76. Benbadis SR. Errors in EEGs and the misdiagnosis of epilepsy: importance, causes, consequences, and proposed remedies. Epilepsy Behav 2007;11(3):257–62.
77. Benbadis SR, Lin K. Errors in EEG interpretation and misdiagnosis of epilepsy. Which EEG patterns are overread? Eur Neurol 2008;59(5):267–71.
78. LaFrance WC Jr, Barry JJ. Update on treatments of psychological nonepileptic seizures. Epilepsy Behav 2005;7(3):364–74.
79. Duncan R. The withdrawal of antiepileptic drugs in patients with non-epileptic seizures: safety considerations. Expert Opin Drug Saf 2006;5(5):609–13.
80. Oto M, Espie C, Pelosi A, et al. The safety of antiepileptic drug withdrawal in patients with non-epileptic seizures. J Neurol Neurosurg Psychiatry 2005;76(12):1682–5.

Ictal Panic and Interictal Panic Attacks: Diagnostic and Therapeutic Principles

Andres M. Kanner, MD[a,b,c,d,*]

KEYWORDS

- Postictal panic • Temporal lobe epilepsy
- Hippocampal sclerosis • Generalized anxiety disorders
- Major depressive episodes

"Is it a panic attack or is it ictal panic?" This question illustrates one of the examples of the borderlands between epilepsy and psychiatric disorders. The similarities of the clinical manifestations of the 2 types of paroxysmal episodes have resulted in frequent diagnostic errors.[1–3] Indeed, it is not infrequent for simple partial seizures of mesial temporal lobe origin presenting as panic episodes to be treated as panic attacks until the patient develops a secondarily generalized tonic-clonic seizure or is witnessed to have a complex partial seizure.

In epilepsy, psychiatric symptoms are classified into periictal and interictal in relation to their temporal occurrence to seizures.[4] Periictal symptoms are of 3 types: preictal (preceding a seizure), ictal (presenting as a seizure), and postictal (occurring within 120 hours of a seizure). Interictal symptoms occur independently of seizures. Often, ictal and postictal panic can be identified in the same patient suffering from interictal panic attacks. Furthermore, interictal symptoms can worsen in severity during the postictal period.

Disclosures: A.M.K. has received research grant funding from Glaxo-Smith-Kline, Novartis, and Pfizer. He has received honoraria for serving as a consultant to Pfizer.
[a] Department of Neurological Sciences, Rush University Medical Center, Rush Medical College at Rush University, 1653 West Congress Parkway, Chicago, IL 60612, USA
[b] Department of Psychiatry, Rush University Medical Center, Rush Medical College at Rush University, 1653 West Congress Parkway, Chicago, IL 60612, USA
[c] Laboratory of EEG and Video-EEG-Telemetry, Rush University Medical Center, 1653 West Congress Parkway, Chicago, IL 60612, USA
[d] Section of Epilepsy and Rush Epilepsy Center, Rush University Medical Center, 1653 West Congress Parkway, Chicago, IL 60612, USA
* Department of Neurologic Sciences, Rush Medical College at Rush University, Rush University Medical Center, 1653 West Congress Parkway, Chicago, IL 60612.
E-mail address: akanner@rush.edu

Neurol Clin 29 (2011) 163–175
doi:10.1016/j.ncl.2010.11.002
0733-8619/11/$ – see front matter © 2011 Elsevier Inc. All rights reserved.

The involvement of common neuroanatomical structures and the pathogenic role played by the same neurotransmitters (serotonin [5-HT], γ-aminobutyric acid [GABA]) probably explain the similar clinical manifestations and relatively high comorbidity between periictal panic symptoms and interictal panic disorders (PDs). This article reviews these data and provides practical strategies that can be used in the differential diagnosis and treatment of ictal and postictal panic episodes and panic attacks.

EPIDEMIOLOGIC ASPECTS

Whereas ictal panic is the classic expression of anxiety symptoms presenting as a simple partial seizure, postictal panic is a seizure-related symptom that often goes unrecognized but is relatively frequent. Ictal panic is the most frequent type of simple partial seizures, presenting primarily with psychiatric symptoms and corresponding to 60% of all psychiatric auras.[5,6] Postictal panic has been identified in 10% of 100 consecutive patients with treatment-resistant partial epilepsy, occurring during the postictal period (defined in this study as the 72 hours following a seizure or cluster of seizures) of more than 50% of their seizures and having a median duration of 24 hours.[7] In that same study, 39% of patients reported postictal symptoms of agoraphobia.

Epileptic patients have been found to suffer more frequently from interictal PD than nonepileptic people. For example, one population-based study performed in Canada found a 12-month prevalence rate of interictal PD to be 5.6%, almost 3-fold higher than in nonepileptic subjects (2%).[8] A prevalence of 5.1% was found in a prospective study of 97 patients with treatment-resistant epilepsy.

Ictal panic has been typically associated with partial seizure disorders of mesial temporal origin.[3,9–12] However, seizures of frontal lobe origin have also been associated with ictal panic.[13] When the seizures involve the orbitofrontal cortex in the nondominant hemisphere, they may present with sudden panic-stricken screams, with nonverbal screams or verbal vocalizations of "help me…help me," or "Oh my God!" These differ from the classic ictal panic in that the ictal panic occurs in the setting of complex partial seizures and patients are not aware of the distressing affect and associated phenomena, which include complex automatisms. Seizures of parietal lobe origin have also been associated with ictal panic on rare occasions. For example, Alemayehu and colleagues[14] reported 2 cases with ictal panic originating from the right parietal lobe where a brain tumor was identified. Intracranial monitoring documented correlations between the symptoms of fear and restricted regional parietal cortical discharges. Surgical resections of the lesions (1 total and 1 subtotal) resulted in either complete recovery or improvement.

PATHOPHYSIOLOGY

Do ictal panic and PDs share common pathogenic mechanisms? The similarity of clinical semiology between these 2 types of paroxysmal events (see later discussion) and the relatively high comorbidity of interictal PD in patients with ictal panic may be explained by the existence of common pathogenic mechanisms operant in both conditions. These conditions include (1) structural and functional abnormalities of common neuroanatomical structures and (2) disturbances of the function of common neurotransmitters, including 5-HT and GABA.

Abnormalities in Common Neuroanatomical Structures

Panicky symptoms are typical of temporal lobe epilepsy (TLE) of mesial temporal origin with particular involvement of the amygdala. In fact, electric stimulation of the amygdala produces many of symptoms of panic attacks (eg, intense fear, dizziness, nausea, tachycardia, chest pain, and depersonalization).[8,9]

In patients with primary PD, volumetric measurements of mesial temporal structures have demonstrated a smaller volume of the amygdala. For example, Massana and colleagues[15] measured the volumes of amygdalae, hippocampi, and temporal lobes in 12 drug-free symptomatic patients with primary PD and 12 case-matched healthy controls. Patients with PD had bilateral smaller volumes of the amygdala than the controls, but no differences were found in either hippocampi or temporal lobes. In a separate study, Cendes and colleagues[16] performed magnetic resonance imaging (MRI) volumetric measurements of amygdala and hippocampus in 50 patients with intractable TLE. Among them, 17 patients (34%) had a clear history of ictal panic accompanied by a rising epigastric sensation as the initial manifestation of their habitual attacks. The amygdala volumes in this group were significantly smaller (mean, 2131.6 mm^3) than the volumes of the 33 patients without these symptoms (mean, 2561.5 mm^3). Both patient groups had smaller mean amygdala volumes when compared with normal controls (mean, 2828.2 mm^3). Postoperative pathology correlated well with volumetric atrophy.

Evidence of a pivotal role of the amygdala in anxiety disorders has been also suggested by data from animal models. For example, the central nucleus of the amygdala has been found to be primarily responsible for mediating fear (emotional reaction to aversive events) and anxiety (the apprehension of an imminent aversive event) in the fear-conditioning animal model of anxiety.[17] Furthermore, stimulation of this nucleus resulted in fearlike responses (reminiscent of symptoms of panic attacks in humans) such as freezing, shivering, and autonomic nervous system activation, including tachycardia and increase in blood pressure. On the other hand, bilateral lesions of the central nucleus of the rabbit amygdala have resulted in loss of the fear-induced tachycardia to a conditioned auditory fear stimulus,[18] whereas lesions of the central nucleus of the rat eliminated a fear-potentiated startle response.[19]

Structural abnormalities of mesial structures are not restricted to the amygdala but have been found in hippocampal formations and parahippocampal gyri and have resulted in smaller total volumes of the temporal lobes. Thus, Massana and colleagues[20] investigated the gray matter density in 18 outpatients with PD and 18 healthy subjects using a voxel-based morphometry approach. They found that gray matter density of the left parahippocampal gyrus was significantly lower in patients with PD compared with healthy subjects. In a separate study, Vythilingam and colleagues[21] measured the volume of the temporal lobes and hippocampi in 13 patients with primary PD and 14 healthy control subjects. They found that the mean volume of both temporal lobes was significantly smaller in PD compared with healthy subjects, but there was no significant difference in the volume of the hippocampi between the 2 groups.

Uchida and colleagues[22] conducted volumetric studies of temporal lobe structures in 11 patients with primary PD and 11 controls matched for age, sex, handedness, socio-economic status, and years of education. They found that in patients with PD, the mean volume of the left temporal lobe was 9% less than that of controls; although the mean volume of the right temporal lobes were also less, the difference only reached a trend (7%, $P = .06$). Furthermore, there was a trend in the difference of the volumes of the right amygdala (8%, t21 = 1.83, $P = .08$), left amygdala (5%, t21 = 1.78, $P = .09$), and left hippocampus (9%, t21 = 1.93, $P = .07$) in patients when compared with controls. Of note, these investigators found a positive correlation between left hippocampal volume and duration of PD (r = 0.67, $P = .025$), with recent cases showing more reduction than older cases.

Functional abnormalities have been demonstrated in temporal and extratemporal lobe structures. First, positron emission tomographic (PET) studies conducted in healthy humans demonstrated increased perfusion in the amygdala when they were shown images of fearful as opposed to happy faces.[23] Likewise, PET studies targeting the 5-HT$_{1A}$ receptor have demonstrated involvement of temporal and extratemporal limbic structures. For example, in one study of 9 symptomatic untreated patients with PD, 7 patients who recovered on selective serotonin reuptake inhibitor (SSRI) medication and 19 healthy volunteers underwent PET scan using the 5-HT$_{1A}$ tracer ^{11}C-WAY-100635.[24] In comparison with controls, both presynaptic and postsynaptic 5-HT$_{1A}$ receptor binding was reduced in patients, with the most significant reductions being in the raphe, orbitofrontal cortex, temporal cortex, and amygdala. In recovered patients, presynaptic binding was reduced but there was no significant reduction in postsynaptic binding. In another study of 16 unmedicated symptomatic outpatients with PD (7 of whom also suffered from a mood disorder of mild severity) and 15 matched healthy controls, PET studies were performed to target the 5-HT$_{1A}$ receptor with the selective 5-HT$_{1A}$R radioligand ^{18}F-trans-4-fluoro-N-2-[4-(2-methoxyphenyl) piperazin-1-yl]ethyl]-N-(2-pyridyl)cyclohexanecarboxamide (FCWAY).[25] A reduction in binding of 5-HT$_{1A}$ receptor was found in the anterior cingulate, posterior cingulated, and raphe in patients compared with controls. The binding of 5-HT$_{1A}$ receptors did not differ between patients with PD and patients with comorbid depression, whereas the latter differed significantly from controls in that 5-HT$_{1A}$ receptor binding was reduced in cingulate and raphe nuclei.

Disturbances of the Function of Some Common Neurotransmitters

5-HT has been found to play an important pathogenic role in PD and epilepsy.[26,27] The role of 5-HT in PD can be appreciated in the data from the PET studies discussed earlier. Furthermore, the prophylactic effect of SSRIs and tricyclic antidepressant imipramine 5-HT in PD is an expression of the pathogenic role of 5-HT.[28,29]

The pathogenic role of 5-HT in epilepsy has been demonstrated in various animal models of epilepsy, illustrated in particular by the genetically epilepsy prone rat whose brain reveals deficits in serotonergic arborization and decreased postsynaptic 5-HT$_{1A}$ receptor density in hippocampus.[30–32] Conversely, drugs that enhance serotonergic transmission, such as the SSRIs sertraline and fluoxetine cause a reduction in seizure frequency in a dose-dependent manner that correlates to the extracellular thalamic serotonergic thalamic concentration. In addition, an antiepileptic effect of 5-HT$_{1A}$ receptors has been correlated to a membrane hyperpolarizing response, which is associated with increased potassium conductance in hippocampus-kindled seizures in cats and in intrahippocampal kainic acid–induced seizures in freely moving rats.[33,34] The pathogenic role of 5-HT in epilepsy has been reviewed in greater detail elsewhere.[35,36]

GABA is another neurotransmitter with important pathogenic roles in PD and epilepsy. It is a neurotransmitter that promotes the inhibition of neuronal excitability through the chloride ion channels. In fact, several of the commonly used antiepileptic drugs (AEDs) such as benzodiazepines, barbiturates, tiagabine, and vigabatrin exert their antiepileptic effect by increasing synaptic GABA concentrations.[37] Furthermore, the convulsant agent pentylenetetrazol (a model for generalized seizures) blocks GABA$_A$ receptor function and facilitates the development of anxiety symptoms.[38] It has been suggested that anxiety disorders may be caused by defective neuroinhibitory processes that are mediated in part through GABA. In patients with PD, the pathogenic role of GABA is suggested by the induction of panic symptoms with the benzodiazepine antagonist flumazenil[39]; these data are also supported by the demonstration of widespread decreased binding of flumazenil to benzodiazepine receptor in patients with PD.[40,41] The question is then raised whether downregulation of these receptors is a consequence of exposure to stress or whether a preexisting low level of benzodiazepine receptor density may be a genetic risk factor for the development of stress-related anxiety disorders.

CLINICAL PRESENTATIONS:(DISTINGUISHING ICTAL PANIC, PANIC ATTACK AND POSTICTAL PANIC)

It is not unusual that patients with ictal and/or postictal panic are mistakenly diagnosed as suffering from a PD. Yet a careful history can usually provide enough clues to reach the correct diagnosis, which are summarized in the following sections.[42,43]

Duration

Ictal panic is a very brief event lasting less than 30 seconds. It may evolve into a complex partial or secondarily generalized tonic-clonic seizure, which may last between 60 and 90 seconds on average. Yet, rarely, partial complex status epilepticus associated with isolated fear has been reported.[44,45] In such cases, panic symptoms may last for hours, intermixed with a confusional state. In contrast, the duration of panic attacks can range between 5 and 20 minutes and at times may persist for several hours. Postictal panic can appear within 120 hours of a seizure or cluster of seizures and was found to have a median duration of 24 hours and to range between 1 and 120 hours.

Intensity of the Panic Experience

The sensation of fear in ictal panic is mild to moderate and rarely reaches the intensity of a panic attack. In fact, Williams[5] described ictal fear as unnatural rather than seeming more reality based. In contrast, panic attacks are characterized by a very intense fear or panic often referred as a "feeling of impending doom."[46] It is not infrequent for patients to become extremely apprehensive about experiencing another panic attack that may then lead to the development of a full-blown agoraphobia. In postictal panic, the intensity of the fear sensation is closer to that of ictal panic.

Timing of Occurrence

Ictal panic can occur in awake and sleep states, whereas panic attacks rarely occur out of sleep.[47–49] Postictal panic is typically reported in awake states.

Stereotypic Features

Ictal panic is a stereotypic paroxysmal event, whereas panic attacks may or may not be stereotypic, with respect to duration and associated symptoms.[50] Likewise, postictal panic episodes may or may not be stereotypic in their clinical manifestations and duration.

Associated Symptoms

Unresponsiveness

Typically, patients with ictal panic may be partially or totally aware of their surroundings; in the former scenario, patients report that their concentration is affected during and around the ictus after which they must exert greater effort to achieve the same cognitive tasks. When ictal panic evolves to a complex partial seizure, patients become unaware of their surroundings. Yet in complex partial seizures of mesial temporal origin in the nondominant hemisphere, responsiveness may be preserved and patients may continue interacting with others in a coherent manner during the ictus but become amnesic to the event when questioned postictally. Conversely, in panic attacks, the patients' awareness of their surroundings and responsiveness is typically preserved; yet, in the case of severe panic attacks, the patients may be overwhelmed by the sensation of impending doom to the point where they may not be able to report what is going on around them.[50] In addition, a panic attack associated with profound hyperventilation could also conceivably lead to a "subjective perception" of loss of consciousness. In postictal panic episodes, patients are fully aware of their surroundings.

Autonomic symptoms

These symptoms are present in panic attacks and ictal panic. Among these symptoms, paroxysmal salivation is a pathognomic autonomic symptom in seizures of mesial temporal or insular origin; it has never been reported in panic attacks or postictal panic. Salivation may often be copious and associated with nausea and vomiting, particularly in ictal panic originating in mesial temporal structures in the nondominant hemisphere. Postictal nausea or vomiting has been reported in some patients.

Chest discomfort including chest pain, palpitations, and hyperventilation is a common symptom in ictal panic and panic attacks.[43,50] Of note, intense hyperventilation in panic attacks can lead to carpal spasms that can be confused with dystonic posturing of seizures of temporal lobe origin. All these symptoms may also be present in postictal panic.

Symptoms of derealization, depersonalization, déjà vu, and jamais vu

These symptoms are characteristic of ictal activity of mesial temporal origin and are often associated with ictal panic. Yet they may also occur in primary or interictal panic and generalized anxiety disorders.

Age of Onset

Ictal fear can begin at any age, although they are more likely to occur after late childhood or early adolescence. On the other hand, PD usually begins in late adolescence or early adulthood, but onset in the 30s and even 40s is common. In fact, PD in childhood presents as school phobia.[51] Symptoms that are suggestive of panic attacks and begin in older age groups should be vigorously investigated for the possibility of a seizure disorder. Data on postictal panic in childhood are not available.

PSYCHIATRIC COMORBIDITIES

Recognition of the semiology of ictal panic, panic attacks, and postictal panic is pivotal to reach an accurate diagnosis. Yet it is important to remember that these episodes do not occur in an isolated manner. For example, patients with ictal panic have a high risk of suffering as well from an interictal PD and generalized anxiety disorder. For example, in a study of 12 consecutive patients with ictal panic, Mintzer and Lopez[52] found a comorbid PD in 4 patients (33%). One of these patients developed panic attacks only after epilepsy surgery and another worsened after surgery, whereas the other 2 had panic attacks that were not related to any surgical procedure. Two patients had other anxiety disorders, and 8 patients (67%) had current or past depression independent of the presence of PD.

Furthermore, ictal panic is associated with an increased risk of postsurgical mood disorders in patients undergoing a temporal lobectomy. For example, Kohler and colleagues[53] compared 22 patients with ictal panic and matched groups with other auras and no auras. Neurologic and neuropsychological evaluations before, 1 to 2 months after, and 1 year after temporal lobectomy were reviewed for mood and anxiety disorders and psychotropic medication treatment. Most patients in the 3 groups experienced mood and anxiety disorders before surgery. Mood and anxiety disorders declined in the control but not in the ictal fear group after surgery. Presence of auras at 1 year after surgery was not related to psychiatric outcome. Postoperative mood and anxiety disorders were more common in patients with persistence of seizures and in those in the ictal panic group who were seizure free.

Likewise, patients with PD are likely to suffer from generalized anxiety and depressive disorders and patients with ictal panic and PD often experience postictal panic episodes, which in addition to the panic symptoms may be associated with other symptoms of anxiety and depression.[50]

DIAGNOSTIC TESTING
Electroencephalographic Studies

Although routine electroencephalographic (EEG) studies can help identify epileptiform activity and suggest the presence of a partial seizure disorder, they still cannot identify whether the panic episodes are the expression of ictal panic, postictal panic episodes, or interictal panic attacks. On the other hand, a normal routine EEG study is not unusual in patients with ictal and postictal panic because epileptogenic areas in the amygdala or mesial frontal regions are characteristic for their small electric field that often fails to be detected with scalp recordings. Clearly, when ordering routine EEG studies in these patients, anterior temporal and basal temporal electrodes should be requested to increase the yield of identifying epileptiform activity.

Clearly, a careful description of the events is the best way to reach a diagnosis. However, when there is still confusion, capturing the events on video-EEG (V-EEG) monitoring study may be a solution. Nonetheless, one of the limitations of V-EEG is that simple partial seizures often fail to be detected with scalp recordings and this is a particular problem of epileptiform activity, originating from amygdala because its electric field is characteristically restricted. It is not rare, therefore, that patients with ictal panic may have repeated routine and interictal V-EEG monitoring devoid of any epileptiform activity. Occasionally, even complex partial seizures in which the ictal activity remains restricted to mesial structures fail to be detected with scalp electrodes.[54] To minimize this problem, it is advised to use sphenoidal electrodes inserted under fluoroscopic guidance to ensure that the recording electrode tip is positioned immediately below the foramen ovale.[55]

Estimation of Prolactin Levels

The measurement of postictal serum prolactin levels has been used in the differential diagnosis of epileptic and psychogenic seizures. One limitation is the need to draw samples no later than 15 to 20 minutes after a seizure. Serum concentrations can increase in 30% to 40% of seizures of mesial temporal origin (even in the absence of any obvious change on the surface EEG recording), but a negative result does not rule out the diagnosis.[56]

A cautionary note is that abrupt or rapid discontinuation of benzodiazepines during the V-EEG study may facilitate the occurrence of panic attacks or epileptic seizures.[57] Thus, the use of this medication should be slowly tapered before performing the V-EEG study or lowered only slightly at the time of admission.

Brain MRI Studies

The presence of a structural lesion in mesial temporal structures or of a hippocampal atrophy should raise suspicion of ictal panic, particularly when the panic episode evolves into a complex partial seizure. However, as with routine EEG studies, these findings do not exclude the possibility of interictal panic attacks and postictal panic episodes in addition to or in the absence of ictal panic.

Some auxiliary tests should be considered when suspecting a diagnosis of PD.[58] These tests include thyroid function tests because hyperthyroid disease should be ruled out. Furthermore, an echocardiography should be considered given the high comorbidity of PD and mitral valve prolapse, which may be associated with the symptoms of pressure in the chest and the bouts of paroxysmal tachycardia. It has been suggested that intravenous sodium lactate infusion could be used as a diagnostic tool to confirm a diagnosis of PD, because this infusion can trigger a panic attack with an 80% to 90% probability in patients with PD, whereas in patients without such history the risk is less than 10%. Yet because a significant percentage of patients with ictal panic may also suffer from comorbid interictal PD, the trigger of a panic attack with sodium lactate may result in the false-negative diagnosis of a seizure disorder.

DIFFERENTIAL DIAGNOSIS

PD and ictal panic should also be distinguished from several medical conditions, particular rare disorders associated with paroxysmal cardiac arrhythmias.[50,58] These conditions include the Romano-Ward syndrome, the prolonged QT syndrome, carcinoid syndrome, hypoglycemia, pheochromocytoma, and Cushing syndrome. Other conditions to consider include alcohol withdrawal or other sedating drug use withdrawal, illicit drug effects (amphetamines, cocaine, and marijuana-induced tachycardia), vertigo-related disorders, and asthma.

TREATMENT OPTIONS

Before any treatment strategy is put into place, the following question need to be addressed: Is the panic event the expression of (1) ictal panic only, (2) ictal and postictal panic episodes, (3) comorbid ictal panic with or without postictal panic and interictal panic attacks, or (4) interictal panic attacks only. In addition, careful assessment for comorbid depressive disorders is of the essence either in primary PD, interictal panic attacks, and/or ictal panic.

Ictal Panic and Postictal Panic

The treatment of ictal and postictal panic consists on the eradication of epileptic seizures, initially with AEDs, and a presurgical evaluation must be considered if seizures persist after 2 monotherapy trials with AEDs at optimal doses. The choice of AED has to factor in the presence of comorbid mood and anxiety disorders, including panic attacks. In such cases, AEDs with positive psychotropic properties should be chosen first (eg, carbamazepine, oxcarbazepine, lamotrigine, valproic acid, and pregabalin). Of these AEDs, pregabalin has been found to be effective in the treatment of generalized anxiety disorders, whereas valproic acid has yielded therapeutic effects in PD.[59,60]

Likewise, AEDs known to have negative psychotropic properties, including barbiturates, topiramate, levetiracetam, zonisamide, and vigabatrin, should be used with extreme caution because these AEDs may worsen the comorbid mood and anxiety disorders.[61] Tiagabine is a GABAergic AED that has been used by psychiatrists in the treatment of anxiety disorders but may be associated with increased risk of depressive episodes.

Anterior temporal lobectomy is the most frequently performed surgical procedure in patients with ictal panic. The therapeutic yield has ranged between 50% and 70% of freedom from disabling seizures (complex partial and secondarily generalized tonic-clonic seizures). However, total seizure freedom that includes no ictal panic has been reported in 30% to 40% of case series. If anterior temporal lobectomies are performed, patients need to be monitored for postsurgical psychiatric complications presenting as mood and anxiety disorders.

Panic Attacks

Either as an expression of primary or interictal PD, panic attacks are treated with antidepressant medications of the SSRI and serotonin-norepinephrine reuptake inhibitor (SNRI) families.[28,29,37] Comorbid mood, generalized anxiety disorders, and various types of phobias, in particular agoraphobia, are relatively frequent in patients with PDs; antidepressant drugs with therapeutic efficacy in panic, generalized, and mood disorders should be considered in the presence of these comorbidities. These drugs and their efficacy are listed in **Table 1**. Cognitive behavior therapy can be effective in any and all of these conditions, and behavior therapy should be recommended in cases of agoraphobia or simple phobias.

Because the therapeutic response of antidepressant drugs may not be apparent for 4 to 6 weeks, the use of a benzodiazepine, such as alprazolam or lorazepam, can be considered as a bridge for a 6-week to 8-week period. The goal of treatment must always be the achievement of total remission of panic attacks (and other types of comorbid anxiety or mood disorders, when present). To that end, clinicians must not hesitate to use effective doses of psychotropic drugs in combination with cognitive behavior therapy or behavior therapy.

Safety of Antidepressant Drugs in Patients with Epilepsy

The concern of a proconvulsant effect of antidepressant drugs has been one of the most frequent causes of undertreatment of patients with epilepsy with a mood or anxiety disorder. Yet antidepressants can cause seizures when given at toxic doses, or in patients in whom the drug metabolism is slow, which can result in high serum

Table 1			
Efficacy of SSRIs and SNRIs in primary depression and anxiety disorders			
	Efficacy		
Antidepressant Drugs	**Depression**	**Panic Disorder**	**Generalized Anxiety**
SSRIs			
Paroxetine	+	+	+
Sertraline	+	+	+
Fluoxetine	+	+	+
Citalopram	+	+	+
Escitalopram	+	+	+
SNRIs			
Venlafaxine	+	+	+
Duloxetine	+	−	+

It should be noted, however, that there are no data on the use of duloxetine in patients with epilepsy, although the author has used it in more than 50 patients with poorly controlled epilepsy without any worsening of seizures (Kanner AM, unpublished data, 2009).

concentrations at standard doses. In fact, among all antidepressant drugs available, only 4 have been found to have a relatively high proconvulsant risk.[61] These drugs include bupropion, maprotiline, clomipramine, and amoxapine, whereas none of the SSRIs and SNRIs have been found to increase this risk.

SUMMARY

The distinction between ictal panic and interictal panic attacks can be difficult to make and can result in diagnostic errors. The presence of comorbid occurrence of all these types of events must be considered. Ictal and postictal panic and interictal and primary panic attacks share common symptoms but differ with respect to duration and association with other symptoms. A careful assessment, including an accurate history of comorbid medical conditions and medications, is often sufficient to distinguish these events. Diagnostic testing including EEG, neuroimaging, and/or estimation of prolactin levels can be of additional help to the clinician to reach an accurate diagnosis, optimize treatment option, and improve outcome.

REFERENCES

1. Hirsch E, Peretti S, Boulay C, et al. Panic attacks misdiagnosed as partial epileptic seizures. Epilepsia 1990;31:636.
2. Laidlaw JD, Khin-Maung-Zaw. Epilepsy mistaken for panic attacks in an adolescent girl. BMJ 1993;306:709–10.
3. Young GB, Chandarana PC, Blume WT, et al. Mesial temporal lobe seizures presenting as anxiety disorders. J Neuropsychiatry Clin Neurosci 1995;7:352–7.
4. Kanner AM. Peri-ictal psychiatric phenomena: clinical characteristics and implications of past and future psychiatric disorders. In: Ettinger A, Kanner AM, editors. Psychiatric issues in epilepsy: a practical guide to diagnosis and treatment. 2nd edition. Philadelphia: Lippincott Williams and Wilkins; 2007. p. 321–45.
5. Williams D. The structure of emotions reflected in epileptic experiences. Brain 1956;79:29–67.
6. Daly D. Ictal affect. Am J Psychiatry 1958;115:97–108.
7. Kanner AM, Soto A, Gross-Kanner H. Prevalence and clinical characteristics of postictal psychiatric symptoms in partial epilepsy. Neurology 2004;62:708–13.
8. Tellez-Zenteno JF, Patten SB, Jetté N, et al. Psychiatric comorbidity in epilepsy: a population-based analysis. Epilepsia 2007;48(12):2336–44.
9. Gloor P, Olivier A, Quesney LF. The role of the limbic system in experiencial phenomena of temporal lobe epilepsy. Ann Neurol 1982;12:129–44.
10. Gloor P. Experiential phenomena of temporal lobe epilepsy: facts and hypotheses. Brain 1990;113:1673–94.
11. Fakhoury T, Abou-Khalil B, Peguero E. Differentiating clinical features of right and left temporal lobe seizures. Epilepsia 1994;35(5):1038–44.
12. Roth M, Harper M. Temporal lobe epilepsy and the phobic anxiety-depersonalisation syndrome: 2. Practical and theoretical considerations. Comprehens Psychiatry 1962;3:215–26.
13. Birabena A, Taussigb D, Thomasd P, et al. Fear as the main feature of epileptic seizures. J Neurol Neurosurg Psychiatry 2001;70:186–91.
14. Alemayehu S, Bergey GK, Barry E, et al. Panic attacks as ictal manifestations of parietal lobe seizures. Epilepsia 1995;36:824–30.
15. Massana G, Serra-Grabulosa JM, Salgado-Pineda P, et al. Amygdalar atrophy in panic disorder patients detected by volumetric MRI. Neuroimage 2003;19:80–90.

16. Cendes F, Andermann F, Gloor P, et al. Relationship between atrophy of the amygdala and ictal fear in temporal lobe epilepsy. Brain 1994;117(Pt 4):739–46.

17. LeDoux JE, Cicchetti P, Xagoraris A, et al. The lateral amygdaloid nucleus: sensory interface of the amygdala in fear conditioning. J Neurosci 1990;10:1062–9.

18. Kapp BS, Frysinger RC, Gallgher M, et al. Amygdala central nucleus lesions: effects on heart rate conditioning in the rabbit. Physiol Behav 1979;23:113.

19. Hitchcock JM, Davis M. Lesions of the amygdala, but not of the cerebellum or red nucleus, block conditioned fear as measured with the potentiated startle paradigm. Behav Neurosci 1986;100:15.

20. Massana G, Serra-Grabulosa JM, Salgado-Pineda P, et al. Parahippocampal gray matter density in panic disorder: a voxel-based morphometric study. Am J Psychiatry 2003;160:566–8.

21. Vythilingam M, Anderson ER, Goddard A, et al. Temporal lobe volume in panic disorder—a quantitative MRI study. Psychiatry Res 2000;99:75–82.

22. Uchida RR, Del-Ben CM, Santos AC, et al. Decreased left temporal lobe volume of panic patients measured by MRI. J Med Biol Res 2003;36:7925–9.

23. Ring HA, Nuri G-C. Epilepsy and panic disorder. In: Trimble MR, Schmitz B, editors. The neuropsychiatry of epilepsy. New York: Cambridge University Press; 2002. p. 226–3.

24. Nash JR, Sargent PA, Rabiner EA, et al. Serotonin 5-HT$_{1A}$ receptor binding in people with panic disorder: positron emission tomography study. Br J Psychiatry 2008;193:229–34.

25. Neumeister A, Bain E, Nugent AC, et al. Reduced serotonin type 1A receptor binding in panic disorder. J Neurosci 2004;24(3):589–91.

26. Bell CJ, Nutt DJ. Serotonin and panic. British J Psychiatry 1998;172:465–71.

27. Maron E, Shlik J. Serotonin function in panic disorder: important, but why? Neuropsychopharmacology 2006;31:1–11.

28. Schatzberg AF, Cole JO, DeBattista C. Antianxiety agents. In: Manual of clinical psychopharmacology. 5th edition. Washington, DC: American Psychiatric Association; 2005. p. 313–30.

29. Montgomery SA, Nil R, Durr-Pal N, et al. A 24-week randomized, double-blind, placebo-controlled study of escitalopram for the prevention of generalized social anxiety disorder. J Clin Psychiatry 2005;66(10):1270–8.

30. Jobe PC, Dailey JW, Wernicke JF. A noradrenergic and serotonergic hypothesis of the linkage between epilepsy and affective disorders. Crit Rev Neurobiol 1999; 13:317–56.

31. Yan QS, Jobe PC, Dailey JW. Further evidence of anticonvulsant role for 5-hydroxytryptamine in genetically epilepsy prone rats. Br J Pharmacol 1995;115: 1314–8.

32. Yan QS, Jobe PC, Dailey JW. Evidence that a serotonergic mechanism is involved in the anticonvulsant effect of fluoxetine in genetically epilepsy-prone rats. Eur J Pharmacol 1993;252(1):105–12.

33. Beck SG, Choi KC. 5-Hydroxytryptamine hyperpolarizes CA3 hippocampal pyramidal cells through an increase in potassium conductance. Neurosci Lett 1991; 133:93–6.

34. Okuhara DY, Beck SG. 5-HT1A receptor linked to inward-rectifying potassium current in hippocampal CA3 pyramidal cells. J Neurophysiol 1994;71:2161–7.

35. Kanner AM. Current review in clinical science: depression in epilepsy: a neurobiologic perspective. Epilepsy Currents 2005;5(1):21–7.

36. Kanner AM. Mood disorder and epilepsy: a neurobiologic perspective of their relationship. Dialogues Clin Neurosci 2008;10(1):39–45.

37. Stahl SM. Anxiolytics and sedative hypnotics. In: Essential psychopharmacology: neuroscientific basis and practical applications. 2nd edition. Cambridge (UK): Cambridge University Press; 2000. p. 297–334.

38. Jung ME, Lal H, Gatch MB. The discriminative stimulus effects of pentylenetetrazol as a model of anxiety: recent developments. Neurosci Biobehav Rev 2002;26:429–39.

39. Nutt DJ, Glue P, Lawson CW, et al. Flumazenil provocation of panic attacks: evidence for altered benzodiazepine receptor sensitivity in panic disorders. Arch Gen Psychiatry 1990;47:917–25.

40. Malizia AL, Cunningham VJ, Bell CJ, et al. Decreased brain GABA(A)-benzodiazepine receptor binding in panic disorder: preliminary results from a quantitative PET study. Arch Gen Psychiatry 1998;55(8):715–20.

41. Cameron OG, Huang GC, Nichols T, et al. Reduced γ-aminobutyric acid(A)–benzodiazepine binding sites in insular cortex of individuals with panic disorder. Arch Gen Psychiatry 2007;64:793–800.

42. Vazquez B, Devinsky O. Epilepsy and anxiety. Epilepsy Behav 2003;4(Suppl 4):S20–5.

43. Ettinger AB, Bird JM, Kanner AM. Panic disorder and hyperventilation syndrome. In: Engel J, Pedley TA, editors. Epilepsy: a comprehensive textbook. 2nd edition. Philadelphia: Lippincott Williams & Wilkins; 2008. p. 2828–36.

44. McLachlan RS, Blume WT. Isolated fear in complex partial status epilepticus. Ann Neurol 1980;8:639–41.

45. Henriksen GF. Status epilepticus partialis wit fear as clinical expression. Report of a case and ictal EEG findings. Epilepsia 1973;14(1):39–46.

46. Kaplan HI, Sadock BJ, Grebb JA. Synopsis of psychiatry. Baltimore (MD): Williams & Wilkins; 1994. p. 574.

47. Craske M, Barlow D. Nocturnal panic. J Nerv Ment Dis 1989;177:160–7.

48. Lesser I, Poland R, Holcomb C, et al. Electroencephalographic study of nighttime panic attacks. J Nerv Ment Dis 1990;173:744–6.

49. Mellman TA, Uhde TW. Sleep panic attacks: new clinical findings and theoretical implications. Am J Psychiatry 1989;146:1204–7.

50. Moore D, Jefferson J. Panic disorder. 2nd edition. St Louis (MO): Mosby; 2004.

51. Klein RG, Kopplewicz HS, Kanner A. Imipramine treatment of children with separation anxiety disorder. J Am Acad Child Adolesc Psychiatry 1992;31:21–8.

52. Mintzer S, Lopez F. Comorbidity of ictal fear and panic disorder. Epilepsy Behav 2002;3(4):330–7.

53. Kohler CG, Carran MA, Bilker W, et al. Association of fear auras with mood and anxiety disorders after temporal lobectomy. Epilepsia 2001;42(5):674–81.

54. Devinsky O, Sato S, Theodore WH, et al. Fear episodes due to limbic seizures with normal scalp EEG: a subdural electrographic study. J Clin Psychiatry 1989;50:28–30.

55. Kanner AM, Jones JC. When do sphenoidal electrodes yield additional data to that obtained with antero-temporal electrodes? Electroencephalogr Clin Neurophysiol 1997;102(1):12–9.

56. Chen DK, So YT, Fisher RS. Use of serum prolactin in diagnosing epileptic seizures: report of the Therapeutics and Technology Assessment Subcommittee of the American Academy of Neurology. Neurology 2005;65(5):668–75.

57. American Psychiatric Association Task Force on Benzodiazepine Dependency. Benzodiazepine dependence, toxicity, and abuse: a task force report of the American Psychiatric Association. Washington, DC: American Psychiatric Association; 1990.

58. Katon W. Panic disorder in the medical setting. Washington, DC: U.S. Government Printing Office; 1989.

59. Pande AC, Crockatt JG, Feltner DE, et al. Pregabalin in generalized anxiety disorder: a placebo-controlled trial. Am J Psychiatry 2003;160:533–40.
60. Baetz M, Bowen RC. Efficacy of divalproex sodium in patients with panic disorder and mood instability who have not responded to conventional therapy. Can J Psychiatry 1998;43:73–7.
61. McConnell HW, Duncan D. Treatment of psychiatric comorbidity in epilepsy. In: McConnell HW, Snyder PJ, editors. Psychiatric comorbidity in epilepsy. Washington, DC: American Psychiatric Press; 1998. p. 245–362.

Diagnosis and Treatment of Major Depressive Disorder

Laili Soleimani, MD, MSc[a], Kyle A.B. Lapidus, MD, PhD[a],
Dan V. Iosifescu, MD, MSc[b,c,d],*

KEYWORDS

- Major depressive disorder • Comorbid medical illness
- Comorbid neurologic illness • Antidepressant treatments
- Pharmacotherapies • Psychotherapies • Somatic treatments

Major depressive disorder (MDD) encompasses a large number of psychobiological syndromes with the core features of depressed mood and/or loss of interest associated with cognitive and somatic disturbances, which causes significant functional impairment. Depressive disorders are classified as mood disorders and are distinguished from bipolar disorders by the absence of manic episodes. According to the American Psychiatric Association (APA) Diagnostic and Statistical Manual of Mental Disorders, fourth edition, Text Revision (DSM-IV-TR), depressive disorders include MDD (**Box 1**), dysthymic disorder (low-grade chronic depression occurring more than 50% of the days for at least 2 years), and minor depression (minimum of 2 depressive symptoms present for at least 2 weeks).[1]

Large epidemiologic studies suggest that major depressive disorder is common,[2,3] with a lifetime prevalence of 16.6%, occurring with approximately twofold higher frequency in women compared with men.[2,3] MDD aggregates in families; it is 1.5 to 3 times more common in individuals with first-degree biologic relatives affected with MDD compared with the general population.[4] The point prevalence of MDD has been reported to be 10% in the primary care setting, 15% to 20% in the nursing home population, and 22% to 33% in medically ill patients.[5–7]

Historically, MDD pathology has been associated with brain monoamine neurotransmitter or receptor abnormalities. Studies of cerebrospinal fluid chemistry,

L. Soleimani and K.A.B Lapidus contributed equally (ie, shared first authorship).
[a] Department of Psychiatry, Mount Sinai School of Medicine, One Gustave L. Levy Place Box 1230, New York, NY 10029, USA
[b] Mood and Anxiety Disorders Program, Mount Sinai School of Medicine, One Gustave L. Levy Place Box 1230, New York, NY 10029, USA
[c] Psychiatry Department, Massachusetts General Hospital, Boston, MA, USA
[d] Harvard Medical School, Boston, MA, USA
* Corresponding author. Mood and Anxiety Disorders Program, Mount Sinai School of Medicine, One Gustave L. Levy Place Box 1230, New York, NY 10029.
E-mail address: dan.iosifescu@mssm.edu

Neurol Clin 29 (2011) 177–193
doi:10.1016/j.ncl.2010.10.010
0733-8619/11/$ – see front matter © 2011 Elsevier Inc. All rights reserved.
neurologic.theclinics.com

Box 1
Criteria for major depressive episode (DSM-IV-TR)[1]

- At least 5 of the following symptoms must be present continuously for 2 weeks; at least 1 should be either depressed mood or lack of interest:

  - depressed mood (or irritability in children and adolescents)

  - lack of interest or pleasure

  - appetite change or weight change

  - insomnia or hypersomnia

  - psychomotor agitation or retardation

  - fatigue or loss of energy

  - feelings of worthlessness or guilt

  - decreased concentration

  - recurrent thoughts of death and suicidal ideation

- No history of bipolar disorder (eg, manic or hypomanic episodes)

- Symptoms should cause clinically significant functional impairment

- Symptoms should not be secondary to a substance (eg, a drug of abuse, a medication) or a general medical condition (eg, hypothyroidism)

- Symptoms are not better accounted for by bereavement

From American Psychiatric Association. Diagnostic and statistical manual of mental disorders (DSMIV-TR). Fourth edition. Washington, DC: American Psychiatric Association; 2000. p. 356; with permission.

---

neuroreceptor, and transporter systems, as well as clinical response to monoaminergic agents, have suggested that serotonergic, noradrenergic, other neurotransmitter, and neuropeptide systems may be abnormal in MDD (reviewed in Refs.[8,9]). However, there has been an increasing focus on the interplay of environmental factors with genetic and neuroendocrine systems and the involvement of intracellular signaling pathways. The hypothalamic-pituitary-adrenal axis has been suggested to mediate environmental stress and contribute to neuronal atrophy. The common cellular abnormality in various forms of depression may be reduced cellular resilience caused by decreased expression of several neurotrophic factors (eg, brain-derived neurotrophic factor, Bcl-2).[8–11]

EVALUATION
Diagnostic Evaluation

Clinical suspicion is key to the diagnosis of MDD. Patients should be asked about depressed mood and/or lack of interest or pleasure when they present with nonspecific symptoms suggestive of depression (**Box 2**). Clinicians should evaluate the patient for the following features: onset, duration, accompanying psychological symptoms, possible psychosocial precipitating factors (eg, relationship problems, work-related stressors, or living conditions), and the effect of these symptoms on the patient's daily life and function. A key component of the evaluation is determining the absence or presence of suicidal ideations and/or homicidal ideations, in which case the clinician should also inquire whether the patient has intent to hurt self or others and whether a plan has been made.

Box 2
Common symptoms of depression
Depressed mood
Anxiety, excessive worrying
Irritable mood
Anger attacks
Crying spells
Loss of interest or pleasure
Distractability
Change in appetite
Change in sleep
Fatigue
Pain (eg, headaches, back pain)
Muscle tension
Heart palpitations
Guilt
Feelings of worthlessness
Recurrent thoughts of death or suicide

Detailed history of past depressive or manic episodes, other psychiatric disorders, and possible use of alcohol or other substances should be obtained because these can significantly influence diagnosis and treatment decisions.

Some depressive disorders may be secondary to medical conditions or medications (**Box 3**); the diagnosis will rest on physical signs and symptoms, medical history, and medication history.

Laboratory testing, including thyroid function tests, B12, and folate levels, may aid in reaching an accurate diagnosis and uncovering medical problems partially or fully responsible for the psychiatric presentation.

Box 3
Examples of medical conditions causing depressive symptoms
Autoimmune disorders (eg, systemic lupus erythematosus, rheumatoid arthritis)
Neurologic disorders (eg, stroke, dementias, multiple sclerosis, seizure disorder, Huntington disease, traumatic brain injury)
Endocrine disorders (eg, hypercalcemia, hypercortisolism, hyperparathyroidism, hyperthyroidism, hypoparathyroidism, hypothyroidism)
Malignancies (eg, gastrointestinal cancer, pancreatic cancer)
Infectious disease (eg, hepatitis, human immunodeficiency virus, mononucleosis)
Medications or substances: antihypertensive medications (eg, propranolol, thiazides, clonidine), anticholinergic agents, anticonvulsant agents, oral contraceptives, sedatives (eg, barbiturates, benzodiazepines), antiparkinsonian medications (eg, methyldopa, amantadine), and alcohol

Measuring Depression Severity with Standardized Scales

Clinician-administered and self-rated scales allow a more objective assessment of depression severity but need to be interpreted in the context of patients' symptoms and medical conditions. Such scales can also be useful in monitoring the effect of treatments. Because multiple well-established and validated scales are available, physicians can choose appropriate measures based on their patient populations and practice settings (**Box 4**).

The Hamilton Rating Scale for Depression (HAM-D), the most widely used clinician-administered instrument, focuses on biologic and somatic symptoms of MDD; the 17-item version is the most frequently used subscale of the original 31-item HAM-D.[13,14] The Montgomery-Asberg Depression Rating Scale (MADRS), has a lower number of items, less overlap with anxiety symptoms, and is one of the most user-friendly observer-rating scales.[15]

Self-administered instruments require less interaction with the clinician. The Quick Inventory of Depressive Symptomatology (QIDS-SR; http://www.ids-qids.org) overlaps well with the *Diagnostic and statistical manual* symptoms of MDD and has been extensively validated.[12] The Beck Depression Inventory (BDI), is an older self-rating scale that preferentially detects and rates cognitive aspects of depression, with an emphasis on self-esteem.[16] The Geriatric Depression Scale (GDS) is a 30-item self-administered scale that includes questions about symptoms such as cognitive complaints, self-image, and loss; these symptoms are believed to be particularly relevant in late-life depression.[17,18]

Safety Evaluation

Suicide is one of the most severe and potentially fatal mental health–related emergencies and is 20 times more common in patients suffering from MDD than in healthy populations. Clinicians play an important role in the screening and prevention of suicide because most suicidal patients have contact with their physicians within the month before suicide.[19] Therefore, physicians should always ask about and document thoughts of death in patients with depression or other mental health problems (**Box 5**). Positive responses should be followed by assessment of the content of the thoughts (plans or intent), history of past attempts, triggering factors, and other associated risk factors. The physician should also work with both patient and family to limit access to lethal means (eg, firearms and large amounts of medications), and, when necessary, consider psychiatric consultation and/or hospitalization.

Box 4
Examples of rating scales for depressive symptoms

Clinician administered

Hamilton Rating Scale for Depression (HAM-D)

Montgomery-Asberg Depression Rating Scale (MADRS)

Self-report scales

Beck Depression Inventory

Quick Inventory of Depressive Symptoms–Self-report (QIDS-SR;[12] http://www.ids-qids.org)

Geriatric Depression Scale (GDS; http://www.stanford.edu/~yesavage/GDS.html)

> **Box 5**
> **Suicidal thought item from Montgomery-Asberg Depression Rating Scale[15]:**
>
> *Clinician's question*
>
> This last week have you had any thoughts that life is not worth living, or that you would be better off dead? What about thoughts of hurting or even killing yourself? If YES: What have you thought about? Have you actually made plans? (Have you told anyone about it?)
>
> *Responses (with anchor points for consistent rating of patient responses)*
>
> 0: Enjoy life or take it as it comes
>
> 1
>
> 2: Weary of life. Only fleeting suicidal thoughts
>
> 3
>
> 4: Probably better off dead. Suicidal thoughts are common, and suicide is considered as a possible solution, but without specific plans or intention
>
> 5
>
> 6: Explicit plans for suicide when there is an opportunity. Active preparation for suicide
>
> *From* Montgomery SA, Asberg M. A new depression scale designed to be sensitive to change. Br J Psychiatry 1979;134:398; with permission.

DIFFERENTIAL DIAGNOSIS

Depression is a common symptom among many psychiatric conditions. **Table 1** lists the most common psychiatric differential diagnoses of MDD.

SPECIAL MDD POPULATIONS
Depression in Patients with General Medical Conditions

Depression is more prevalent among patients with medical illness (including cardio-vascular disease, diabetes, and other conditions listed in **Box 3**) and has been suggested to increase mortality by as much as 4.3 times.[20] Major depression itself is harder to treat in medically ill patients.[21] It is important to understand the relationship between depressive symptoms and the underlying medical conditions. For example, in patients with depression and chronic pain, controlling the pain often results in significant improvement of mood symptoms. Treating both medical and depressive symptoms can improve the outcome of medical treatment and adherence to medical therapy and rehabilitation. Atypical depressive symptoms and associated positive laboratory findings for a nonprimary depressive disorder warrant a full medical work-up.

Depression in Patients with Stroke

About one-third of all patients with stroke develop poststroke depression (PSD).[22] PSD can contribute to the disability caused by the stroke and can increase mortality. A meta-analysis of 51 population-, hospital-, and rehabilitation-based stroke studies conducted between 1977 and 2002 showed that depression was associated with physical disability, stroke severity, and cognitive impairment.[22] A prospective, randomized controlled trial of 448 patients with stroke evaluated for depression 1 month after stroke and followed up at 12 and 24 months showed that mood symptoms were associated with increased 12- and 24-month mortality after adjustment for other

Table 1
Psychiatric differential diagnoses of major depression

Differential Diagnoses	Characteristic Feature
Nonpathologic periods of sadness	Short duration, few associated symptoms, and lack of significant functional impairment or distress
Bereavement	In response to the loss of a loved one, usually ameliorating within 2 months and not lasting more than 6 months
Adjustment disorder with depressed mood	In response to an immediate stressor; does not meet full criteria for a major depressive episode
Seasonal depression	Recurrent episodes with clear seasonal pattern (onset in fall or winter and full remission usually by the spring)
Premenstrual dysphoric disorder	Characterized by significant depressed mood, anxiety, and irritability during the 1–2 weeks before menses and resolving with menses
Postpartum depressive disorder	Full depressive episode with an onset within a few months after delivery. To be differentiated from postpartum blues (fewer symptoms, onset shortly after delivery, and subsides usually within 3 weeks)
Bipolar I or bipolar II disorder	History of 1 or more manic, mixed, or hypomanic episodes
Mood disorder caused by a general medical condition	Direct physiologic effect of a general medical condition
Substance-induced mood disorder	Caused by the direct physiologic effect of a substance (including medication); symptoms develop within a month of substance use
Dysthymic disorder	Depressed mood present more than 50% of days in a 2-year period, in the absence of major depressive episodes
Schizoaffective disorder	Recurrent periods of at least 2 weeks of delusions or hallucinations; at least some of these periods occur in the absence of prominent mood symptoms
Schizophrenia, delusional disorder, psychotic disorder not otherwise specified	Depressive symptoms are brief relative to the total duration of the psychotic disturbance (eg, delusions, hallucinations)
Posttraumatic stress disorder	Occurs within the 6 months following a stressful event; characterized by hyperarousal, episodes of flashbacks, nightmares, detachment, numbness, maladaptive coping responses, and excessive use of alcohol and drugs
Dementia	Characterized by a progressive history of declining cognitive functioning (usually before depressive symptoms). Low scores (usually <23) on the mini–mental status examination

identified risk factors.[23] The incidence of PSD peaks 3 to 6 months after the stroke; risk factors include severity of disability, poor social support, personal and family history of depression, and the development of aphasia. Numerous studies have reported increased risk of PSD in left anterior hemisphere strokes or basal ganglia (reviewed in Refs.[24,25]).

Although multiple studies support the use of selective serotonin reuptake inhibitors (SSRIs) and tri/tetracyclic antidepressants (TCAs) in PSD, there are no well-designed studies that guide therapeutic decision making for patients with PSD.[26,27] More than 60% of patients with PSD respond to antidepressants, with no particular class of antidepressant showing a clear advantage in treatment efficacy. The data are less conclusive regarding psychostimulants because of a lack of randomized controlled trials. Overall, antidepressants and stimulants are well tolerated in patients with stroke (reviewed in Ref.[28]). In a recent randomized controlled study both the SSRI escitalopram and problem-solving therapy (a form of cognitive-behavioral therapy [CBT]) were more effective than placebo in preventing development of PSD in 176 at-risk patients.[29]

Depression in Patients with Multiple Sclerosis

Cross-sectional studies estimate that almost half of patients with multiple sclerosis (MS) develop depression during the course of their disease.[30] Based on a large-scale Canadian national survey, the 12-month prevalence of MDD is 15% in this population of patients with MS.[31–33] Multiple studies have shown a lower quality of life, increased risk of suicidal ideation, and impaired cognitive function in patients with MS with depression (reviewed in Ref.[31]).

The consensus from research suggests that the development of depression in patients with MS is multifactorial: psychosocial stress related to the diagnosis and exacerbation or progression of disability, as well as MS-related brain changes (eg, neuroinflammatory and neurodegenerative changes) and underlying preexisting psychiatric comorbidities, can predispose patients to depression (reviewed in Ref.[34]). A recent multicenter, observational study of 798 patients suggested that past history of depression (rather than specific MS treatments, ie, interferon or glatiramer acetate) predicted emergence of depressed mood.[35]

Screening and detection of depression in patients with MS is particularly important because depression has also been identified as one of the 3 most significant factors contributing to noncompliance with immune-modulatory treatment.[36] A follow-up study of 85 patients with MS who developed depression after initiation of interferon therapy showed improved treatment adherence with both psychotherapy and antidepressants.[37] The general consensus is that the combination therapy is the best approach to treatment of depression in this population.[38,39]

SSRIs are often the first-line treatment option because of their safer side effect profile, fewer contraindications, and significantly lower chance of negative drug interactions. Based on tolerability rather than any evidence for differences in efficacy, TCAs and monoamine oxidase inhibitors (MAOIs) are generally used in patients in whom SSRIs have been ineffective. However, for patients experiencing chronic pain or sleep disturbance, TCAs (eg, nortriptyline, amitriptyline) may be the treatment of choice because of their ability to reduce pain and because of their sedative effects.[40] Counseling and social support have also been found to be helpful in the treatment of depression in these chronically ill patients.[34,41]

Depression in Patients with Parkinson Disease

Depression is the most common psychiatric disturbance in patients with Parkinson disease (PD) and, although the prevalence varies across different studies, depression is estimated to occur in approximately half of all patients with PD.[42,43] Despite its high prevalence, depression is frequently underdiagnosed and undertreated in these patients. This is most likely because of the challenge of distinguishing PD symptoms, such as psychomotor slowing and blunted affect, from depressive symptoms. Degeneration of monoaminergic neurotransmitter systems and frontocortical dysfunction have been suggested as the underlying mechanism of depression in PD.[44,45]

Randomized controlled studies have shown that TCAs and bupropion are efficacious for the treatment of depression in Parkinson disease.[46–48] SSRIs have shown similar efficacy compared with TCAs, but show a different profile of adverse effects, which may be particularly favorable in elderly patients.[49] A recent double-blind, randomized, placebo-controlled study showed that desipramine and citalopram each improved depressive symptoms after 30 days, but that mild adverse events were twice as frequent in the desipramine-treated group.[50] A randomized multicenter national study showed that pramipexole improved motor symptoms but also had antidepressant efficacy that was comparable with sertraline and specifically improved anhedonia.[49,51] Although based on this single study, pramipexole could be recommended as a first-line treatment in patients with PD and depression. Lithium, a commonly used augmentation agent with antidepressant drugs, should be avoided in patients with PD because of the risk of tremor induction.[49]

TREATMENT OF MDD

Useful treatments for depression include pharmacotherapy, focused psychotherapies, somatic treatments, and lifestyle changes.

Pharmacotherapy

Commonly used antidepressants and doses are listed in **Table 2**. Although several pharmacologic agents are approved by the US Food and Drug Administration (FDA), none are clearly superior in efficacy. They differ in pharmacologic and side effect profile (**Table 3**). Although onset of antidepressant efficacy may vary for individual patients, onset of efficacy may require 4 to 6 weeks of treatment with most currently available agents, whereas full efficacy may require 8 to 12 weeks.[52,53] As a general rule, antidepressant side effects can be minimized by slowly increasing dosage (especially in the elderly), although this strategy may also delay the onset of efficacy.

SSRIs

SSRIs are frequently used as a first-line treatment of depressive disorders because their specificity results in fewer drug-drug interactions, safety in overdose, and a favorable side effect profile.[54] They also effectively treat anxiety disorders and other psychiatric comorbidities frequently associated with depression.[55,56]

Serotonin and norepinephrine reuptake inhibitors

Serotonin-norepinephrine reuptake inhibitors (SNRIs) are also effective in treating depression and anxiety. They may be particularly useful in SSRI nonresponders and in specific chronic pain conditions.[57] However, they tend to be more expensive.

TCAs

TCAs are older, inexpensive agents that also act primarily by inhibiting serotonin and norepinephrine reuptake, are effective as antidepressants, and effectively treat chronic pain.[58] They also interact with many other receptors, which may contribute to their efficacy, but produces side effects that may limit tolerability and compliance.[59] TCAs block muscarinic acetylcholine receptors, leading to anticholinergic side effects (see **Table 3**). The risk of confusion and disorientation is most significant in elderly patients, and delirium has been reported in 5% of elderly patients taking TCAs.[60] TCAs also antagonize histamine H1 receptors and α_1 adrenergic receptors; caution is advised in patients with narrow angle glaucoma, prostatic hypertrophy, or low blood pressure. Because TCAs prolong cardiac repolarization, they can act similarly to class I antiarrhythmic agents. Their toxic effects on cardiac conduction, which make TCAs

Table 2
Recommended dosages for commonly prescribed antidepressants

Drug	Usual Dose (mg/d)	Initial Dose (mg/d)	Notes
SSRIs			
Citalopram (Celexa)	20–60	10–20	Few drug interactions
Escitalopram (Lexapro)	10–20	5–10	Few drug interactions
Paroxetine (Paxil and Paxil CR)	10–50	10–20	Short half-life
Sertraline (Zoloft)	25–200	25–50	
Fluvoxamine (Luvox)	50–300	25–50	
Fluoxetine (Prozac)	10–60	10–20	Longest half-life
SNRIs			
Venlafaxine (Effexor and Effexor XR)	75–225	37.5	
Desvenlafaxine (Pristiq)	50–100	50	
Duloxetine (Cymbalta)	40–120	20–40	
Tricyclic/Tetracyclic Antidepressants			
Amitriptyline (Elavil)	100–300	10–50	
Clomipramine (Anafranil)	100–250	25	
Doxepin (Adapin)	100–300	25–50	
Imipramine (Tofranil)	100–300	10–25	
Trimipramine (Surmontil)	100–300	25–50	
Desipramine (Norpramin)	100–300	25–50	Favorable tolerability
Nortriptyline (Pamelor)	50–150	10–25	Favorable safety, tolerability
Protriptyline (Vivactil)	15–60	10	Activating
Amoxapine (Asendin)	100–400	50	
Maprotiline (Ludiomil)	100–225	50	
MAOIs			
Phenelzine (Nardil)	45–90	15	
Tranylcypromine (Parnate)	30–60	10	
Isocarboxazid (Marplan)	30–60	20	
Selegiline (Eldepryl)	30–40	10	Selective MAO-B Inhibitor at low doses
Selegiline transdermal (Emsam)	6–12	6	
Other Antidepressants			
Bupropion (Wellbutrin)	300–450	75–150	Available as SR and XL/XR
Mirtazapine (Remeron)	15–45	15	

Abbreviations: MAOI, monoamine oxidase inhibitor; SNRI, serotonin-norepinephrine reuptake inhibitor; SSRI, selective serotonin reuptake inhibitor.

Table 3
Important side effects of antidepressants

Drug Class	Important Side Effects
SSRIs and SNRIs	Nausea, decreased appetite, weight loss, diaphoresis, insomnia, sedation, nervousness, sexual dysfunction, headache, dizziness
TCAs	Anticholinergic: dry mouth, constipation, hyperthermia, sinus tachycardia, blurred vision, urinary retention, cognitive/memory impairment Antihistaminic: sedation, increased appetite, weight gain, hypotension Antiadrenergic: postural hypotension, dizziness, tachycardia Reduced seizure threshold, sexual dysfunction, cardiac conduction effects similar to class 1A antiarrhythmics, cardiotoxicity in overdose
MAOIs	Insomnia, sedation, weight gain, orthostatic hypotension, sexual dysfunction Less common: pyridoxine deficiency with parasthesias, tremor, anticholinergic effects Hypertensive crisis: occurs with tyramine ingestion (eg, aged cheese and meats, fava beans, soy sauce) Serotonin syndrome: life threatening with rapid onset of hyperthermia, hypertension, tachycardia, shock
Bupropion (Wellbutrin)	Agitation, dry mouth, insomnia, nausea, constipation, tremor, headache Increased seizure risk
Mirtazapine (Remeron)	Antihistaminic: sedation, increased appetite, weight gain, hypotension, dry mouth, constipation, dizziness

potentially lethal in overdose, can be detected by QT_C prolongation. Therefore, obtaining an electrocardiogram is advisable before and 4 weeks after initiating TCA treatment.[61] Plasma levels can help guide dosage adjustments.[62] In PD, a controlled trial showed superiority of TCA treatment, with a response rate of 53%.[63]

MAOIs

MAOIs are most often used in patients with atypical depression or in treatment-resistant patients who fail trials of other medications. In patients with atypical depression, MAOI response rates of 59% to 71% have been reported.[64,65] MAOIs can also be effective in PD, and may be particularly suited for treating depression in these patients. They act by inhibiting monoamine oxidase (MAO)-A and -B, enzymes that break down monoamines including serotonin, dopamine, and norepinephrine. These MAO enzymes are widely distributed throughout the body and can be found throughout the gastrointestinal tract and liver, and in platelets, as well as in neurons and glia. Several MAOIs available in the United States (eg, phenelzine, tranylcypromine) irreversibly inhibit both MAO-A and MAO-B, so their effects persist through several drug-free days until enzyme stores are replenished. Intake of foods containing the sympathomimetic amine tyramine can result in potentially lethal hypertensive crises. Serotonin syndrome is also possible with MAOIs, TCAs, and SSRIs; it involves cognitive changes such as confusion or agitation, autonomic dysregulation such as fever, changes in blood pressure, diarrhea, flushing, and diaphoresis, as well as hyperreflexia, myoclonus, and tremor.[66] Tryptophan-containing foods also pose a risk for serotonin syndrome. To avoid serotonin syndrome, a washout period of at least 2 weeks (5 weeks for fluoxetine, because of its longer half-life) is recommended when switching to or from an MAOI.[67] Other medications that may react with MAOIs to cause hypertensive crises or serotonin syndrome include meperidine, tramadol, dextromethorphan, and SSRIs.

Other agents

Additional antidepressants include bupropion and mirtazapine. These agents are generally safer in overdose than TCAs, and mirtazapine has a particularly favorable safety profile, with a large study reporting no fatalities in 2599 suicidal ingestions.[68] Bupropion has dopaminergic properties and energizing effects; it is used as an aid for smoking cessation and has few sexual side effects. Because of increased seizure risk, bupropion is contraindicated in patients with seizure disorders or bulimia. Mirtazapine can be easily combined with other agents because of limited drug-drug interactions. Its side effects, such as weight gain and sedation, result mainly from histamine H1 receptor blockade.[69]

Augmenting standard antidepressants with atypical antipsychotics is the best shown augmentation strategy in treatment-resistant depression.[70,71] Many high-quality studies also support antidepressant augmentation with lithium[72] or thyroid hormones,[73] although most of those studies were carried out with tricyclic antidepressants, and few of those studies included modern antidepressants.[74] Smaller studies also support the role of certain natural remedies (eg, S-adenosyl-methionine),[75] and psychostimulants as augmentation strategies in cases of partial or nonresponse to an antidepressant agent.

Psychotherapy

CBT (including mindfulness and relaxation techniques), behavioral therapy, and interpersonal therapy are efficacious in treating MDD. Although short-term dynamic and emotion-focused psychotherapies may also be efficacious, less evidence supports these strategies for the treatment of depressed patients.[76] Although remission rates with cognitive therapy or medication alone have been reported to reach 40% to 46%, patients with moderate or severe depression may benefit more from a combination of pharmacotherapy and psychotherapy.[77]

Somatic Treatments

Electroconvulsive therapy (ECT) is well established and highly effective in resistant depression.[78,79] Electrical stimulation is applied bilaterally or unilaterally to the head to induce a seizure. ECT requires anesthesia and can cause transient cognitive side effects or amnesia and is therefore generally used after patients have failed pharmacologic trials and/or in very severe forms of depression.[80] Hypertension and arrhythmias have also been noted, but these complications occur more frequently in patients with preexisting cardiac complications and can be well managed in clinical contexts.[81] Hence, there are no absolute contraindications, although relative contraindications include coronary artery disease, arrhythmia, and increased intracranial pressure or lesions.

Other FDA-approved treatments for resistant depression include transcranial magnetic stimulation (TMS) and vagus nerve stimulation (VNS). TMS (a noninvasive brain depolarization induced by a magnetic field) has shown modest efficacy (14% remission rates) but few adverse effects in subjects with MDD with mild to moderate levels of treatment resistance.[82] A recent meta-analysis of more than 34 randomized, sham-controlled trials, including more than 1000 patients, supports the efficacy of TMS as both monotherapy and as an adjunctive treatment to pharmacotherapy.[83] VNS requires a surgically implanted device sending electrical impulses to ascending fibers of the vagus nerve, and has shown no significant efficacy compared with placebo after 3 months, but increasing efficacy in open treatment up to 1 year in populations with severe treatment-resistant depression.[84] Phototherapy, which involves the application of bright light, may be particularly useful in seasonal depression.[85]

Lifestyle changes and alternative remedies with some efficacy in the treatment of depression include physical exercise, and some dietary supplements (eg, ω-3 fatty acids, S-adenosyl methionine, St John's wort).[86]

PHASES OF TREATMENT

The recently published APA *Practice guidelines for the treatment of patients with major depressive disorder*, 3rd edition[87] incorporates insights from large studies in MDD in the last decade, including the large National Institute of Mental Health–sponsored Sequenced Treatment Alternatives to Relieve Depression (STAR*D) study. According to the APA guidelines, management of the patient with MDD can be framed in the context of 3 phases.

The acute phase of treatment is focused on the acutely depressed patient and begins with tailoring a strategy that is based on the severity of the symptoms, history of prior positive responses, presence of other psychiatric symptoms, side effect profile of the medication, and the patient's preference (eg, pharmacotherapy without/with psychotherapy for the mild/moderate symptoms, ECT for severe depression, and presence of psychotic features or catatonia). In cases of treatment failure (ie, no improvement after 4–8 weeks of treatment), raising antidepressant doses to the optimal tolerable level (optimization) should be considered before switching to another drug within the same class or in another class of drugs. For partial responders, combination of antidepressant medications (adding buproprion, low-dose TCA, mirtazapine, or buspirone) or augmentation strategies (with atypical antipsychotics, lithium, triiodothyronine, psychostimulants, or dopaminergic agents) can be used before switching medications.

Box 6
Helpful clinical recommendations

- Explain depression as an illness associated with neurochemical dysregulation in the brain, rather than a personal weakness or fault

- More than 60% of patients with MDD are at risk for recurrence; patients with recurrent depression should be educated about the early signs of depression; some may require lifelong antidepressant therapy

- Education about the anticipated side effects of the medications will improve patient compliance

When to refer to, or consult with, a psychiatrist:

- Significant risk for suicide or homicide (acute suicidal risk may require a psychiatric hospitalization)

- Current or plans for future pregnancy

- Poor social support

- Disability caused by depression

- Suboptimal response to 1 or 2 adequate treatments

- Comorbid psychiatric problems (psychosis, mania, severe anxiety, substance abuse, panic attacks, posttraumatic stress disorder, dementia)

- Need for alcohol or illicit drug detoxification

The continuation treatment refers to the phase after the initial remission of symptoms. The antidepressant treatment that led to remission in the acute phase should be continued for an additional 6 to 9 months with full antidepressant doses to decrease the risk of relapse.

The maintenance treatment is the phase during which patients with high risk of relapse (ie, patients with a history of 3 or more major depressive episodes) might benefit from indefinite maintenance therapy to prevent the risk of recurrence.

SUMMARY

MDD is a common illness associated with significant morbidity and mortality. The prevalence of MDD is even higher in medically ill patients. It is important for clinicians to suspect the diagnosis of MDD in patients with suggestive symptoms or risk factors. Such suspicion should be followed by a review of diagnostic symptoms (possibly through the administration of standardized scales) with an emphasis on the presence of suicidal thinking, and by laboratory tests to differentiate from medical causes of depression. Although several pharmacotherapies, psychotherapies, and somatic treatments have been shown to effectively treat MDD, a large number of patients do not improve sufficiently with any single treatment and can benefit from switching or combining different antidepressant modalities. Patients with severe depression and/or suicidal ideation, and those having failed several antidepressant treatments, would benefit from consultation with, or referral to, a psychiatrist (**Box 6**).

REFERENCES

1. American Psychiatric Association. Diagnostic and statistical manual of mental disorders fourth edition (text revision) DSM-IV-TR. Washington, DC: American Psychiatric Association; 2000.
2. Kessler RC, Chiu WT, Demler O, et al. Prevalence, severity, and comorbidity of 12-month DSM-IV disorders in the National Comorbidity Survey Replication. Arch Gen Psychiatry 2005;62(6):617–27.
3. Weissman MM, Olfson M. Depression in women: implications for health care research. Science 1995;269(5225):799–801.
4. Pincus HA, Zarin DA, Tanielian TL, et al. Psychiatric patients and treatments in 1997: findings from the American Psychiatric Practice Research Network. Arch Gen Psychiatry 1999;56(5):441–9.
5. Ustun TB, Sartorius N, editors. Mental illness in general health practice: an international study. New York: Wiley; 1995.
6. Teresi J, Abrams R, Holmes D, et al. Prevalence of depression and depression recognition in nursing homes. Soc Psychiatry Psychiatr Epidemiol 2001;36(12): 613–20.
7. World Psychiatric Association. International Committee for Diagnosis and Treatment of Depression. Educational program on depressive disorders, module II. Depressive disorders in physical illness, part I: 2. New York: NCM Publishers; 1998.
8. Manji HK, Drevets WC, Charney DS. The cellular neurobiology of depression. Nat Med 2001;7(5):541–7.
9. Charney DS, Manji HK. Life stress, genes, and depression: multiple pathways lead to increased risk and new opportunities for intervention. Sci STKE 2004; 2004(225):re5.
10. Mann JJ, Currier D. Effects of genes and stress on the neurobiology of depression. Int Rev Neurobiol 2006;73:153–89.

11. Nestler EJ, Barrot M, DiLeone RJ, et al. Neurobiology of depression. Neuron 2002;34(1):13–25.
12. Rush AJ, Trivedi MH, Ibrahim HM, et al. The 16-Item Quick Inventory of Depressive Symptomatology (QIDS), clinician rating (QIDS-C), and self-report (QIDS-SR): a psychometric evaluation in patients with chronic major depression. Biol Psychiatry 2003;54(5):573–83.
13. Hamilton M. A rating scale for depression. J Neurol Neurosurg Psychiatr 1960;23: 56–62.
14. Hamilton M. Development of a rating scale for primary depressive illness. Br J Soc Clin Psychol 1967;6(4):278–96.
15. Montgomery SA, Asberg M. A new depression scale designed to be sensitive to change. Br J Psychiatry 1979;134:382–9.
16. Beck AT, Ward CH, Mendelson M, et al. An inventory for measuring depression. Arch Gen Psychiatry 1961;4:561–71.
17. Yesavage JA, Brink TL, Rose TL, et al. Development and validation of a geriatric depression screening scale: a preliminary report. J Psychiatr Res 1982;17(1): 37–49.
18. Hybels CF, Blazer DG, Pieper CF, et al. Profiles of depressive symptoms in older adults diagnosed with major depression: latent cluster analysis. Am J Geriatr Psychiatry 2009;17(5):387–96.
19. Mann JJ, Apter A, Bertolote J, et al. Suicide prevention strategies: a systematic review. JAMA 2005;294(16):2064–74.
20. Bruce ML, Leaf PJ. Psychiatric disorders and 15-month mortality in a community sample of older adults. Am J Public Health 1989;79(6):727–30.
21. Iosifescu DV. Treating depression in the medically ill. Psychiatr Clin North Am 2007;30(1):77–90.
22. Hackett ML, Yapa C, Parag V, et al. Frequency of depression after stroke: a systematic review of observational studies. Stroke 2005;36(6):1330–40.
23. House A, Knapp P, Bamford J, et al. Mortality at 12 and 24 months after stroke may be associated with depressive symptoms at 1 month. Stroke 2001;32(3): 696–701.
24. Robinson RG. Poststroke depression: prevalence, diagnosis, treatment, and disease progression. Biol Psychiatry 2003;54(3):376–87.
25. Robinson RG, Price TR. Post-stroke depressive disorders: a follow-up study of 103 patients. Stroke 1982;13(5):635–41.
26. Robinson RG, Schultz SK, Castillo C, et al. Nortriptyline versus fluoxetine in the treatment of depression and in short-term recovery after stroke: a placebo-controlled, double-blind study. Am J Psychiatry 2000;157(3):351–9.
27. Wiart L, Petit H, Joseph PA, et al. Fluoxetine in early poststroke depression: a double-blind placebo-controlled study. Stroke 2000;31(8):1829–32.
28. Whyte EM, Mulsant BH. Post stroke depression: epidemiology, pathophysiology, and biological treatment. Biol Psychiatry 2002;52(3):253–64.
29. Robinson RG, Jorge RE, Moser DJ, et al. Escitalopram and problem-solving therapy for prevention of poststroke depression: a randomized controlled trial. JAMA 2008;299(20):2391–400.
30. Sadovnick AD, Remick RA, Allen J, et al. Depression and multiple sclerosis. Neurology 1996;46(3):628–32.
31. Ziemssen T. Multiple sclerosis beyond EDSS: depression and fatigue. J Neurol Sci 2009;277(Suppl 1):S37–41.
32. Kargiotis O, Geka A, Rao JS, et al. Quality of life in multiple sclerosis: effects of current treatment options. Int Rev Psychiatry 2010;22(1):67–82.

33. Patten SB, Beck CA, Williams JV, et al. Major depression in multiple sclerosis: a population-based perspective. Neurology 2003;61(11):1524–7.
34. Wilken JA, Sullivan C. Recognizing and treating common psychiatric disorders in multiple sclerosis. Neurologist 2007;13(6):343–54.
35. Treadaway K, Cutter G, Salter A, et al. Factors that influence adherence with disease-modifying therapy in MS. J Neurol 2009;256(4):568–76.
36. Mohr DC, Goodkin DE, Likosky W, et al. Therapeutic expectations of patients with multiple sclerosis upon initiating interferon beta-1b: relationship to adherence to treatment. Mult Scler 1996;2(5):222–6.
37. Mohr DC, Goodkin DE, Likosky W, et al. Treatment of depression improves adherence to interferon beta-1b therapy for multiple sclerosis. Arch Neurol 1997;54(5): 531–3.
38. The Goldman Consensus statement on depression in multiple sclerosis. Mult Scler 2005;11(3):328–37.
39. Mohr DC, Goodkin DE. Treatment of depression in multiple sclerosis: review and meta-analysis. Clin Psychol Sci Pract 1999;6:1–9.
40. Sindrup SH, Jensen TS. Efficacy of pharmacological treatments of neuropathic pain: an update and effect related to mechanism of drug action. Pain 1999; 83(3):389–400.
41. Minden SL. Mood disorders in multiple sclerosis: diagnosis and treatment. J Neurovirol 2000;6(Suppl 2):S160–7.
42. Ravina B, Camicioli R, Como PG, et al. The impact of depressive symptoms in early Parkinson disease. Neurology 2007;69(4):342–7.
43. Cummings JL. Depression and Parkinson's disease: a review. Am J Psychiatry 1992;149(4):443–54.
44. Mayberg HS, Solomon DH. Depression in Parkinson's disease: a biochemical and organic viewpoint. Adv Neurol 1995;65:49–60.
45. Remy P, Doder M, Lees A, et al. Depression in Parkinson's disease: loss of dopamine and noradrenaline innervation in the limbic system. Brain 2005;128(Pt 6):1314–22.
46. Andersen J, Aabro E, Gulmann N, et al. Anti-depressive treatment in Parkinson's disease. A controlled trial of the effect of nortriptyline in patients with Parkinson's disease treated with L-DOPA. Acta Neurol Scand 1980;62(4):210–9.
47. Laitinen L. Desipramine in treatment of Parkinson's disease. A placebo-controlled study. Acta Neurol Scand 1969;45(1):109–13.
48. Goetz CG, Tanner CM, Klawans HL. Bupropion in Parkinson's disease. Neurology 1984;34(8):1092–4.
49. Lemke MR, Brecht HM, Koester J, et al. Anhedonia, depression, and motor functioning in Parkinson's disease during treatment with pramipexole. J Neuropsychiatry Clin Neurosci 2005;17(2):214–20.
50. Devos D, Dujardin K, Poirot I, et al. Comparison of desipramine and citalopram treatments for depression in Parkinson's disease: a double-blind, randomized, placebo-controlled study. Mov Disord 2008;23(6):850–7.
51. Barone P, Scarzella L, Marconi R, et al. Pramipexole versus sertraline in the treatment of depression in Parkinson's disease: a national multicenter parallel-group randomized study. J Neurol 2006;253(5):601–7.
52. Watanabe N, Omori IM, Nakagawa A, et al. Mirtazapine versus other antidepressants in the acute-phase treatment of adults with major depression: systematic review and meta-analysis. J Clin Psychiatry 2008;69(9):1404–15.
53. Trivedi MH, Rush AJ, Wisniewski SR, et al. Evaluation of outcomes with citalopram for depression using measurement-based care in STAR*D: implications for clinical practice. Am J Psychiatry 2006;163(1):28–40.

54. Papakostas GI. The efficacy, tolerability, and safety of contemporary antidepressants. J Clin Psychiatry 2010;71(Suppl E1):e03.
55. Fava M, Alpert JE, Carmin CN, et al. Clinical correlates and symptom patterns of anxious depression among patients with major depressive disorder in STAR*D. Psychol Med 2004;34(7):1299–308.
56. Ravindran LN, Stein MB. The pharmacologic treatment of anxiety disorders: a review of progress. J Clin Psychiatry 2010;71(7):839–54.
57. Stahl SM, Grady MM, Moret C, et al. SNRIs: their pharmacology, clinical efficacy, and tolerability in comparison with other classes of antidepressants. CNS Spectr 2005;10(9):732–47.
58. Atkinson JH, Slater MA, Williams RA, et al. A placebo-controlled randomized clinical trial of nortriptyline for chronic low back pain. Pain 1998;76(3):287–96.
59. Snyder SH, Yamamura HI. Antidepressants and the muscarinic acetylcholine receptor. Arch Gen Psychiatry 1977;34(2):236–9.
60. Moore AR, O'Keeffe ST. Drug-induced cognitive impairment in the elderly. Drugs Aging 1999;15(1):15–28.
61. Lavoie FW, Gansert GG, Weiss RE. Value of initial ECG findings and plasma drug levels in cyclic antidepressant overdose. Ann Emerg Med 1990;19(6):696–700.
62. Preskorn SH, Simpson S. Tricyclic-antidepressant-induced delirium and plasma drug concentration. Am J Psychiatry 1982;139(6):822–3.
63. Menza M, Dobkin RD, Marin H, et al. A controlled trial of antidepressants in patients with Parkinson disease and depression. Neurology 2009;72(10):886–92.
64. Quitkin FM, et al. L-Deprenyl in atypical depressives. Arch Gen Psychiatry 1984;41(8):777–81.
65. Quitkin FM, Stewart JW, McGrath PJ, et al. Phenelzine versus imipramine in the treatment of probable atypical depression: defining syndrome boundaries of selective MAOI responders. Am J Psychiatry 1988;145(3):306–11.
66. Lane R, Baldwin D. Selective serotonin reuptake inhibitor-induced serotonin syndrome: review. J Clin Psychopharmacol 1997;17(3):208–21.
67. American Psychiatric Association. American Psychiatric Association practice guidelines for the treatment of psychiatric disorders. Compendium 2006. Arlington (VA): American Psychiatric Association; 2006. p. 1600, xii.
68. White N, Litovitz T, Clancy C. Suicidal antidepressant overdoses: a comparative analysis by antidepressant type. J Med Toxicol 2008;4(4):238–50.
69. Holm KJ, Markham A. Mirtazapine: a review of its use in major depression. Drugs 1999;57(4):607–31.
70. Papakostas GI, Shelton RC, Smith J, et al. Augmentation of antidepressants with atypical antipsychotic medications for treatment-resistant major depressive disorder: a meta-analysis. J Clin Psychiatry 2007;68(6):826–31.
71. Valenstein M, McCarthy JF, Austin KL, et al. What happened to lithium? Antidepressant augmentation in clinical settings. Am J Psychiatry 2006;163(7):1219–25.
72. Bauer M, Dopfmer S. Lithium augmentation in treatment-resistant depression: meta-analysis of placebo-controlled studies. J Clin Psychopharmacol 1999;19(5):427–34.
73. Aronson R, Offman HJ, Joffe RT, et al. Triiodothyronine augmentation in the treatment of refractory depression. A meta-analysis. Arch Gen Psychiatry 1996;53(9):842–8.
74. Nierenberg AA, Fava M, Trivedi MH, et al. A comparison of lithium and T(3) augmentation following two failed medication treatments for depression: a STAR*D report. Am J Psychiatry 2006;163(9):1519–30 [quiz: 1665].

75. Papakostas GI, Mischoulon D, Shyu I, et al. S-Adenosyl methionine (SAMe) augmentation of serotonin reuptake inhibitors for antidepressant nonresponders with major depressive disorder: a double-blind, randomized clinical trial. Am J Psychiatry 2010;167(8):942–8.
76. Hollon SD, Ponniah K. A review of empirically supported psychological therapies for mood disorders in adults. Depress Anxiety 2010;27(10):891–932.
77. DeRubeis RJ, Hollon SD, Amsterdam JD, et al. Cognitive therapy vs medications in the treatment of moderate to severe depression. Arch Gen Psychiatry 2005; 62(4):409–16.
78. Paul SM, Extein I, Calil HM, et al. Use of ECT with treatment-resistant depressed patients at the National Institute of Mental Health. Am J Psychiatry 1981;138(4): 486–9.
79. Prudic J, Haskett RF, Mulsant B, et al. Resistance to antidepressant medications and short-term clinical response to ECT. Am J Psychiatry 1996;153(8):985–92.
80. Semkovska M, McLoughlin DM. Objective cognitive performance associated with electroconvulsive therapy for depression: a systematic review and meta-analysis. Biol Psychiatry 2010;68(6):568–77.
81. Zielinski RJ, Roose SP, Devanand DP, et al. Cardiovascular complications of ECT in depressed patients with cardiac disease. Am J Psychiatry 1993;150(6):904–9.
82. George MS, Lisanby SP, Avery D, et al. Daily left prefrontal transcranial magnetic stimulation therapy for major depressive disorder: a sham-controlled randomized trial. Arch Gen Psychiatry 2010;67(5):507–16.
83. Slotema CW, Blom JD, Hoek HW, et al. Should we expand the toolbox of psychiatric treatment methods to include repetitive transcranial magnetic stimulation (rTMS)? A meta-analysis of the efficacy of rTMS in psychiatric disorders. J Clin Psychiatry 2010;71(7):873–84.
84. Rush AJ, Marangell LB, Sackeim HA, et al. Vagus nerve stimulation for treatment-resistant depression: a randomized, controlled acute phase trial. Biol Psychiatry 2005;58(5):347–54.
85. Rosenthal NE, Sack DA, Carpenter CJ, et al. Antidepressant effects of light in seasonal affective disorder. Am J Psychiatry 1985;142(2):163–70.
86. Shelton RC, Osuntokun O, Heinloth AN, et al. Therapeutic options for treatment-resistant depression. CNS Drugs 2010;24(2):131–61.
87. American Psychiatric Association. Practice guidelines for the treatment of patients with major depressive disorder. 3rd edition (supplement to American Journal of Psychiatry, Volume 167, Number 10, October 2010).

Index

Note: Page numbers of article titles are in **boldface** type.

A

Neurol Clin 29 (2011) 195–206
doi:10.1016/S0733-8619(10)00149-0
0733-8619/11/$ – see front matter © 2011 Elsevier Inc. All rights reserved.

Moving?

Make sure your subscription moves with you!

To notify us of your new address, find your **Clinics Account Number** (located on your mailing label above your name), and contact customer service at:

Email: journalscustomerservice-usa@elsevier.com

800-654-2452 (subscribers in the U.S. & Canada)
314-447-8871 (subscribers outside of the U.S. & Canada)

Fax number: 314-447-8029

Elsevier Health Sciences Division
Subscription Customer Service
3251 Riverport Lane
Maryland Heights, MO 63043

*To ensure uninterrupted delivery of your subscription, please notify us at least 4 weeks in advance of move.

Printed and bound by CPI Group (UK) Ltd, Croydon, CR0 4YY

03/10/2024

01040445-0001